The Infection-Prone Hospital Patient

The Infection-Prone Hospital Patient

Edited by John F. Burke, M.D.

Helen Andrus Benedict Professor of Surgery, Harvard Medical School;
Chief of Staff, Shriners Burns Institute, Boston;
Visiting Surgeon, Massachusetts General Hospital

and Gavin Y. Hildick-Smith, M.D.

Director of Medical Affairs, Johnson & Johnson, New Brunswick;
Clinical Assistant Professor, Department of Pediatrics, College of Medicine
and Dentistry, New Jersey Rutgers Medical School, Piscataway

Little, Brown and Company Boston

Preface

Infection is a constant problem in clinical medicine. Until recently, the main emphasis was placed on control of the bacteria to treat the infection. The discoveries of Pasteur and Lister led over the years to the development of efficient aseptic control measures and the widespread use of sterilized materials. The development of antibiotics revolutionized the treatment of bacterial disease, and the eventual complete control of bacterial diseases was predicted. The fact remains, however, that in spite of the aseptic measures, the use of sterile materials and the availability of myriad antibiotics, patients continue to suffer from serious infection, particularly when it is associated with other disease.

It is clear from the information available that a large fraction of the patients who suffer from bacterial diseases have an altered resistance to bacterial infections. Further improvement in our ability to prevent these diseases will probably not be completely dependent on aseptic technique and antibacterial substances but will come in greatest measure through a thorough understanding of host resistance mechanisms. It is our hope that the new knowledge being amassed in this field will suggest measures that will enhance and restore natural host factors in patients who are deficient in resistance or who, because of treatment itself, are placed at great risk of bacterial invasion and subsequent infection. During the coming decade, we can look for the growth of research in this important phase of medicine. In our optimistic view, this information will afford the possibility of controlling infection and, even more important, preventing infection.

The chapters in this book are papers that were presented at a symposium designed to highlight the state of knowledge in an important field of medicine and to stimulate further research in it. The symposium was held under the auspices of the Shriners Burns Institute and the Harvard Medical School and was supported by a grant from the Patient Care Division of Johnson & Johnson, New Brunswick, New Jersey.

J. F. B.
G. Y. H-S.

Contents

Contributing Authors

J. Wesley Alexander, M.D.
Professor of Surgery, University of Cincinnati College of Medicine; Director, Transplantation Division, Department of Surgery, University of Cincinnati Medical Center, Cincinnati

Demetrius H. Bagley, M.D.
Fellow, Section of Urology, Yale University School of Medicine, New Haven

Lee L. Bernardis, Ph.D.
Research Professor of Surgery, State University of New York at Buffalo School of Medicine, Buffalo

Ronald H. Birkhahn, Ph.D.
Assistant Professor of Surgery and Biochemistry, Medical College of Ohio at Toledo

Gerald P. Bodey, M.D.
Professor of Medicine, Medical Director, Cancer Clinical Research Center, and Chief, Chemotherapy Branch and Infectious Diseases Section, Department of Developmental Therapeutics, University of Texas System Cancer Center, M. D. Anderson Hospital and Tumor Institute, Houston

John R. Border, M.D.
Professor of Surgery, State University of New York at Buffalo School of Medicine; Attending Surgeon, Edward J. Meyer Memorial Hospital, Buffalo

John F. Burke, M.D.
Helen Andrus Benedict Professor of Surgery, Harvard Medical School; Chief of Staff, Shriners Burns Institute; Visiting Surgeon, Massachusetts General Hospital, Boston

Zanvil A. Cohn, M.D.
Professor and Senior Physician, Laboratory of Cellular Physiology and Immunology, The Rockefeller University, New York

Starkey D. Davis, M.D.
Professor of Pediatrics and Microbiology, The Medical College of Wisconsin, Milwaukee; Director of Infectious Disease, Milwaukee Children's Hospital, Milwaukee

Renzo Dionigi, M.D.
Associate Professor of Surgery, University of Pavia; Attending Surgeon, Istituto di Patologia Chirurgica, Policlinico S. Matteo, Pavia, Italy

Robert Edelman, M.D.
Chief, Clinical Studies Branch, Microbiology and Infectious Disease Program, National Institute of Allergy and Infectious Diseases, Bethesda, Maryland

Emil J Freireich, M.D.

Professor of Medicine and Chief, Division of Oncology, Department of Medicine, University of Texas Medical School at Houston, Health Science Center at Houston; Head, Department of Developmental Therapeutics, University of Texas System Cancer Center, M. D. Anderson Hospital and Tumor Institute, Houston

Vincent A. Fulginiti, M.D.

Professor and Head, Department of Pediatrics, and Director, Department of Clinical Pediatrics, Arizona Health Sciences Center, University of Arizona College of Medicine, Tucson

Richard A. Gatti, M.D.

Professor of Pediatrics, University of California, Los Angeles (UCLA), School of Medicine; Director, Pediatric Oncology and Immunology, Cedars-Sinai Medical Center, Los Angeles

A. Arthur Gottlieb, M.D.

Chairman, Department of Microbiology and Immunology, and Professor of Medicine, Tulane University School of Medicine, New Orleans

William H. Harris, M.D.

Clinical Professor of Orthopaedic Surgery, Harvard Medical School; Chief, Hip and Implant Unit, Department of Orthopaedic Surgery, Massachusetts General Hospital, Boston

Gavin Y. Hildick-Smith, M.D.

Director of Medical Affairs, Johnson & Johnson, New Brunswick; Clinical Assistant Professor of Pediatrics, College of Medicine and Dentistry, New Jersey Rutgers Medical School, Piscataway

Alfred S. Ketcham, M.D.

Professor of Surgery, University of Miami School of Medicine; Chief, Division of Surgical Oncology, Jackson Memorial Hospital, Miami

Panja Kulapongs, M.D.

Department of Pediatrics, Faculty of Medicine, Chiang Mai University; Anemia and Malnutrition Research Center, Chiang Mai, Thailand

John LaDuca, M.D.

Assistant Professor of Surgery, State University of New York at Buffalo School of Medicine; Attending Surgeon, Edward J. Meyer Memorial Hospital, Buffalo

Claus Leitzmann, Ph.D.

Institut für Ernährungswissenschaft I der Justus Liebig-Universität, Giessen, Germany

R. H. McMenamy, Ph.D.

Professor of Biochemistry, State University of New York at Buffalo School of Medicine; Attending Scientist, Edward J. Meyer Memorial Hospital, Buffalo

Michael A. Medici, M.D.
Immunology Fellow, Department of Pediatric Oncology and Immunology, Cedars-Sinai Medical Center, Los Angeles

Peter J. Morris, Ph.D.
Nuffield Professor of Surgery and Fellow of Balliol, Oxford University; Honorary Consultant in Surgery, Radcliffe Infirmary and Churchill Hospital, Oxford, England

Sir Gustav Nossal, M.B., B.S.
Director, Walter & Eliza Hall Institute of Medical Research; Physician, Royal Melbourne Hospital, Melbourne, Australia

Robert E. Olson, M.D., Ph.D.
Chairman, Department of Biochemistry, St. Louis University School of Medicine, St. Louis

Paul G. Quie, M.D.
Professor of Pediatrics and Microbiology, University of Minnesota Medical School —Minneapolis; Infectious Disease Division, University of Minnesota Hospitals of the University of Minnesota Health Sciences Center, Minneapolis

Victorio Rodriguez, M.D.
Associate Professor of Medicine and Associate Internist, Department of Developmental Therapeutics, University of Texas System Cancer Center, M. D. Anderson Hospital and Tumor Institute, Houston

Roger Seibel, M.D.
Assistant Professor of Surgery, State University of New York at Buffalo School of Medicine; Attending Surgeon, Edward J. Meyer Memorial Hospital, Buffalo

Stitaya Sirisinha, D.M.D., Ph.D.
Associate Professor, Department of Microbiology, Faculty of Science, Mahidol University, Bangkok, Thailand

Ronald Sorkness, M.S.
Clinical Assistant Professor of Pharmacy, State University of New York at Buffalo School of Pharmacy; Pharmacist, Edward J. Meyer Memorial Hospital, Buffalo

J. Dwight Stinnett, Ph.D.
Assistant Professor of Research Surgery and Microbiology, University of Cincinnati College of Medicine, Cincinnati

Robert M. Suskind, M.D.
Associate Professor of Pediatrics and Clinical Nutrition, Nutrition and Food Science, Massachusetts Institute of Technology, Cambridge; Nutrition Support Service, Children's Hospital Medical Center, Boston

Vicharn Vithayasai, M.D., Ph.D.
Assistant Professor of Microbiology and Pediatrics, Chiang Mai Medical School, Chiang Mai University; Deputy Director and Head of Immunology Section, Anemia and Malnutrition Research Center, Chiang Mai University, Chiang Mai, Thailand

The Infection-Prone Hospital Patient

1. The Contribution of Polymorphonuclear Neutrophils to Host Resistance

Paul G. Quie

Patients with deficient numbers of polymorphonuclear neutrophils and patients with neutrophils that do not function properly are remarkably susceptible to severe disease from a variety of microbial agents, especially staphylococci, enteric bacteria, and fungal species. In clinical situations with insufficient numbers or deficient neutrophils or in pathologic conditions in which phagocytic cells cannot reach sequestered organisms (i.e., around foreign bodies), high-dose antibiotic therapy is often incapable of eradicating the infecting microorganisms in spite of the susceptibility of these microbes to the antibiotics used. On the basis of this clinical evidence, a critical role for circulating phagocytic cells, primarily polymorphonuclear neutrophils, in host defense against bacterial illness is now fully appreciated.

Until relatively recently, clinical investigations have concentrated on situations in which numbers of mature neutrophils are not adequate, i.e., in the various forms of neutropenia and in leukemia. In the past decade, however, since discovery of defective phagocyte function in certain patients with recurrent, severe infections, intense interest has developed in the function of neutrophils. This discussion is confined to human polymorphonuclear neutrophil function in relation to host defense against microbial disease and does not include a discussion of the other leukocytes. The other leukocytes include eosinophils and basophils, which are not discussed; monocytes and macrophages, which are discussed in Chapter 2; and lymphocytes, which are discussed in Chapter 3.

Development and Morphology of Polymorphonuclear Neutrophils

There is evidence that neutrophils develop from the same pluripotent stem cells that differentiate into monocytes, lymphocytes, erythrocytes, or megakaryocytes under different environmental conditions. The stem cells destined to become neutrophils differentiate into cells that have cytoplasmic granules at the promyelocyte stage of development, and by the myelocyte stage the cytoplasmic granules are prominent. As neutrophils mature, they lose mitochondria, become capable of phagocytosis, acquire oxidative metabolic capacity, and become mobile. It is this combination of capacity for rapid mobility, rich supply of microbicidal factors in granules, and unique oxidative response that makes these cells such excellent defenders of the host and has led to the expression "professional phagocytes" when describing neutrophils.

The studies reported from the author's laboratories were supported in part by U.S. Public Health Service Grants AI 08821, AI 06931, and AI 12402. Support from the Minnesota Medical Foundation is also acknowledged.

The bone marrow produces approximately as many neutrophils (an estimated 120 billion) each day as erythrocytes, but the neutrophils have a much shorter life (approximately 6 to 7 hours) in the circulation than do erythrocytes, so there is normally only one circulating neutrophil for every 2,000 erythrocytes. Mature neutrophils collect along the walls of capillaries — i.e., marginate — and there are large stores of mature cells in the bone marrow, so there is a "ready reserve" of neutrophils that can be instantly mobilized when invasion of tissue by microbes occurs. Under normal conditions neutrophils migrate at a steady rate through the spaces between endothelial cells into the tissues and body spaces [7]. The life span of the cells in tissue is a few hours to several days, but mature neutrophils never reenter the circulation.

The identification of factors regulating production of neutrophils has been made possible by in vivo cultivation of bone marrow neutrophil precursor cells. It appears that a soluble factor, termed *colony stimulating factor,* released by monocytes and macrophages as well as by neutrophils, stimulates proliferation of neutrophils [10, 55]. Although the factors that stimulate neutrophil proliferation in vitro have not been proved to be neutrophil regulators in vivo, it seems logical that phagocytic leukocytes that are present at the interface of tissue and its environment would regulate the supply of professional phagocytes. During an infectious process the supply of neutrophils can be dramatically increased by release of mature reserve cells; in addition, there is a shortening of maturation time and increased activity in the mitotic pool [49].

Neutrophil Locomotion and Chemotaxis

Neutrophils in the circulation are concentrated in the area of inflammation because of increased stickiness of endothelial surfaces, and cells diapede through vessel walls into the tissue. The kinin system is involved in the change of capillary permeability, but once in the tissues, neutrophils are attracted in a unidirectional fashion toward the site of microbial invasion by chemotactic factors. Chemotactic factors involved in the attraction of leukocytes include complement components C3a, C5a, and $\overline{C567}$ and factors released from disrupted leukocytes and tissue cells. In addition, bacteria and fungi release potent chemotactic substances. It is the gradient of these chemotactic substances, which are at highest concentration at the center of the inflammatory process, that brings about unidirectional locomotion of neutrophils toward the site of inflammation (Figure 1-1).

Neutrophil locomotion can be measured in vivo by producing an inflammatory site on the skin and placing a glass coverslip or chambers on the site. Large numbers of neutrophils are present on coverslips after 2 to 4 hours, and this neutrophil influx is followed after several hours by infiltration with mononuclear cells. In experimental animals, it has been demonstrated that a delay of influx of neutrophils into an inflammatory site of as

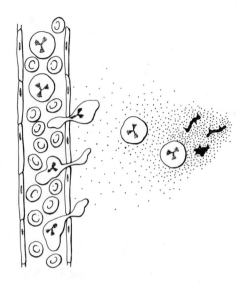

Figure 1-1. Inflammation. Neutrophil locomotion during the first stages of an inflammatory response. Neutrophils adhere to the surface of capillaries and venules, diapede through spaces between endothelial cells, and migrate toward microbial invaders. Directional locomotion occurs because of the gradient of chemotactic factors. Chemotactic factors are depicted by small dots around bacteria and cells outside the capillary lumen.

little as 2 hours severely compromises the animal's ability to localize an infectious process [37]. These experimental data and the finding of defective neutrophil chemotactic responsiveness in several clinical conditions characterized by recurrent bacterial infections are compelling evidence for a direct association between the capacity of neutrophils for rapid locomotion and directional response to chemotactic stimulation with normal host defense against bacterial disease.

In 1971 several patients were described with defective neutrophil chemotactic activity. Miller, Oski, and Harris described two children from unrelated families with recurrent infections and defective neutrophil chemotaxis [38]. Steerman et al. described another patient with recurrent infections whose neutrophils did not respond in vitro to known chemotactic stimulation [54]. This patient also had hypogammaglobulinemia. Clark and Kimball described defective chemotaxis in children with Chediak-Higashi syndrome [6]. These defective neutrophils are also defective in bacterial killing [51].

A marked defect in neutrophil chemotaxis occurs in patients with measles [2]. The defect lasts for approximately 10 days, and neutrophil chemotaxis returns to normal when the rash and clinical symptoms disappear. Patients with Down's syndrome have a variety of immunologic abnormalities, and defective neutrophil chemotaxis has recently been added to the list of compromised host-defense factors in patients with this syndrome [28].

Defective neutrophil chemotaxis may also be an acquired defect in host defense [11]. We have found that patients with greater than 30% second- and third-degree burns have defective neutrophil chemotaxis that persists for several weeks, and there is return to normal neutrophil function as patients are grafted and return to a normal clinical state [11]. Patients with severe bacterial infections with a high percentage of toxic neutrophils are defective in neutrophil chemotactic responsiveness [35]. We have also observed that patients with chronic renal failure and uremia have moderately depressed chemotactic responsiveness and, paradoxically, after prolonged hemodialysis (after 7 to 10 hemodialysis treatments), the neutrophil chemotactic responsiveness is even further depressed [12].

Certain patients with extremely elevated levels of serum IgE and recurrent, severe disease from staphylococci and *Candida albicans* have neutrophils that react slowly to chemotactic stimulation [17, 18, 60]. Patients with Job's syndrome (characterized by severe early-onset eczema, nearly constant staphylococcal skin lesions, and adenitis) have extremely elevated levels of IgE and defective neutrophil chemotactic responsiveness [19]. The association between allergic manifestations, such as eczema or urticaria, and extreme hyperimmunoglobulin E and defective neutrophil chemotaxis suggests that abnormal metabolism of histamine or other circulating amines in these patients may be responsible for neutrophil abnormalities. The serum from patients with extremely elevated IgE produces chemotactic factors normally, and inhibitors of chemotaxis could not be identified. Furthermore, the neutrophils had normal bactericidal activity. Defective neutrophil chemotactic responsiveness appeared to be the only measurable cellular defect in these patients. However, it seems probable that more sensitive methods may have detected a depressed rate of phagocytosis. All these pieces of clinical evidence point to an important role for prompt neutrophil chemotactic responsiveness for normal host defense against severe disease from invading bacteria.

The cellular machinery necessary for neutrophil locomotion and the energy required to fuel this machinery is similar to that found in other contractile cells, such as muscle cells. In muscles, of course, the individual cells are closely ordered by matrix for organ function, while neutrophils are single cells and can be considered as only slightly disciplined, "adolescent" individualists. When viewed by phase contrast microscopy, migrating neutrophils have a leading edge of hyaline ectoplasm that appears to contract and relax, and the rest of the cell contents are pulled along by this activity. Electron microscopic magnification has revealed that this ectoplasm contains microfilaments. It is believed that these filaments, composed of actin and myocin, relax and contract by action of ATP and ATPase and by a shift in the compartmentalization of calcium ions [58]. A role for actin is suggested by the report of Boxer, Hedley-White, and Stossel, who described

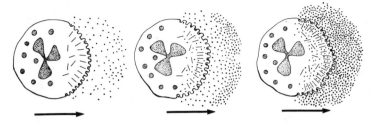

Figure 1-2. Chemotaxis. Directional locomotion of a neutrophil in response to a gradient of chemotactic substances. The receptors on the neutrophil membrane must be considered hypothetical, since a wide variety of factors are capable of attracting neutrophils. A change at the membrane level in response to stimulation by chemotactic factors activates contractile structures (microfilaments and microtubules), shown here as parallel lines just within the neutrophil membrane.

a patient with recurrent infections with neutrophils that completely lacked the capacity for locomotion. These neutrophils were found to have abnormal actin [5].

In addition to microfilaments, there are microtubules composed of the protein tubulin that are also able to polymerize and depolymerize. These structures are larger and more stable and may serve as a support for the contracting microfilaments [44]. Receptors for chemotactically active substances are present on the surface membrane of neutrophils, and the activation of these receptors brings about contraction and directional movement. The increased concentration of chemotactically active substances on one side of the cell may bring about increased microtubule activity on that side and hence directional movement, as shown diagrammatically in Figure 1-2.

We are presently investigating the possible role of histamine and other factors on the cyclic nucleotide metabolism of neutrophils [16]. Factors that stimulate adenylate cyclase and increase levels of intracellular cyclic adenosine monophosphate (cyclic AMP) depress chemotactic responsiveness of neutrophils. It is speculative but interesting to consider the possibility that abnormal membrane regulation of cyclic nucleotide metabolism may be related to defective neutrophil function. If such proves to be the case, pharmacologic manipulation of this host defense parameter may be possible.

Attachment and Engulfment of Microbes by Neutrophils

Once neutrophils reach the microbial invaders, a complex interaction of humoral and cellular responses occur. For there to be attachment of microorganisms to phagocytes, potent antiphagocytic factors on the microbial surface must be neutralized. Examples of these microbial factors are the M protein of group A streptococci, the polyribose phosphate of *Hemophilus influenzae* type B, and the capsular factors of *Escherichia coli*. The humoral factors that coat the microbial surfaces, termed *opsonins,* in addition to neutralizing antiphagocytic factors on microbes, act as ligands between the microbe and the phagocyte. The two major opsonins that produce a tight bond between microbe and neutrophils are antibacterial antibodies and the C3b fragment of complement component C3.

There is a great variation in the opsonic requirement of different microbial species and of strains within species, which is related to the virulence of the microbes, i.e., the more resistant to phagocytosis, the more virulent. Therefore the availability of opsonins is critically important for rapid, efficient phagocytosis of and host resistance against microbial disease.

In the nonimmune host, i.e., when antibodies have not developed, complement may be activated by direct action of microbial surfaces on humoral factors that are known as the alternative, or properdin, pathway of complement activation. Activation of complement with the production of C3b via the alternative pathway may be the most important mechanism of opsonization in the nonimmune host, i.e., during the first encounter with a particular microorganism. There will be extensive discussion of the role and function of opsonins in host defense in subsequent chapters; this section concentrates on the response of neutrophils once microbial attachment has occurred.

Neutrophils have receptors for the Fc part of IgG antibodies and for the C3b component of complement on the surface, or plasma, membrane [39]. There are undoubtedly other receptors on neutrophil membranes since certain bacterial species, such as *Staphylococcus epidermidis* and rough strains of pneumococci, are phagocytized in the absence of opsonins. The nature of these receptors is unknown. If there are only a few opsonic configurations on the microbes that match receptors on the phagocyte plasma membrane, attachment alone occurs. However, when the microbe is thoroughly opsonized with antibody and C3b, the machinery of locomotion is set into action, and the neutrophil moves around microbes with an embrace that encloses the microbes inside a phagocytic pouch (Figure 1-3).

There is a requirement for the divalent cations calcium and magnesium during phagocytosis; and a shift in the concentration of these ions around the neutrophil surface is related somehow with activation of the phagocytic process [57]. This may have clinical application since the kinetics of engulfment of bacteria is severely compromised when hypertonic conditions are present. There is also evidence of depressed neutrophil locomotion when there is severe hypophosphatemia [8].

The energy for the neutrophil engulfment process involves ATP generated glycolysis, and the movement of pseudopodia around microbes requires actin and myosin microfilament activity similar to that required for locomotion in response to chemotactic stimulation [57]. When the neutrophil plasma membrane fuses, the "inside-out" membrane that surrounds the engulfed microbes buds off and becomes a new organelle in the cytoplasm, termed a *phagosome.*

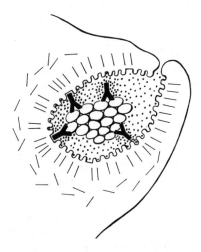

Figure 1-3. Phagocytosis. A portion of a neutrophil engulfing an opsonized clump of bacteria. The Y-shaped structures are specific antibacterial antibodies and the small dots, C3b molecules. Antibodies are opsonic, since neutrophils have receptors for the Fc part of IgG molecules. The presence of complement greatly amplifies the opsonic potential of antibacterial antibodies.

Degranulation

Neutrophils contain a rich collection of granules in the cytoplasm that have specialized functions. The two types that have been most carefully characterized are the azurophilic granules, which contain acid phosphatase and other hydrolases, and specific granules, which contain the antibacterial factors lysozyme and lactoferrin [4]. There is fusion of these granules with the newly formed phagosome, accompanied by vigorous degranulation and discharge of granule contents into the phagosomes, which become phagocytic vacuoles [20]. The environment within the vacuole is highly lethal for the microbes and most organisms are killed with great rapidity. Digestion of the killed organism proceeds with nearly unbelievable speed.

The effect of certain pharmacologic agents on the membrane function of neutrophils is of interest, since several of these agents are associated with increased susceptibility to infection. Corticosteroids in high concentrations impair the process of ingestion by neutrophils [13]. Similar effects have also been observed with phenylbutazone and levorphanol, a derivative of morphine [56, 59]. Other compounds, such as colchicine, vinblastine, and cytochalasin B, have an effect on neutrophils that involves several cellular mechanisms, including ion transport and inhibition of ingestion of particles [56]. The pharmacologic agents that inhibit engulfment of microbes by neutrophils also inhibit chemotaxis of these cells and therefore profoundly interfere with the neutrophils' contribution to host defense.

The fusion of cytoplasmic granules and degranulation of lysosomal contents into phagocytic vacuoles occurs within seconds when microbes are engulfed by neutrophils, and nearly simultaneously there is a sudden burst in the oxidative metabolic activity of the neutrophils. Under anerobic conditions the capacity of neutrophils to kill intracellular microbes is markedly decreased, suggesting that the oxygen-dependent antimicrobial systems are highly important for neutrophil microbicidal function [29, 30].

Chronic Granulomatous Disease

Clinical evidence of the fundamental importance of oxygen-dependent microbicidal systems in neutrophils was the discovery of the clinical chronic granulomatous disease of childhood (CGD) in which the neutrophils are morphologically normal and engulf microbes normally but cannot effectively kill most bacterial and fungal species [46]. The neutrophils from patients with CGD do not respond to phagocytosis with the typical burst of oxidative metabolism and, as a result, hydrogen peroxide and other oxidative products are not produced.

Since the clinical presentation of patients with neutrophil abnormalities of several etiologies are similar, the nature of the infections in children with CGD are described in some detail. Infections in children with CGD involve primarily those tissues that receive constant challenge from bacteria, i.e., skin, lungs, and perianal tissue. Infections begin to occur in the first few months of life, and the earliest lesions are typically eczematoid reactions of the skin around the ears and nose. These progress to purulent skin lesions and enlarged local lymph nodes. There are frequent recurrences, producing tissue necrosis, granuloma formation, and suppurative adenopathy. Hepatosplenomegaly is a constant finding, suggesting spread of viable bacteria to the reticuloendothelial system. Abscesses of the liver, spleen, lungs, and bones with bacteria are frequent and severe [45].

Pulmonary involvement is present in nearly all children with CGD. There is hilar enlargement, bronchopneumonia, and empyema, as well as lung abscess. The rapid clearing of symptoms usually associated with antibiotic treatment of bacterial pneumonia is seldom observed, and the lung infiltrates persist for several weeks in spite of appropriate antibiotic therapy. There is x-ray evidence of reticulonodular densities in the lung fields that represent granulomas. In certain patients, areas of bronchopneumonia resolve into discrete areas of consolidation, termed *encapsulating pneumonia,* which are considered to be distinctive and diagnostic of CGD [62].

Osteomyelitis occurs with great frequency in patients with CGD, and the small bones of the hands or feet are typically involved. The bones become enlarged, and although considerable destruction occurs, there is minimal sclerosis, presumably because the cellular response is that of granuloma. The bacteria recovered from bone lesions are similar to those recovered from suppurative lymph nodes or abscesses. Osteomyelitis may develop in different bones while the patient is receiving antibiotic therapy, but eventually, after many weeks of therapy, complete healing of affected bones occurs [61].

The diagnosis of CGD depends on demonstration of normal phagocytosis of bacteria, intracellular survival of bacteria in large numbers, and abnormal metabolic response during phagocytosis as measured by NBT dye reduction or oxygen uptake.

Assays utilizing differential centrifugation for separating viable leukocyte-associated bacteria from nonphagocytized bacteria show that approximately 80 to 100% of *Staphylococcus aureus* inside the polymorphonuclear leukocytes of patients with CGD are viable after 120 min of incubation [47]. Polymorphonuclear leukocytes from controls kill 99% of intracellular staphylococci under similar conditions. Leukocytes from patients with CGD also lack fungicidal capacity [43]. Abnormal function of eosinophils and mononuclear leukocytes has also been demonstrated in these patients [32, 50].

Nitroblue tetrazolium dye (NBT) is used in a histochemical test to identify leukocytes with oxidase activity during phagocytosis. Oxidized NBT is colorless, but when reduced, NBT precipitates in the cytoplasm as blue formazan. Approximately 80 to 90% of normal leukocytes reduce NBT during phagocytosis. In contrast, less than 10% of leukocytes from patients with CGD reduce NBT during phagocytosis. This test has become highly useful in screening patients with CGD, although demonstration of neutrophil bactericidal deficiency remains the final diagnostic test for the disease.

Neutrophils from patients with chronic granulomatous disease do not respond with respiratory oxidative metabolic activity during phagocytosis. There is not the burst of oxygen consumption, shift to hexose monophosphate shunt, glucose metabolism, or accumulation of hydrogen peroxide that is present in control neutrophils [22].

Streptococcus faecalis, Streptococcus viridans, and *Streptococcus pyogenes* (all hydrogen peroxide producing bacteria) are killed normally by CGD leukocytes [25]. Streptococci produce hydrogen peroxide within the phagocytic vacuoles of neutrophils, thereby contributing to their own death by supplying the reagent that the defective neutrophils cannot produce. There is a remarkable absence of infections due to hydrogen peroxide–producing bacteria, such as streptococci or pneumococci, in patients with CGD, and this correlation between clinical and laboratory observations is strong evidence that hydrogen peroxide or other oxygen radicals are essential bactericidal factors in neutrophils.

Certain female patients with CGD are deficient in glutathione peroxidase activity during phagocytosis. This enzyme is not deficient in boys with CGD. The most important aspect of this observation is the concept that there may be several different enzymatic abnormalities, involving the oxidative metabolic response, that limit production of hydrogen peroxide and other oxygen radicals and hence bacterial killing in neutrophils.

Oxidative Metabolism Associated with Antimicrobial Activity

In normal neutrophils, there is a rapid increase in oxygen consumption, a shift to hexose monophosphate shunt activity, and hydrogen peroxide production during phagocytosis, which occurs within a few seconds after there is attachment and beginning engulfment of microbes by neutrophils [26, 31, 52, 53]. Indeed, the reaction is so rapid that the enzyme systems responsible for oxygen consumption are probably located in the neutrophil plasma membrane. This location would allow continued production of hydrogen peroxide and other active oxygen radicals by phagosomes. The inside-out plasma membrane around the encased microbes would be ideally suited for this function.

Hydrogen peroxide reacts with the granular enzyme myeloperoxidase that is discharged into phagosomes during fusion of cytoplasmic granules with phagosomes and forms a strong oxidizing complex that reacts with halides, such as iodine and chloride. Iodination of bacteria has been demonstrated in phagocytic vacuoles [31], and there is good evidence that chloride, which is in high concentrations in neutrophils, participates in the myeloperoxidase-hydrogen peroxide-halogen antimicrobial system [53].

There are other highly reactive oxygen molecules, such as superoxide (O_2^-), singlet oxygen (O_2), hydroxyl radical $(OH\cdot)$, and hydrogen peroxide (H_2O_2) produced by neutrophils during phagocytosis. Superoxide is a reactive oxygen radical that is formed by the univalent reduction of oxygen. It is produced by normal neutrophils during phagocytosis and is not produced by CGD neutrophils [10]. This oxygen radical can be converted to hydrogen peroxide and O_2, i.e., dismutated by an enzyme superoxide dismutase. Bacteria that are resistant to oxygen (aerobes) have high levels of superoxide dismutase and bacteria susceptible to oxygen (anaerobes) do not have superoxide dismutase. Therefore superoxide dismutase is a control mechanism, or antagonist, of superoxide and accelerates the conversion of superoxide to hydrogen peroxide and oxygen by the following formula:

$$2\,O_2^- + 2\,H^+ \longrightarrow H_2O_2 + O_2$$

It has recently been shown that superoxide dismutase complexed onto latex particles that are phagocytized along with *E. coli* can strikingly inhibit the bactericidal capacity of neutrophils [23]. This suggests that superoxide may be an important antimicrobial factor in neutrophils. Both superoxide dismutase, which converts O_2^- to H_2O_2, and catalase, which detoxifies hydrogen peroxide into H_2O and O_2, have been identified in the cytosol of neutrophils [24]. Therefore these enzymes do not interfere with the microbicidal action of superoxide and hydrogen peroxide within the phagosome but do protect the neutrophil cytoplasm from these freely diffusible toxic oxygen radicals.

Singlet oxygen is another electronically excitable oxygen molecule produced during phagocytosis by normal neutrophils. It emits light (chemiluminescense), which can be measured in a liquid scintillation counter. Production of this oxygen radical is also impaired in CGD neutrophils [55]. Singlet oxygen is formed during the spontaneous dismutation of superoxide and also during the reaction of myeloperoxidase, hypochlorite, and hydrogen peroxide, all of which are known to be present in phagosomes during phagocytosis. The high energy of singlet oxygen is believed to be capable of disrupting double carbon bonds in the membranes of microorganisms and therefore this oxygen radical may be microbicidal [1].

Still another oxygen radical produced in phagosomes during phagocytosis is the hydroxyl radical. The formula for its production is

$$O_2^- + H_2O_2 \longrightarrow O_2 + OH^- + OH$$

The reagents necessary for formation of hydroxyl radical, i.e., superoxide and singlet oxygen, are present in phagosomes and a role for hydroxyl radicals in microbial killing is suggested by the observation that bacterial killing is inhibited by hydroxyl scavengers, ethanol, mannitol, and benzoate [14]. The measurable changes in metabolism of human neutrophils during phagocytosis are outlined as follows:

1. There is increased NADH/NADPH oxidase activity.
2. Oxygen is converted to superoxide.
3. A shift to HMP shunt activity occurs.
4. Hydrogen peroxide is produced.
5. Singlet oxygen and hydroxyl radicals are produced.
6. Chemiluminescence is produced.
7. NBT dye is reduced.

Neutrophils from patients with CGD and neutrophils without glucose 6-phosphate dehydrogenase do not have an oxidative metabolic response during phagocytosis, and the laboratory differences between these neutrophils and normal neutrophils is outlined as follows:

1. Oxygen is not converted to superoxide.
2. There is no increase in NADH/NADPH oxidase activity.
3. H_2O_2 is not produced.
4. NBT dye is not reduced.
5. There is no shift to HMP shunt.
6. There is no chemiluminescence response.
7. Iodination of particles does not occur.
8. Catalase producing microbes are not killed.

For the past decade there has been intense investigation in several laboratories to determine what triggers the observed burst in oxidative metabolism during phagocytosis in normal neutrophils and why this does not occur when neutrophils from CGD phagocytize bacteria. If this puzzle could be solved, we would know which enzyme or enzyme systems are responsible for the burst of oxidative metabolism.

The rate-limiting factors in the oxidative response of neutrophils during phagocytosis may be the puridine nucleotides NADH and NADPH, which provide electrons for conversion of oxygen into hydrogen peroxide and other oxygen radicals [40]. This concept was recently confirmed when it was found that NADPH was the primary electron donor for superoxide production in homogenates of human neutrophils [3]. There was also contribution of electrons by NADH but none by glucose 6-phosphate, lactate, gluta-thione, or ascorbic acid. There was no superoxide produced by intact CGD neutrophils, but superoxide was produced by the homogenates of neutro-phils from two patients with CGD. These findings were in accord with an earlier report by Nathan, Baehner, and Weaner, who found normal NBT reduction by homogenates of CGD neutrophils and no reduction by intact phagocytizing neutrophils [41]. Johnston et al. found that separated gran-ules from CGD neutrophils produced superoxide while intact neutrophils do not [24]. In contrast, Curnutte, Kipnes, and Babior found no NADPH oxidase activity in granules from patients with CGD [9].

These observations support the suggestions that puridine nucleotide oxidases or the enzyme(s) that activate the puridine nucleotide oxidases are critical factors missing in CGD [21, 27].

There are antimicrobial systems in neutrophils that do not require oxygen or oxygen metabolites, including acid, lysozyme, lactoferrin, and cationic proteins. Certain bacteria such as *S. edipermidis* and *Pseudomonas aeruginosa* are killed by neutrophils in the absence of oxygen [34]. Further-more, certain *Candida* species are killed normally by CGD neutrophils and by myeloperoxidase deficient neutrophils [33]. Therefore in addition to the oxidative metabolic activity discussed above, neutrophils also have backup systems that are effective in killing certain microorganisms.

The pH of phagosome contents during phagocytosis becomes increasingly acid because of lactic acid production, and this alone may inhibit microbial replication. For example, pneumococci are highly sensitive to an acid pH. Most other bacteria, however, survive under these conditions.

Lysozyme is present in neutrophil granules and is discharged into phago-somes during degranulation. Most bacteria and fungi are resistant to the lytic action of lysozyme but per se several species become sensitive when acted on by antibody and complement of hydrogen peroxide [30]. Lysozyme therefore may act synergistically with other antimicrobial systems in the phagosome, but its primary role appears to be digestive rather than cidal. Specific granules of neutrophils contain lactoferrin, which inhibits micro-bial growth by binding iron, an essential nutrient for most microbes. Lacto-ferrin may also react with hydrogen peroxide in the oxygen-dependent bactericidal activity of neutrophils. Cationic proteins extracted from human neutrophil granules can be separated into fractions and each fraction demonstrates specificity of antibacterial activity [42, 63]. These cationic proteins are believed to be toxic for microbes by interfering with acidic groups on the microbial membranes. The cationic proteins in human neutrophils are greatly amplified by the addition of hydrogen peroxide and halide [30]. Therefore they may be cofactors rather than a primary microbicidal mechanism. Rabbit neutrophils are particularly rich in cationic proteins; human neutrophils are not.

Summary and Conclusion

This chapter is a brief report of recent advances in our understanding of the role of neutrophils in host defense against microbial disease. Abnormality of neutrophil locomotion and chemotactic responsiveness has been identified in several clinical syndromes, most of which are characterized by increased susceptibility to infection. Correlation between defective neutrophil chemotaxis with pathologic processes in vivo is necessary to evaluate the role of chemotaxis deficiency in the pathogenesis of infection. However, there is accumulating evidence that rapid directional locomotion of neutrophils is important for adequate host defense. The cellular factors required for locomotion of neutrophils and regulation of locomotion in response to chemotactic stimulation are better understood than before; however, the molecular trigger for activating this system remains a mystery. Regulation of function appears to be related to the cyclic nucleotide system, which suggests that neutrophil function may be responsive to pharmacologic manipulation.

The greatest advance in knowledge of neutrophil function has been in identification of factors in neutrophils contributing to the microbicidal function of these cells. It can be stated with some certainty that the primary antimicrobial systems of human neutrophils are dependent on oxygen metabolism, and several reactive oxygen radicals contribute to the microbicidal armamentarium of the neutrophils. There are other factors, such as lysozyme and cationic proteins that are microbicidal, but these factors have a limited spectrum, and neutrophils need the products of oxidative metabolism together with myeloperoxidase and halides to kill a wide spectrum of microbes with amazing rapidity. Thus understanding has come from intense investigation of neutrophils without oxidative metabolism and with defective microbicidal function, i.e., neutrophils from CGD patients. The factor or factors that activate this burst of oxidative metabolism during phagocytosis has not been identified with certainty, but most likely resides in the neutrophil plasma membrane.

Several new methods for studying the metabolic response of neutrophils during phagocytosis have evolved during the past decade. For example, hydrogen peroxide can be measured by scopolatin; superoxide, by reduction of cytochrome C; and singlet oxygen, by measurement of chemiluminescense. These methods may reveal subtle defects of metabolic response in neutrophils from patients with increased susceptibility to infection, such as infants and patients with protein-calorie malnutrition.

Stored leukocytes that have been separated from erythrocytes and plasma of healthy blood donors and stored under standard blood bank conditions maintain normal function for at least 24 hours [36]. Therefore leukocyte transfusions as adjunct therapy for sepsis in patients with neutrophils or with dysfunctional neutrophils is practical.

References

1. Allen, R. C., Stjernholm, R. L., and Steele, R. H. Evidence for the generation of an electronic excitation state in human polymorphonuclear leukocytes and its participation in bactericidal activity. *Biochem. Biophys. Res. Commun.* 47:679, 1972.
2. Anderson, R., et al. Defective chemotaxis in measles patients. *S. Afr. Med. J.* 48:1819, 1974.
3. Babior, B. M., Curnutte, J. T., and Kipnes, R. S. Pyridine nucleotide-dependent superoxide production by a cell-free system from human granulocytes. *J. Clin. Invest.* 56:1035, 1975.
4. Bainton, D. F., and Ferquhar, M. G. Differences in enzyme content of azurophil and specific granules of polymorphonuclear leukocytes. I. and II. *J. Cell Biol.* 39:286, 1968.
5. Boxer, L. A., Hedley-Whyte, E. T., and Stossel, T. P. Neutrophil actin dysfunction and abnormal neutrophil behavior. *N. Engl. J. Med.* 291:1093, 1974.
6. Clark, R. A., and Kimball, H. R. Defective granulocyte chemotaxis in the Chediak-Higashi syndrome. *J. Clin. Invest.* 50:2645, 1971.
7. Craddock, C. G. Production, distribution and fate of granulocytes. In W. J. Williams et al. (Eds.), *Hematology.* New York: McGraw-Hill, 1972.
8. Craddock, M. B., et al. Acquired phagocyte dysfunction: A complication of hypophosphatemia of parental hyperalimentation. *N. Engl. J. Med.* 290:1403, 1974.
9. Curnutte, J. T., Kipnes, R. S., and Babior, B. M. Defect in pyridine nucleotide dependent superoxide production by a particulate fraction from the granulocytes of patients with chronic granulomatous disease. *N. Engl. J. Med.* 293:628, 1975.
10. Curnutte, J. T., Whitten, D. M., and Babior, B. M. Defective leukocyte superoxide production in chronic granulomatous disease. *N. Engl. J. Med.* 290:593, 1974.
11. Faville, R. J., and Quie, P. G. Unpublished observations.
12. Greene, W. H., et al. The effect of hemodialysis on neutrophil chemotactic responsiveness. *J. Lab. Clin. Med.* 88:971, 1976.
13. Greendyke, R. M., Bradley, E. M., and Swisher, S. N. Studies of the effects of administration of SCTH and adrenal corticosteroids on erythrophagocytosis. *J. Clin. Invest.* 44:746, 1965.
14. Gregory, E. M., and Fridovich, I. Oxygen metabolism in *Lactobacillus plantarum.* *J. Bacteriol.* 117:166, 1974.
15. Golde, D. W., Finley, R. N., and Cline, M. J. Production of colony stimulating factor by human macrophages. *Lancet* II:1397, 1972.
16. Hill, J. R., et al. Modulation of human neutrophil chemotactic responses by cyclic 3'5' guanosine monophosphate and cyclic 3'5' adenosine monophosphate. *Metabolism* 24:447, 1975.
17. Hill, R. H., and Quie, P. G. Association of eczema, hyperimmunoglobulin E,

defective neutrophil chemotaxis and recurrent bacterial infections. *Lancet* I:183, 1974.

18. Hill, H. R., and Quie, P. G.   Defective neutrophil chemotaxis associated with hyperimmunoglobulinemia E. In J. A. Bellanti, and D. H. Dayton (Eds.), *The Phagocytic Cell in Host Resistance*. New York: Raven Press, 1975.

19. Hill, H. R., et al.   Defect in neutrophil granulocyte chemotaxis in Job's syndrome of recurrent "cold" staphylococcal abscesses. *Lancet* II:617, 1974.

20. Hirsch, J. G.   Cinemicrophotographic observations on granule lysis in polymorphonuclear leukocytes during phagocytosis. *J. Exp. Med.* 116:827, 1962.

21. Hohn, D. C., and Lehrer, R. I.   NADPH oxidase deficiency in X-linked chronic granulomatous disease. *J. Clin. Invest.* 55:707, 1975.

22. Holmes, C., Page, A. R., and Good, R. A.   Studies of the metabolic activity of leukocytes from patients with a genetic abnormality of phagocytic function. *J Clin. Invest.* 46:1422, 1967.

23. Johnston, R. B., Jr.   The mechanism of bacterial killing by normal and chronic granulomatous disease leukocyte. *Birth Defects* XI:71, 1975.

24. Johnston, R. B., et al.   Inhibition of phagocytic bactericidal activity by superoxide dismutase. A possible role of superoxide anion in killing of phagocytized bacteria. *J. Clin. Invest.* 52:44a, 1973.

25. Kaplan, E. L., Laxdal, T., and Quie, P. G.   Studies of polymorphonuclear leukocytes from patients with chronic granulomatous disease of childhood: Bactericidal capacity for streptococci. *Pediatrics* 41:591, 1968.

26. Karnovsky, M. L.   The metabolism of leukocytes. *Semin. Hematol.* 5:156, 1968.

27. Karnovsky, M. L.   Chronic granulomatous disease—pieces of a cellular and molecular puzzle. *Fed. Proc.* 32:1527, 1973.

28. Khan, A. F., et al.   Defective neutrophil chemotaxis in patients with Down's syndrome. *J. Pediatr.* 87:87, 1975.

29. Klebanoff, S. J., Clem, W. H., and Leubke, R. G.   The peroxidase-thiocyanate-hydrogen peroxide antimicrobial system. *Biochim. Biophys. Acta* 117:63, 1972.

30. Klebanoff, S. J.   Antimicrobial mechanisms in neutrophilic polymorphonuclear leukocytes. *Semin. Hematol.* 12:117, 1975.

31. Klebanoff, S. J.   Intraleukocytic microbicidal defects. *Annu. Rev. Med.* 22:39, 1975.

32. Lehrer, R. I.   Measurement of candidacidal activity of specific leukocyte types in mixed cell populations. II. Normal and chronic granulomatous disease eosinophils. *Infect. Immun.* 3:800, 1971.

33. Lehrer, R. I.   Functional aspects of a second mechanism of candidacidal activity by human neutrophils. *J. Clin. Invest.* 51:2566, 1972.

34. Mandell, G. L.   Bactericidal activity of aerobic and anaerobic polymorphonuclear neutrophils. *Infect. Immun.* 93:37, 1974.

35. McCall, C. E., et al.   Functional characteristics of human toxic neutrophils. *J. Infect. Dis.* 124:68, 1971.

36. McCullough, J., et al.   Effect of blood bank storage on leukocyte function. *Lancet* II:1333, 1969.

37. Miles, A. A., Miles, E. M., and Burke, J.   The value and duration of defense reactions of the skin to primary lodgement of bacteria. *Br. J. Exp. Pathol.* 38:79, 1957.

38. Miller, M. E., Oski, F. A., and Harris, M. B.   Lazy leukocyte syndrome, a new disorder of neutrophil function. *Lancet* I:665, 1971.

39. Messner, R. R., and Jelinek, J.   Receptors for human gamma G globulin on human neutrophils. *J. Clin. Invest.* 49:2165, 1970.

40. Nathan, D. G., and Baehner, R. L.   Disorders of phagocytic cell function. *Prog. Hematol.* 7:235, 1971.

41. Nathan, D. G., Baehner, R. L., and Weaner, D. K.   Failure of nitroblue tetra-

zolium reduction in the phagocytic vacuoles of leukocytes in chronic granulomatous disease. *J. Clin. Invest.* 48:1895, 1969.

42. Odeberg, H., Olsson, I., and Benge, P. Antibacterial and esterase activity of cationic proteins of human granulocytes. *Int. Res. Communic. System.* 2:1355, 1974.
43. Oh, M. H. K., et al. Defective candidacidal capacity of polymorphonuclear leukocytes in chronic granulomatous disease of childhood. *J. Pediatr.* 75:300, 1969.
44. Olmstead, J. B., and Borisy, G. G. Microtubules. *Annu. Rev. Biochem.* 42:507, 1967.
45. Quie, P. G. Chronic granulomatous disease in childhood. In I. Schulman (Ed.), *Advances in Pediatrics* 16:287, 1969.
46. Quie, P. G. Bactericidal function of human polymorphonuclear leukocytes. *Pediatrics* 50:264, 1972.
47. Quie, P. G., et al. *In vitro* bactericidal capacity of human polymorphonuclear leukocytes: Diminished activity in chronic granulomatous disease of childhood. *J. Clin. Invest.* 46:668, 1967.
48. Robinson, W. A., and Mangalik, A. Regulation of granulopoiesis: Positive feedback. *Lancet* II:742, 1972.
49. Robinson, W. A., and Mangalik, A. The kinetics and regulation of granulopoiesis. *Semin. Hematol.* 12:7, 1975.
50. Rodey, G. E., et al. Defective bactericidal activity of monocytes in fatal granulomatous disease. *Blood* 33:813, 1969.
51. Root, R. K., Rosenthal, A. S., and Balestra, D. J. Abnormal bactericidal, metabolism and lysosomal functions of Chediak-Higashi syndrome leukocytes. *J. Clin. Invest.* 51:649, 1972.
52. Rossi, F., Romeo, D., and Patriarca, P. Mechanism of phagocytosis-associated oxidative metabolism in polymorphonuclear leukocytes and macrophages. *J. Reticuloendothel. Soc.* 12:127, 1972.
53. Sbarra, A. J., et al. Biochemical aspects of phagocytic cells as related to bactericidal function. *J. Reticuloendothel. Soc.* 11:492, 1972.
54. Steerman, R. L., et al. Intrinsic defect of the polymorphonuclear leukocytes resulting in impaired chemotaxis and phagocytosis. *Clin. Exp. Immunol.* 9:939, 1971.
55. Stjernholm, R. L., et al. Impaired chemiluminescence during phagocytosis of opsonized bacteria. *Infect. Immun.* 7:313, 1973.
56. Stossel, T. P. Phagocytosis. *N. Engl. J. Med.* 290:717, 774, 833, 1974.
57. Stossel, T. P. Phagocytosis: Recognition and ingestion. *Semin. Hematol.* 12:83, 1975.
58. Stossel, T. P., and Pollard, T. D. Myosin in polymorphonuclear leukocytes. *J. Biol. Chem.* 248:8288, 1973.
59. Strauss, R. R., Paul, B. B., and Sbarra, A. J. Effect of phenylbutazone on phagocytosis and intracellular killing by guinea pig polymorphonuclear leukocytes. *J. Bacteriol.* 96:1982, 1968.
60. Van Scoy, R. E., et al. Familial neutrophil chemotaxis defect, recurrent bacterial infections, mucocutaneous candidiasis and hyperimmunoglobulinemia E. *Ann. Intern. Med.* 82:766, 1975.
61. Wolfson, J. J., et al. Bone findings in chronic granulomatous disease of childhood. *J Bone Joint Surg.* [A] 51:1573, 1969.
62. Wolfson, J. J., et al. Roentgenologic manifestations in children with a genetic defect of polymorphonuclear leukocyte function: Chronic granulomatous disease of children. *Radiology* 91:37, 1968.
63. Zeya, H. I., and Spitznagel, J. K. Arginine-rich proteins of polymorphonuclear leukocyte lysosomes. Antimicrobial specificity and biochemical heterogenecity. *J. Exp. Med.* 127:927, 1968.

2. The Role of Macrophages in Infectious Processes

Zanvil A. Cohn

The role of mononuclear phagocytes in resistance to infection and in inflammatory processes in general has been recognized since the classic studies of Metchinkoff. Wandering and sessile cells throughout the organism, either in direct contact with the bloodstream or in the extravascular compartment, play an important part in the recognition, ingestion, and destruction of foreign microbes or tissue cells. Within the past decade considerable progress has been made in understanding both the cellular and humoral factors involved in their physiology, and this has led to more rational approaches in delineating the basic mechanisms whereby they influence the economy of mammals in both normal and pathologic states.

Although I am unaware of a body of knowledge concerning their specific role in human infections, it is nevertheless worthwhile reviewing the biology of these cells and pointing out areas that might have relevance. We will therefore review the sequence of events leading to their effector role in the tissues and discuss factors that either enhance or depress these properties. For those of you unfamiliar with recent advances in the field, a number of reviews [5, 17, 19] will serve as background information.

Populations and Dynamics

The mononuclear phagocytes constitute a group of morphologically heterogeneous cells of common lineage that are widely distributed throughout the body. Most of our information concerning their kinetics and maturation comes from studies of small rodents, whereas our knowledge in man is still rather rudimentary. Like many blood-borne cells, this series is thought to arise from multipotent bone marrow stem cells, which through a series of cell divisions give rise to more mature and functionally active effector cells. The earliest recognizable members of the series have been referred to as monoblasts and promonocytes [18, 20]. They have been distinguished on the basis of substrate adherence, endocytosis, morphology, and cytochemical characteristics. It appears that the promonocyte is the immediate precursor of the monocyte and is the last member that actively divides under steady-state situations. In the mouse, promonocytes constitute only a small fraction of the bone marrow population and the 25 to 30 gm animal has about 5×10^5 cells. From thymidine labeling studies it has been determined that they have a generation time of approximately 16 hours and a 12-hour period of DNA synthesis.

Following division promonocytes give rise to monocytes, which spend a short time in the marrow before being released into the circulation. The general scheme of mononuclear phagocyte differentiation differs markedly from that of the granulocyte series in that no large reserve of mature cells is available in the marrow. Once in the bloodstream monocytes represent a nondividing population that constitutes only 3 to 5% of the total circulating white cells. In the mouse the total monocyte pool is approximately 1 to 2×10^6 cells, which, under steady-state conditions, has an intravascular half-life of about 22 hours. The monocytes leave the circulation randomly and presumably enter all tissue compartments, where they mature into typical macrophages. Data on man [21] suggest a generation time of 19 to 25 hours and a circulation time of 30 to 100 hours.

Under conditions of inflammation, the kinetics of this series may be markedly changed [20]. The production rate of monocytes increases from 0.65×10^5 per hour to 1.06×10^5 per hour, and this is correlated with a decrease in both the cell cycle and the DNA synthesis time. Preliminary evidence suggests that a humoral factor may govern the production rate [20]. Depending on the site of inflammation or infection, monocytes are focused into the lesion and as much as 50% of the total production may accumulate in these sites. In contrast, glucocorticoids reduce the production rate, yield a striking monocytopenia, and severely depress the accumulation of monocytes in local lesions [20].

The tissue stores of macrophages are very large when compared to the number of cells present in the bone marrow and intravascular compartments. Most of these cells are thought to be derived from circulating monocytes that either attach to the wall of sinusoids in the liver and spleen or emigrate between endothelial cells of post-capillary venules, thereby gaining access to the tissue spaces. Here they appear to have a relatively long life span, a slow turnover rate, and in most circumstances are nondividing cells arrested in a go state. Under some situations, however, these cells do demonstrate restricted cell division and this may lead to elevated local populations. It is reasonably certain, however, that the majority of macrophages that accumulate in inflammatory lesions are of monocyte origin.

Emigration and Focusing

It is apparent that to adequately control microbial multiplication, sufficient numbers of cells must be able to enter the lesion promptly and continuously. The factors responsible for the directed localization of monocytes are still imperfectly understood. Much of our knowledge comes from in vitro assays utilizing the Boyden chamber technique to study the directional migration of macrophages on monocytes along a concentration gradient of an attractant. Under these conditions agents such as C5A have potent chemotactic activity. This split product of C5 may be generated with immune complexes, endotoxin, or through the action of leukocyte proteases. A number of less well defined agents have been discussed that are present in either serum or plasma or may be the products of stimulated bone marrow derived lymphocytes, i.e., lymphokines [14]. It seems likely, however, that many attractants can be generated via the complement, kinin, or clotting systems and can act in concert to focus the circulating monocyte into local lesions. The relative potency, temporal production, and specificity of these agents under in vivo conditions is an important area for future research. Furthermore, recent observations suggest the presence of chemotactic inhibitors in serum as well as depressed chemotactic responsiveness of cells from patients with malignancies [15].

Endocytosis

One of the primary roles of macrophages in controlling infections is the recognition and interiorization of microbial agents. In most instances humoral factors, such as antibody and complement, are either required or greatly enhance the rate of phagocytosis. This is largely the result of opsonization of the organism's surface followed by the attachment of the particle to the macrophage's plasma membrane. In this regard, macrophages have functional "receptors" on their plasmalemmas, as yet uncharacterized, which aid in this process. The first has been termed the Fc receptor and represents a trypsin insensitive domain that interacts with the Fc piece of IgG and is present on both monocytes and macrophages. Particles bound through the Fc receptor are rapidly interiorized and are then contained within a phagocytic vacuole, the membrane of which is derived from the plasma membrane. The factors that control the fusion of membranes to form the vacuole are largely unknown. Recent evidence by Silverstein and his colleagues suggests that circumferential attachment must occur prior to interiorization. This implies that the macrophage membrane flows around the particle, making continual receptor-ligand contacts until it reaches the apex and fuses. Although contractile elements beneath the plasma membrane are thought to play a role in the phagocytic process, their nature, attachment sites, and triggers remain as areas for future study.

A second important receptor recognizes activated complement components, particularly a cleavage product of C3, i.e., C3B. This combining site on the membrane is readily removed with trypsin in contrast to the Fc receptor. In unstimulated monocytes and macrophages it leads only to the attachment of the particle to the macrophage surface (EA IgM-C3B) and is not followed by ingestion. However, stimulated macrophages, evoked by a variety of inflammatory agents, do have the capacity to readily ingest these particles [2].

Less well defined attachment sites exist for a number of particles that do not require the presence of either antibody or complement. These include polystyrene latex beads, zymosan, aldehyde-fixed erythrocytes, and a number of bacterial species of low virulence. These sites are distinct from the Fc receptor since an antimacrophage antibody blocks the ingestion of Ig coated particles. Therefore the Fc receptor does not influence the phagocytosis of this group [10].

Post-phagocytic Events

Once a microorganism is contained within a phagocytic vacuole, a series of events ensues that may lead to its ultimate inactivation and degradation. The vacuole itself, or phagosome, enters the cytoplasm and is often transported toward the region of the Golgi apparatus. In this locus it fuses with a group of organelles called lysosomes, which contain a variety of hydrolytic enzymes and perhaps bactericidal components. This fusion forms a composite structure known as the phagolysosome, or digestive body, thereby mixing within the same membrane-bounded vacuole enzymes of macrophage origin and exogenous organisms taken up by phagocytosis. Depending on the susceptibility of the microorganism to the contents of this vacuole, it may either be killed or in some instances survive and multiply, leading to an intracellular infection.

The mechanisms involved in the killing of bacteria, viruses, and protozoa within the macrophage are poorly understood as compared to the events within the granulocyte. A number of factors have been defined but their relative potency and importance are not clear. The first to be considered is the acid condition that prevails within the phagolysosome — the milieu in which the lysosomal hydrolases have their most efficient activity. This may reach levels of pH 4 to 5.5, a hydrogen ion concentration that is sufficient to kill a restricted group of saprophytes and pathogens. A second agent present within both monocytes and macrophages is the aminopolysaccharidase lysozyme, or muramidase. This enzyme by itself or when present with antibody and complement has the ability to degrade the cell walls of a number of species. A third component consists of the metabolic intermediates hydrogen peroxide (H_2O_2) and superoxide anion O_2^-. Peroxide by itself at an acid pH and in the absence of peroxidases has intrinsic bactericidal activity as reviewed by Klebanoff and Hammon [11]. The role of superoxide is less clear-cut but may, through the intervention of superoxide dismutase, be converted to H_2O_2 with resulting bactericidal activity. Hydrogen peroxide may also have a greater microbicidal effect in the presence of either myeloperoxidase and/or catalase. In this respect, myeloperoxidase is only demonstrable in circulating monocytes, not in tissue macrophages, whereas catalase is present in the more mature cell type.

Subsequent to the microbicidal event many organisms are partially or totally degraded within the phagocytic vacuole as the result of the concerted efforts of the lysosomal hydrolases. Proteins, lipids, nucleic acids, and polysaccharides are all attached, although at different rates. Some polysaccharides, because of unusual chemical linkages, may persist for long periods of time, whereas other components are rapidly digested. Studies employing labeled macromolecules have given some weight to the rate and extent of intralysosomal hydrolysis [16]. In the case of proteins, these are degraded to amino acids and dipeptides, which then permeate through the lysosomal membrane and are either excreted or utilized for protein synthesis.

Aberrations in Post-phagocytic Events

There are a number of examples in which specific microorganisms influence the train of intracytoplasmic events discussed previously. The first to be mentioned are those instances in which the organism is able to escape the confines of the vacuolar system and subsequently replicate in the cytosol. Perhaps the best studied example is the interaction of vaccinia virus in mouse macrophages [13]. Here, the virus enters by endocytosis, is partially uncoated by lysosomal enzymes, but then escapes from the phagolysosome. In this instance, coating the virus with specific antibody blocks the escape mechanism and the vision is completely degraded within the lysosome. More recently Nadia Noguiero in our laboratory has extended this analysis to *Trypanosoma cruzi*, the causative agent of Chaga's disease. In this instance the trypanosome also escapes from the phagocytic vacuole and replicates in the extravacuolar space.

A different mechanism is employed by the *Chlamydia*, virulent tubercle bacilli, and *Toxoplasma* [1, 9]. These organisms modify the phagocytic vacuole in as yet unknown ways and block the fusion with primary and secondary lysosomes, thereby avoiding bactericidins and digestive enzymes. A similar situation exists when macrophages are treated with the plant lectin concanavalin A (Con A) [3, 4]. Con A, after binding to mannose-containing glycoproteins on the plasma membrane, inhibits the fusion between pinocytic vesicles and lysosomes, inhibiting the intracellular digestion of the vesicles' contents. In this system, Con A can be removed from intracellular membranes with the competitive sugar α-methyl mannoside, thereby allowing fusion to occur and digestion to proceed.

Acquired Antibacterial Immunity

Within the past decade there has been considerable progress in our understanding of acquired resistance to a group of intracellular bacterial parasites, e.g., *Listeria* and *Salmonella*, that produce chronic infections. These organisms persist and multiply in organs such as liver and spleen, in part within the resident macrophages. Largely through the studies of George Mackaness and his colleagues at the Trudeau Institute, many aspects of this complicated sequence have been unraveled. Two cell types appear to be involved — the macrophage as a nonspecific effector and the T lymphocyte as the immunologically specific component. During a chronic infection T lymphocytes are activated by as yet unknown products from the viable organism. These cells in turn are thought to either produce lymphokines or, through some other form of close cell contact, modulate the bactericidal activity of macrophages. A number of results ensue that lead to the control of infection and the eventual destruction of the bacterium. Coincident with the acquisition of host resistance, macrophages display enhanced listericidal activity and are altered morphologically in terms of cell surface ruffling, endocytosis, and a variety of metabolic parameters. This then suggests modification of the effector on a cellular level. There are, however, other important concomitants that have to do with population dynamics. In particular, as demonstrated by North [12], the critical requirement is for circulating monocytes to enter the parenchymatous lesions. Presumably large numbers of fresh cells are necessary to control bacterial replication and it seems likely that lymphocyte products may aid the focusing system. Little is known about this form of host resistance in man largely because of the difficulty of devising appropriate clinical models.

Extracellular Products and the Role of Macrophages as Secretory Cells

We have so far stressed intracellular mechanisms for the uptake and destruction of infectious agents by macrophages. There are, however, other routes by which macrophages may influence their milieu and that are pertinent to a discussion of both specific infections and inflammation in general. This is through the liberation of products into their extracellular environment — products that can alter the connective tissue matrix, microorganisms, and other neighboring cells. These products fall into at least three categories. The first is the extracellular release of lysosomal hydrolases during the process of phagocytosis. This may, in part, be the result of the fusion of lysosomes with partially interiorized particles and the release of enzymes from the imperfectly closed phagocytic vacuole. These enzymes would then find themselves in an environment quite different in terms of pH from the secondary lysosome. A second mechanism, which has been appreciated only recently, is the active biosynthesis and secretion of enzymes with neutral pH optima. These may well have important physiologic roles in tissue remodeling. The first to be described is the enzyme lysozyme [6]. This enzyme appears to be the major secretory product of monocytes and macrophages and is secreted by both unstimulated and stimulated cells. It is in a sense a "constitutive" product whose formation is not influenced by a variety of perturbations, including endocytosis. Another group of enzymes, all of which are neutral proteinases, are actively secreted only by the stimulated, or "activated," macrophage. These include a plasminogen activator, a specific collagenase, and an elastase that differs from the granulocyte elastase in its substrate specificity. It is of interest that with certain of these enzymes, the uptake and storage of a nondigestible particle leads to continual, long-term release, whereas the uptake of a rapidly digestible particle leads to a brief increase in secretion [7].

There are, in addition, a large number of factors, released by macrophages in an unspecified manner, that have important biological effects. These include a bactericidal agent that kills *Listeria monocytogenes;* a colony-stimulating factor that promotes the growth of bone marrow cells in soft agar, endogenous pyrogen, and interferon; and factors that stimulate the growth of lymphocytes and fibroblasts in vitro. None of these agents has been characterized in a chemical sense; and such characterization awaits future investigation. Much of this area has recently been reviewed by Gordon, Unkeless, and Cohn [8].

Conclusion

It is apparent that we are only beginning to appreciate the diverse roles played by mononuclear phagocytes in homeostatic mechanisms. Modulated by humoral and cellular factors, they are able to adapt to microenvironments, thereby altering their functional properties. These properties, although becoming delineated in experimental animals, are largely unstudied in man, partly because it is difficult to obtain tissue populations in homogeneous form. Nevertheless, through the use of appropriate sources, such as the circulating monocyte, alveolar macrophages, and those cells that accumulate in serous cavities, significant progress can be made. Such concerted effort should, within a reasonable period of time, give us a means to evaluate their activities in the infection-prone patient and in other pathologic states.

References

1. Armstrong, J. A., and Hart, P. D. Response of cultured macrophages to *Mycobacterium tuberculosis*, with observations on fusion of lysosomes with phagosomes. *J. Exp. Med.* 134:713, 1973.
2. Bianco, C., Griffin, R. M., Jr., and Silverstein, S. C. Studies of the macrophage complement receptor. Alteration of receptor function upon macrophage activation. *J. Exp. Med.* 141:1278, 1975.
3. Edelson, P. J., and Cohn, Z. A. Effects of concanavalin A on mouse peritoneal macrophages. I. Stimulation of endocytic activity and inhibition of phagolysosome formation. *J. Exp. Med.* 140:1364, 1974.
4. Edelson, P. J., and Cohn, Z. A. Effects of concanavalin A on mouse peritoneal macrophages. II. Metabolism of endocytized proteins and reversibility of the effects of mannose. *J. Exp. Med.* 140:1387, 1974.
5. Gordon, S. and Cohn, Z. A. The macrophage. *Int. Rev. Cytol.* 36:171, 1973.
6. Gordon, S., Todd, J., and Cohn, Z. A. *In vitro* synthesis and secretion of lysozyme by mononuclear phagocytes. *J. Exp. Med.* 139:1228, 1974.
7. Gordon, S., Unkeless, J. C., and Cohn, Z. A. Induction of macrophage plasminogen activator by endotoxin stimulation and phagocytosis. Evidence of a two-stage process. *J. Exp. Med.* 140:995, 1974.
8. Gordon, S., Unkeless, J. C., and Cohn, Z. A. The Macrophage as Secretory Cell. In A. Rosenthal (Ed.), *Immune Recognition.* New York: Academic, 1975.
9. Jones, T. C., and Hirsch, J. G. The interaction between *Toxoplasma gondii* and mammalian cells. II. The absence of lysosomal fusion with phagocytic vacuoles containing living parasites. *J. Exp. Med.* 136:1173, 1972.
10. Holland, P., Holland, N., and Cohn, Z. A. The selective inhibition of macrophage phagocytic receptors by anti-membrane antibodies. *J. Exp. Med.* 135:458, 1972.
11. Klebanoff, S. J., and Hammon, C. B. Antimicrobial Systems of Mononuclear Phagocytes. In R. van Furth (Ed.), *Mononuclear Phagocytes in Immunity, Infection and Pathology.* London: Blackwell Scientific, 1975.

12. North, R. J. Suppression of cell-mediated immunity to infection by an anti-mitotic drug: Further evidence that migrant macrophages express immunity. *J. Exp. Med.* 132:535, 1970.
13. Silverstein, S. Macrophages and viral immunity. *Sem. Hematol.* 7:185, 1969.
14. Snyderman, R., and Stohl, C. Chemotaxis of Mononuclear Leukocytes. In E. Sorkin et al. (Eds.), *Biology and Chemistry of Chemotaxis.* White Plains, N.Y.: Phiebig, 1974.
15. Snyderman, R., and Stohl, C. Defective Immune Effector Function in Patients with Neoplastic and Immune Deficiency Diseases. In J. A. Bellanti and D. H. Dayton (Eds.), *The Phagocytic Cell in Host Resistance.* New York: Raven, 1975.
16. Steinman, R. M., and Cohn, Z. A. The interaction of soluble horseradish peroxidase with mouse peritoneal macrophages *in vitro. J. Cell Biol.* 55:186, 1972.
17. Steinman, R. M., and Cohn, Z. A. The Metabolism and Physiology of the Mononuclear Phagocytes. In B. W. Zweifach, L. Grant, and R. T. McCloskey (Eds.), *The Inflammatory Process.* New York: Academic, 1974.
18. Van Furth, R., and Cohn, Z. A. The origin and kinetics of mononuclear phagocytes. *J. Exp. Med.* 128:415, 1968.
19. Van Furth, R. Origin and Kinetics of Monocytes and Macrophages. *Sem. Hematol.* 7:125, 1970.
20. Van Furth, R. Modulation of Monocyte Production. In R. van Furth (Ed.), *Mononuclear Phagocytes in Immunity, Infection and Pathology.* London: Blackwell Scientific, 1975.
21. Whitelaw, D. M., and Batho, H. F. Kinetics of Monocytes. In R. van Furth (Ed.), *Mononuclear Phagocytes in Immunity, Infection and Pathology.* London: Blackwell Scientific, 1975.

3. The Role of the Lymphocyte in Preventing Bacterial and Viral Infection

Sir Gustav Nossal

This paper surveys the chief mechanisms by which antibody (manufactured following B lymphocyte activation) and cell-mediated immunity (through activated T lymphocytes) guard against bacterial and viral infection. First, the physiology of T and B lymphocytes is briefly described. Then some of the means by which microbes can evade immune destruction are summarized. Mention is made of illuminating models of T or B lymphocyte deficiency in experimental animals.

More detailed attention is given to establishing the validity of the clonal selection theory of antibody formation as a prelude to explaining many of the antigen-activated mechanisms and feedback loops to *depress*, rather than stimulate, immune responses. These include immunologic tolerance; negative feedback by antibody; blockade of lymphocyte receptors by antigen, or, more efficiently, by antigen-antibody complexes; suppressor T cells; and anti-idiotype networks.

As soon as semiquantitative methods became available for the measurement of immune responses in the early part of this century, a vision of immunity of a rather oversimplified character became widespread. It is schematized in Figure 3-1. Here, the immune response is seen as a kind of all-conquering avalanche, with a latent period, an exponential phase, and a plateau and decline, together with a heightened response to booster immunization. Although quantitation is more difficult for delayed hypersensitivity than for antibody formation, the pattern is broadly similar, with perhaps an even longer duration of immunity.

The model is an accurate description of responses to many artificial vaccines, but the real-life situation in natural infections may be much more complex. Thus we find situations where infection persists in the face of a mounting immune response, or where infections with microorganisms, usually of low pathogenicity, occur following even relatively minor changes in the integrity of the immune defense system. In other words, the immune response to an antigenic load is really the result of a complex network of regulatory processes and feedback loops and far from an all-or-none event.

Three Interacting Cells in the Immune System

My role in this symposium is to delineate the function of lymphocytes in im-

This is Publication No. 2166 from The Walter and Eliza Hall Institute.
This work was supported by the National Health and Medical Research Council, Canberra, Australia, by Grant AI 03958 and Contract No. 1-23889 from NIH, U.S. Public Health Service, and by the Volkswagen Foundation Grant No. 112147.

26.

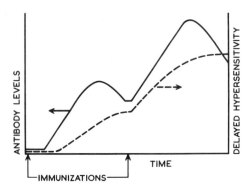

Figure 3-1. A stereotyped version of typical immune responses.

munity, but this can only be addressed by admitting that the cellular basis of immunity depends centrally on three kinds of interacting cells, namely B lymphocytes, T lymphocytes, and macrophages (Figure 3-2) and, for various effector functions, also on other collaborating cells such as neutrophils, eosinophils, and mast cells.

The B lymphocyte is the ancestor of antibody-forming cells [18]. It is made in the fetal liver and later in the adult bone marrow [15] and, by an as yet mysterious process of somatic diversification, different B lymphocytes come to possess immunoglobulin (Ig) receptors of differing specificity. One cell only shows one kind of receptor [2, 11], and when an antigen enters the body, it only stimulates those subsets of B lymphocytes with receptors that are capable of uniting with the antigen (Figure 3-3). Some evidence for this clonal selection theory of antibody formation is presented later in this chapter.

T lymphocytes are made in the thymus. They recognize antigen by means of receptors; but for reasons that are not clear, the receptors are much more difficult to identify and characterize. There is now good evidence for an IgM-like molecule on the T cell surface [10], and it is possible that T cells also have other receptors, perhaps involved in lymphocyte collaboration [9]. The T cell can help the B cell to form antibody, probably by

 B LYMPHOCYTE. MADE IN BONE MARROW. HAS IgM RECEPTORS FOR ANTIGEN; 'ONE CELL, ONE RECEPTOR;' TRIGGERING GIVES RISE TO AFC.

Figure 3-2. Some characteristics of B cells, T cells, and macrophages.

 T LYMPHOCYTE. MADE IN THE THYMUS. HAS 'BURIED' Ig RECEPTORS AND MAY HAVE ANOTHER KIND OF RECEPTOR. HELPS B CELLS MAKE ANTIBODY. MEDIATES CELLULAR IMMUNITY.

 MACROPHAGE. ITS RECEPTORS FOR ANTIGEN ARE PASSIVELY ACQUIRED; ONE MACROPHAGE 'SEES' MANY ANTIGENS. IT IS INVOLVED IN T−B COLLABORATION AND IN INITIATION OF CELLULAR IMMUNITY.

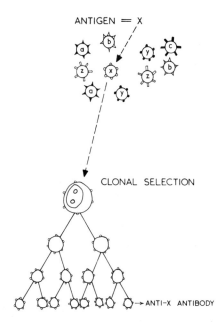

ANTIGEN = X

CLONAL SELECTION

ANTI-X ANTIBODY

Figure 3-3. Burnet's clonal selection theory of antibody formation.

secreting factors that facilitate B lymphocyte triggering by antigen. They are also the key cells in the various forms of cell-mediated immunity.

Macrophages are important accessory cells in antibody formation. In many models, lymphocyte activation and T-B lymphocyte collaboration cannot proceed without macrophages. As well as concentrating antigen and presenting it to lymphocytes, macrophages can, when suitably activated, secrete products that aid B cell triggering. Indeed, it is possible that the observed T cell effects are mediated through the activation of macrophages.

Some Central Concepts in Immunity to Infections

How can some infections persist chronically in the face of an effective immune attack? It must be recalled that intracellular microorganisms, such as facultative intracellular bacteria or intracytoplasmic viruses, are inaccessible either to antibody or to T cells. It is only when the infected cell bears antigens on its surface, as in the case of a cell infected with budding viruses, that it becomes susceptible to T cell killing [1]. This process may limit the spread of infection, but it may also cause considerable cellular damage [3]. As far as antibody is concerned, it alone is usually not able to kill bacteria but requires collaboration of complement or macrophages; thus defects in either of these may facilitate chronicity. Equally important in limiting the efficacy of the immune attack may be various antigen-activated mechanisms to *depress* rather than stimulate immunity. We consider these separately.

Antibody is uniquely useful in preventing infection and, as the early experiments with pneumonia showed, can also play a major role in controlling the spread of infection. In bacterial infections, antibody can have bacteriolytic effects through classic complement-dependent pathways. It can opsonize bacteria and aid phagocytosis and elimination; and it can neutralize bacterial endotoxins and exotoxins, thus limiting host damage. In viral infections, antibodies to viral surface macromolecules, important in the attachment of a virus to a host cell, can prevent viral entry and thus limit the spread of infection. Virus opsonization is also important, and there is some evidence in favor of complement-dependent virus neutralization.

T lymphocytes are at least equally important in controlling infection. First, in many experimental situations, T lymphocytes are essential for B lymphocytes to make antibody, especially the IgG antibodies responsible for most antitoxin activity. Second, activated T lymphocytes release lymphokines, which are responsible for attracting monocytes and for activating them, as is more fully discussed in Chapter 2. Further, T lymphocytes make interferon (important in viral infections) and also can kill cells bearing viral antigens on their surface by direct cytotoxic action [6].

These concepts explain why the immunodeficient patient is infection-prone. In the laboratory, two classic models show the role of lymphocytes most dramatically. These are the congenitally athymic (nu/nu or nude) mouse, which lacks functional T cells, and the "bursaless" chicken, which lacks B cells and antibodies [24]. Both these experimental types of immunodeficiency lead to failure to thrive and death at an early age from overwhelming infection. The nude mouse can be kept in good health by germ-free isolation or strict, specific pathogen-free conditions. In man, as discussed in Chapter 8, there are also somewhat similar types of immunodeficiency. Agammaglobulinemia, which is frequently incomplete, represents a B cell deficiency. Such patients are very susceptible to pyogenic infections. They usually display normal recovery from virus infections or smallpox vaccination but have been shown to be more susceptible to reinfection. Also, they may suffer a higher incidence of paralysis when infected with poliomyelitis virus [22], since prevention of entry from the gut probably depends on intestinal IgA antibody, and spread to the nervous system depends on serum antibodies. The normal recovery from many virus infections highlights the importance of T cell immunity. In T cell deficiencies with normal or near-normal globulin levels, progressive vaccinia has been noted after smallpox vaccination, and infections with herpes simplex, cytomegalovirus, varicella, and measles are often extremely severe. Also, infections with bacteria that are not usually of great pathogenicity, fungi, or yeasts can occur. Patients on immunosuppressive treatment after renal transplantation show similar tendencies.

Evidence for Specialization among B Lymphocytes

The rest of this chapter concentrates on B lymphocyte function. Evidence is shown that these are indeed highly specialized, as the clonal selection theory predicts, and that complex, antigen-dependent mechanisms exist to "silence," as well as activate, these cells.

It has been known for some time that B lymphocyte populations can be deprived of their capacity to react to a given antigen by passing them over affinity columns containing that antigen [25]. In other words, to react to an antigen, lymphocytes must have receptors for it. However, it has only recently proved possible to utilize this technology of specific binding to actually *enrich* a cell's capacity to react to antigen. In our laboratory, a simple technology has recently been developed [6, 7, 17] that allows the isolation of cells that respond 1,000 times better than the original starting population to challenge in tissue culture with a particular hapten. The principle of this technique is to bind mouse lymphoid cells onto a mono-layer of hapten-gelatin at 4°C in the presence of free soluble gelatin to avoid binding of gelatin-specific cells; to wash off nonadherent cells; to warm to 37°C, melting the monolayer; to recover the bound cells by centrifugation; and to remove adherent antigen by collagenase treatment. However, such cells are not completely pure hapten-specific cells, since some problems of nonspecific adherence remain. However, a second cycle of similar fractionation raises the percent of genuine hapten-binding cells from 37 to 67%. Alternatively, a first cycle of hapten-gelatin fractionation can be followed by a second cycle, whereby the cells are rosetted with hapten-coated sheep erythrocytes, separated from nonrosetted cells, and freed of adherent erythrocytes by osmotic shock and trypsin treatment. In this case, cells with up to 90% capacity to bind the hapten are provided.

The capacity of these fractionated lymphocytes, 90% of which are B cells, to form antibody to the given hapten can be tested by specialized microculture techniques [17, 23]. When normal adult mouse spleen cells are used without fractionation, only about 1 cell in 20,000 can be induced to form antibody to a given hapten. The first fractionation step produces a 500-fold enrichment so that an average of 1 in 40 cells can, on appropriate stimulation, give a clone of about 20 antibody-secreting cells within 3 days of tissue culture. A second cycle of hapten-gelatin fractionation raises this to an average of 1 in 21 cells, and the best results are obtained with combined hapten-gelatin binding and rosetting, which yields 1 in 13.5 cells capable of giving an antibody-producing clone. Bearing in mind the high death rate of lymphocytes when placed into artificial tissue culture conditions, this is indeed a remarkable enrichment.

Availability of these fractionated cells allows tests of the validity of the clonal selection theory in two ways. First, the fractionated cells can be tested for their capacity to respond to haptens other than the one used for fractionation. Here, they show only minimal activity, reflecting minor degrees of cross-reactivity between haptens. In other words, the enrichment is specific. Second, using immunofluorescence techniques, one can ask whether all the Ig receptors on the lymphocyte can react with the given hapten used for the fractionation procedure. This is done by attaching the hapten to a polymeric protein carrier that also carries a fluorescent dye, e.g., rhodamine, and then reacting the fractionated cells with this at 37°C for 15 min. The result is that the hapten-specific Ig receptors are pulled into a "cap" at one pole of the cell. Subsequently, the cells can be fixed, preventing further receptor movement, and stained with an antiglobulin reagent carrying a different fluorescent dye, e.g., fluorescein. This will stain the cap but will also stain residual, uncapped Ig receptors as a smooth, linear ring of fluorescence. It has recently been shown [14, 21] that in the majority of cases, all the Ig detectable on the surface of hapten-specific B cells can be capped by hapten-polymer conjugates. In other words, the receptors appear to have uniform specificity: one cell, one antibody.

How Prolonged, Heavy Antigen Loads in Chronic Infections
May Eventually Depress Immunity

Although we know less about receptors for antigen on T cells, it is likely that they, too, are specialized [11]. In other words, there is diversity among T cells but we cannot yet say "one T cell, one specificity." Therefore any antigen-specific suppression of the immune response must depend on suppression or elimination of specific B or T cell clones.

There are various ways in which antigen can be effective in suppressing immunity [13]. The following six are among the most important: (1) immunologic tolerance, (2) negative feedback by antibody, (3) antigen-antibody complex-mediated blockade of lymphocyte receptors, (4) blockade by antigen of lymphocyte receptors, (5) suppressor T cells, and (6) anti-idiotype networks.

Immunologic tolerance can be defined as a specific acquired central failure of immune responsiveness due to prior exposure to antigen. It is specific and thus differs from the immune suppression due to drugs. It is acquired through exposure to antigen, and thus it is different from the specific poor immune responses that go with the possession of certain immune response genes; and it is central in the sense of being a property of the lymphocyte population. It is due to the elimination or functional silencing of all or a proportion of the T or B lymphocytes of a given specificity.

While there are certainly different mechanisms for achieving this goal, one of them is of special interest to my laboratory. Figures 3-4 and 3-5 describe our present understanding of lymphocyte differentiation. As far as B cell neogenesis is concerned, this occurs in the fetal liver, newborn spleen, or adult bone marrow [15, 20]. Stem cells, which are inherently multipotent, differentiate by a series of poorly understood steps into large lymphocytes. These, by a series of mitotic divisions, give rise to medium and small lymphocytes, which can be thought of as pre-B cells because they do not yet possess Ig and other receptors characteristic of the immunologically competent cell. Then, during a critical 2-day nonmitotic maturation phase, which can occur either within the marrow or immediately after seeding to the secondary lymphoid organs, receptors appear in increasing numbers and the cells are ready to respond.

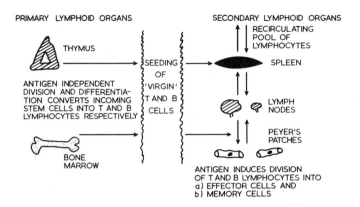

Figure 3-4. Differences between primary and secondary lymphoid organs.

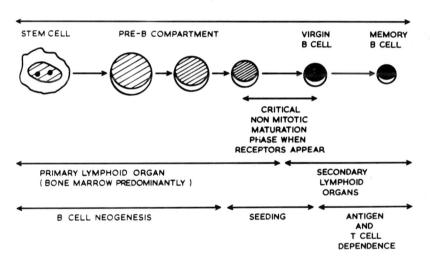

Figure 3-5. Differentiation of B lymphocytes.

We have recently gathered substantial evidence [16] that if cells are exposed to antigen during this critical maturation phase, i.e., when they have some receptors but are not yet mature, the contact may lead to a functional elimination of that cell. We term this process *clonal abortion* — the cell is switched off or eliminated before it differentiates far enough to be able to respond to antigen. One relevant experiment is shown in Figure 3-6. Here, adult mouse bone marrow or adult spleen cells were cultured for 3 days with various concentrations of haptenated antigen, DNP-HGG. At the end of the period, the cells were washed and their capacity to mount an immune response was measured in an adoptive immune assay. Specificity controls are not shown, but both spleen and bone marrow cells responded normally to an irrelevant hapten. Surprisingly low concentrations of the specific anti-

32.

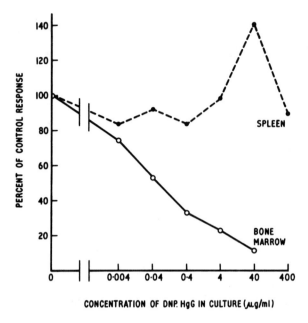

Figure 3-6. The effect of 3 days' incubation with antigen on bone marrow B cell competence.

gen present in culture caused tolerance in the bone marrow, but not the splenic, B cells. The residual 20% reactivity not eliminated by the tolerance treatment is probably due to the presence within bone marrow of a proportion of mature, nontolerizable B lymphocytes (J. W. Stocker, paper in preparation).

Negative feedback by antibody acts in part through the neutralization of antigen, which is needed to drive the immune response along, and in part through a more subtle mechanism. It turns out that antigen-antibody complexes, even at low concentration, are powerfully suppressive for both T and B lymphocytes [5], probably because of a blockade and modulation of surface receptors. Even antigen alone can achieve this effect if present in sufficiently high concentration, and particularly if it is present in multivalent form. This is thought to be behind some of the failure of immune reactivity in metastatic cancer [21]. Suppressor T cells are still poorly understood, but it appears there are circumstances under which antigen can activate T cells to *lower* B cell responses to antigens rather than to help them. This may be a function of a particular subset of T cells. Anti-idiotype networks are a recent, fascinating byway of immunology [4, 8]. The general idea is explained in Figure 3-7. An antibody molecule has a combining site (made up of the V regions of an immunoglobulin heavy chain and light chain), and this in its own right constitutes an antigen. The antigenic specificity of this

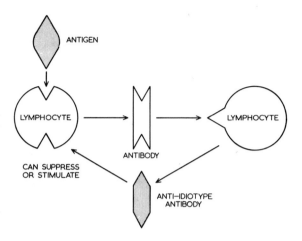

Figure 3-7. Anti-idiotype formation.

antibody is termed its *idiotype*. Anti-idiotype antibodies appear under some circumstances. These can react with the antibody evoking their formation as well as with the originally stimulated T or B lymphocytes. Similarly, anti-idiotype T cells can be generated. Depending on experimental circumstances, this generation can stimulate the cell (the anti-idiotype acts like an antigen) or suppress the cell (the anti-idiotype acts like a tolerogen, or the anti-idiotype T cell kills the idiotype-bearing cell).

This brief analysis has shown that the immune response is indeed subject to a myriad of important control and feedback loops. It should be clear that the "avalanche" paradigm is not always accurate and that a chronic antigenic load may result in a balanced immunity with plateau levels, sometimes set rather low, as an end result.

In the infection-prone patient, congenital or acquired defects in the immune apparatus can affect this delicate network, as can transient stresses (through neuroendocrine mechanisms), malnutrition, uremia, advanced malignancy, aging, and a host of other factors. Thus some insight into the normal physiology of T and B lymphocytes is necessary to develop a more rational understanding and a better management of infection-proneness.

References
1. Blanden, R. V. T cell response to viral and bacterial infection. *Transplant. Rev.* 19:56, 1974.
2. Burnet, F. M. *The Clonal Selection Theory of Acquired Immunity.* London: Cambridge University Press, 1959.
3. Doherty, P. C., and Zinkernagel, R. M. T-cell-mediated immunopathology in viral infection. *Transplant. Rev.* 19:89, 1974.
4. Eichmann, K., and Rajewsky, K. Induction of T and B cell immunity by anti-idiotypic antibody. *Eur. J. Immunol.* 5:661, 1975.

5. Feldmann, M., and Nossal, G. J. V.   Tolerance, enhancement and the regulation of interactions between b cells, B cells and macrophages. *Transplant. Rev.* 13:3, 1972.
6. Haas, W., and Layton, J. E.   Separation of antigen-specific lymphocytes. I. Enrichment of antigen-binding cells. *J. Exp. Med.* 141:1004, 1975.
7. Haas, W.   Separation of antigen-specific lymphocytes. II. Enrichment of hapten-specific antibody-forming cell precursors. *J. Exp. Med.* 141:1015, 1975.
8. Jerne, N. K.   Towards a network theory of the immune system. *Ann. Immunol.* (Paris) [c], 125:373, 1974.
9. Katz, D. H., and Benacerraf, B.   The function and interrelationships of T-cell receptors, Ir genes and other histocompatibility gene products. *Transplant. Rev.* 22:175, 1975.
10. Marchalonis, J. J.   Lymphocyte receptors for antigen. *J. Med.* 5:329, 1974.
11. Nossal, G. J. V.   Various forms of specialization in cells which synthesize immunoglobulins. *Ann. Immunol.* (Paris) [c] 125:239, 1974.
12. Nossal, G. J. V.   Principles of immunological tolerance and immunocyte receptor blockade. *Adv. Cancer Res.* 20:93, 1974.
13. Nossal, G. J. V., and Ada, G. L.   *Antigens, Lymphoid Cells and the Immune Response.* New York, London: Academic, 1971.
14. Nossal, G. J. V., and Layton, J. E.   Antigen-induced aggregation and modulation of receptors on hapten-specific B lymphocytes. *J. Exp. Med.* 143:511, 1976.
15. Nossal, G. J. V., and Pike, B. P.   Studies on the differentiation of B lymphocytes in the mouse. *Immunology* 25:33, 1973.
16. Nossal, G. J. V., and Pike, B. P.   Evidence for the clonal abortion theory of B lymphocyte tolerance. *J. Exp. Med.* 141:904, 1975.
17. Nossal, G. J. V., and Pike, B. P.   Single cell studies on the antibody-forming potential of fractionated, hapten-specific B lymphocytes. *Immunology* 30:189, 1976.
18. Nossal, G. J. V., et al.   Cell to cell interaction in the immune response. III. Chromosomal marker analysis of single antibody forming cells in reconstituted, irradiated or thymectomized mice. *J. Exp. Med.* 128:839, 1968.
19. Nossal, G. J. V., Pike, B. P., and Katz, D. H.   Induction of B cell tolerance in vitro to 2,4-dinitrophenyl coupled to a copolymer of D-glutamic acid and D-lysine (DNP-D-GL). *J. Exp. Med.* 138:312, 1973.
20. Osmond, D. G., and Nossal, G. J. V.   Differentiation of lymphocytes in mouse bone marrow. 2. Kinetics of maturation and renewal of antiglobulin-binding cells studied by double labelling. *Cell Immunol.* 13:132, 1974.
21. Raff, M. C., Feldmann, M., and de Petris, S.   Monospecificity of bone marrow-derived lymphocytes. *J. Exp. Med.* 137:1024, 1973.
22. Schur, P. H., et al.   Selective gamma-G globulin deficiencies in patients with recurrent pyogenic infections. *N. Engl. J. Med.* 283:631, 1970.
23. Stocker, J. W.   Estimation of hapten-specific antibody forming cell precursors in microcultures. *Immunology* 30:187, 1976.
24. Warner, N. L., and Szenberg, A.   The immunological functions of the Bursa of Facricius in chickens. *Annu. Rev. Microbiol.* 18:253, 1964.
25. Wigzell, H., and Andersson, B.   Cell separation on antigen-coated columns; elimination of high rate antibody-forming cells and immunological memory cells. *J. Exp. Med.* 129:23, 1969.

4. The Role of Antibody in Resistance to Infection with Pseudomonas aeruginosa

Starkey D. Davis

Pseudomonas aeruginosa has only recently become a significant hospital problem. Although the organism was recognized in 1872, it was not listed in Osler and McCrae's textbook of medicine published in 1913 [28]. The only reference to this organism in a 1949 bacteriology textbook of 728 pages is the statement that it is "a mildly pathogenic organism that develops bluish-green pigments" [8].

Pseudomonas infection is now one of the most serious common bacterial infections in hospital patients [7, 15, 16, 21, 30]. Infections tend to occur in patients with complex conditions and the results of therapy are poor. The mortality rate is higher for *Pseudomonas* infections than perhaps any other common bacterial infection except *Serratia*.

It is useful to examine the problem of *Pseudomonas* infection with the perspective provided by the germ theory of disease as revised by Stewart, here slightly modified [37]. The relation of the germ to other factors can be written as follows:

$$\text{Severity of disease} = \frac{\text{Inoculum} \times \text{Pathogenicity} \times \text{Virulence}}{\text{Host defense}}.$$

Inoculum refers to the number of bacteria and their physiologic state. Pathogenicity is defined as the capacity to cause disease. For example, the typhoid bacillus is pathogenic for man but *Bacillus subtilis* is not. Virulence is defined here as the degree of pathogenicity of a strain in man. Some strains of *Staphylococcus aureus* are more virulent than others in man.

Many hospital control measures, such as decontamination of respirator equipment, are designed to decrease the inoculum. *Pseudomonas* is essentially nonpathogenic for healthy persons. There is no evidence that strains of *Pseudomonas* differ significantly in their virulence for man, except some strains seem to have a greater capacity to cause disease in the cornea [6].

Major host defense mechanisms against *Pseudomonas* include the skin and mucous membranes, cough mechanism, free urine flow, antibody and complement, and phagocytic cells [3, 4, 5, 42]. Virtually all human infections with *Pseudomonas* follow some insult to one or more of these mechanisms. Common factors that predispose to *Pseudomonas* infection include accidental trauma, surgery, burns, foreign body, antibody deficiency, and neutropenia. The host factor that can be manipulated most easily is antibody, which is the subject of this review.

Supported in part by NIH Grants AI 11641 and EY 01010.

Several consequences may follow the combination of antibody with bacteria or their products. Antibody may neutralize toxin, produce bacterial agglutination, activate complement, initiate immune adherence, and opsonize organisms for phagocytosis. Although many gram-negative bacteria may be killed by antibody and complement, most clinical isolates of *Pseudomonas* are resistant to serum bactericidal activity [42]. The significance of *Pseudomonas* toxins in humans is uncertain and the importance of the antitoxin role for antibody is unknown [24]. The most important role for antibody is that of opsonization.

Opsonins

Research during the past 15 years has clarified our understanding of the mechanism of opsonization of *Pseudomonas*. Hirsch and Strauss in 1964 examined the role of heat-labile opsonins in rabbit serum [19]. They concluded that bacteria can be divided into three general classes in regard to their requirement for serum factors for phagocytosis. Some bacteria require no serum factor for uptake: Rough pneumococcus is an example. Other bacteria are ingested when either heat-labile opsonin or antibody is present. Some encapsulated bacteria are engulfed only in the presence of antibody and heat-labile factors: An encapsulated type III pneumococcus is an example.

Bjornson and Michael recently examined the requirement of serum opsonins for phagocytosis of *Pseudomonas* [4]. In studies with normal human serum and human polymorphonuclear leukocytes, the activity of normal human serum was substantially reduced following absorption with a homologous strain of *Pseudomonas* or with zymosan, which absorbs properdin. Absorption of serum with heterologous *Pseudomonas* did not change the activity. Normal IgG restored the activity of normal human serum that had been absorbed with bacteria but did not restore the activity of serum absorbed with zymosan, indicating that antibodies were involved in the opsonization of *Pseudomonas*. When normal human serum was absorbed with zymosan and then supplemented with properdin, the normal opsonic activity was also restored. Further studies indicated that C3 proactivator also contributed to optimal opsonization.

Immune IgG promoted opsonization of *Pseudomonas* in the absence of heat-labile serum factors and enhanced the opsonization of bacteria by normal human serum. This finding indicated that immune IgG antibody probably opsonized the bacteria by the classic complement pathway.

Although additional studies will be required to fully understand the role of the various serum factors in the opsonization of *Pseudomonas,* the following summary accords with most of the data now available. Natural IgG antibody requires the alternate complement pathway for opsonization. Immune IgG antibody alone can opsonize *Pseudomonas* for phagocytosis. Optimal opsonization probably requires the presence of immune IgG antibody, the classic complement pathway, and the alternate complement pathway [4, 22, 27, 31, 32, 39, 40, 42].

Bjornson and Michael also presented evidence that cytophilic IgG antibodies act as receptors for bacteria-antibody-complement complexes on the surface of human polymorphonuclear leukocytes [5].

Reynolds et al. studied the specificity of opsonic activity of IgA and IgG antibodies with human alveolar macrophages. IgG antibody was more effective in opsonization of *Pseudomonas* than was IgA antibody [29]. IgG coated bacteria were ingested more rapidly and were killed faster than secretory IgA opsonized bacteria. While both IgA and IgG antibodies are found in respiratory secretions, IgG opsonic antibody is probably more effective in enhancing phagocytosis and may be more important in defense to infection with *Pseudomonas*.

Wollman et al. determined the occurrence of heat-stable opsonins in children with acute leukemia [41]. To eliminate the possible deficiency of complement or other heat-labile opsonic factors, fresh human serum absorbed with *Pseudomonas* to remove specific antibody was added in excess to each test. Sera were assayed in an opsonophagocytic system using human polymorphonuclear leukocytes from a healthy adult donor. Tests were carried out against a strain of *Pseudomonas* and one of *Staphylococcus epidermidis*.

At the time of diagnosis of leukemia, most children had normal opsonic activity. After induction of remission, three of 12 patients had deficient anti-*Pseudomonas* activity when tested at 10% serum concentration, and eight patients had defective opsonic activity when tested at 1.25% serum concentration. Children on maintenance therapy and those who were considered preterminal also had opsonic defects. The difference between the pretreatment group and the preterminal group was statistically significant at the 1.25% serum concentration. The decline in specific anti-*Pseudomonas* opsonic antibody may contribute to the increased susceptibility of these children to *Pseudomonas* infections.

It seems possible that these patients may well have defects involving other heat-stable and heat-labile opsonic factors that have not been subjected to systematic study.

Pseudomonas Vaccines

There is controversy over the identity of the protective antigens of *Pseudomonas*. A large body of evidence indicates that immunization with cell wall "O" or lipopolysaccharide antigen is protective against infection with *Pseudomonas* [1, 2, 11, 18, 20, 25, 44]. Other reports suggest the slime layer is the protective antigen [26, 34]. Injection of animals with purified slime caused leukopenia and death. Purified slime prevented phagocytosis when added to mixtures of polymorphonuclear leukocytes and staphylococci. Antiserum to purified slime gave passive protection against experimental infection [34].

Liu and Hsieh have suggested exotoxin A as the lethal factor, and antiserum added to it gave passive protection against infection [24]. Proteases may play an important role in infection, especially in corneal infection [6].

The conflicting claims as to the significance of the various antigens of *Pseudomonas* are not necessarily mutually exclusive. To be most effective in patients, it may be necessary for the vaccine to stimulate antibody to many antigens and toxins.

The *Pseudomonas* vaccine that has had the most extensive laboratory and clinical trials was developed by Fisher, Devlin, and Gnabasik [11]. The vaccine contains lipopolysaccharide antigens of the cell wall from all seven immunotypes of *Pseudomonas* [18]. Immunization with the vaccine gave good protection in experimentally burned animals against *Pseudomonas* infection. It apparently provided protection against fatal *Pseudomonas* infection in uncontrolled clinical trials in burn patients [1, 2].

There have been two controlled trials of the vaccine in patients with leukemia or cancer. In the first, by Haghbin, Armstrong, and Murphy, children under 15 years of age with acute leukemia were enrolled in the study [17]. Thirteen patients received immunizations initially as a pilot study. The remaining 61 were randomized into vaccine [31] and control [30] groups. There were four weekly injections initially and boosters were given at 3-month intervals. About 85% of the vaccinees produced hemagglutinating antibody in response to immunization, but the antibody levels tended to decline rapidly. Opsonizing antibody was not measured. There were five *Pseudomonas* infections in the vaccine group and three in the control group. It was concluded that the immunologic control of *Pseudomonas* infection could not be achieved by vaccination alone in children with acute leukemia. The dose of vaccine was limited in this trial by untoward reactions that were dose related. Adverse effects included tenderness at the site of injection, fever, nausea, vomiting, malaise, and myalgia. A limiting factor in this study is that patients with leukemia under immunosuppressive therapy are not good candidates for vaccination.

The second study was carried out at a cancer center in 361 adults, who were randomized into vaccine and control groups [44]. The two groups did not differ significantly in underlying disease, antibiotic therapy, or antineoplastic treatment. Fatal bacteremia with *Pseudomonas* occurred in 19 control subjects and in 10 vaccinees. Nonbacteremic *Pseudomonas* infections associated with death occurred in 12 control subjects and 3 vaccinees. The mortality rate associated with *Pseudomonas* infection was 13 out of 176 for the vaccinees versus 31 out of 185 in the control group ($P < 0.01$). Use of the vaccine in this trial was associated with a significant but limited reduction in fatal *Pseudomonas* infection. Administration of the vaccine was accompanied by a high frequency of adverse reactions, including redness and tenderness at the local site, fever, malaise, headache, and myalgia. Adverse reactions of some type occurred in 92% of 50 patients, who were carefully followed for reactions.

Research based on a different rationale is also being carried out on developing a vaccine against gram-negative infections. The lipopolysaccharide of *Pseudomonas* appears to be similar to the lipopolysaccharides of other gram-negative enterobacteria and has a comparable side chain and core structure [33]. The serologic specificity of the "O" antigen resides in the chemical structure of the side chains. Analysis of *Pseudomonas* lipopolysaccharide demonstrated major differences in amino compounds in the side chains, which is in contrast to the other lipopolysaccharides in which the variation is normally in neutral sugars. The lipopolysaccharide core of *Pseudomonas* appears to be similar to that of other gram-negative enteric bacteria. Antibody directed against this common core of lipopolysaccharide may be protective against infection with *Pseudomonas*.

In a recent study Young, Stevens, and Ingram made antibodies against the core glycolipid or lipopolysaccharide of a mutant *Salmonella minnesota* prepared by chemical extraction [43]. In dogs, immunization with the glycolipid provided protection against shock and death after challenge with *Escherichia coli* 085:H9 or *Serratia marcescens* 03. It was of particular interest that no significant difference was noted in the bloodstream clearance of these organisms over a 4- to 6-hour interval. Clearance of bacteria from the bloodstream was accelerated in animals immunized with the homologous challenge strain or in animals challenged with the highly serum-sensitive strain of *E. coli*. The results in this study are similar to those previously reported, which indicated a protection against hypotension and death by immunization with core lipopolysaccharide. Several studies indicate that such cross-reactive antibody is not as effective as specific antibody. However, ISG (immune serum globulin) containing cross-reactive antibody may prove to be effective in protecting high-risk patients from infection with gram-negative bacteria.

Immune Serum Globulins

Many investigators have demonstrated that gammaglobulin or human immune serum globulin (ISG) protects against experimental infections with many organisms, including *Pseudomonas* [12, 13, 14, 35]. Fisher and Manning showed the specific antibody nature of this protection by cross-absorption experiments [12]. ISG gave good protection against infection with *Pseudomonas*. ISG absorbed with a heterologous *Pseudomonas* strain, with *S. aureus*, or with *Streptococcus salivarius* also gave good protection against *Pseudomonas* infection. However, ISG absorbed with the homologous *Pseudomonas* did not protect against the lethal infection. In a series of studies Fisher and Manning analyzed some factors that influence the efficacy of ISG [10, 13, 14]. There was a pronounced inoculum effect, in that larger doses of ISG were needed to control infections established by larger numbers of bacteria. Intravenous injection of ISG was superior to intramuscular injection. For a localized infection, local injection of ISG was more effective than systemic injection. In general, ISG was more active against experimental infections established with bacteria that are part of the normal flora.

Since these earlier studies were done, Fisher, Devlin, and Gnabasik developed a typing scheme, based on lipopolysaccharide antigens, which recognizes seven types, as mentioned above [11]. A study was done to determine whether a single lot of ISG would protect against experimental infections with all seven types [9]. Mice were infected intraperitoneally and were given graded doses of ISG intravenously. A single lot of ISG had good activity against five of the seven types and some activity against a sixth. It was essentially inactive against one type. Intravenous injection of ISG was followed by prompt and persistent decline in the numbers of intraperitoneal bacteria, which is compatible with the concept that ISG acted as an opsonin, not as an antitoxin.

The few clinical trials with ISG have reported contradictory results. Kefalides and associates found that children with burns involving 10 to 30% of the body's surface area experienced a lower delayed mortality when treated with plasma or large intramuscular doses of ISG than groups given saline alone or saline and albumin [23]. The reduction in mortality was observed in children under 6 years of age. Beyond this age the early and late mortality was low in all therapy groups. The reduction in delayed mortality from the use of plasma or ISG was due primarily to a decrease in the frequency of septicemia, chiefly by *Pseudomonas*.

In a later trial on burn wound infections, Stone et al. had 60 experimental and 40 control subjects [38]. The experimental patients were given 0.2 to 0.6 ml (average 0.4 ml) of ISG per kilogram of body weight intravenously or intramuscularly every third day until complete skin coverage was achieved, the patient had been discharged or died, or 3 months had elapsed. Strict isolation techniques were maintained from the outset. There was no difference between the two groups with respect to frequency of septicemia, mortality, or length of hospital stay.

Additional controlled trials are needed to assess the value of ISG in the prevention and treatment of infection [35]. Should it prove to be useful, human ISG offers some advantages as a therapeutic agent. Many patients with *Pseudomonas* bacteremia are frankly hypogammaglobulinemic [15, 36]. For these patients ISG would simply be replacement therapy. ISG has a very long half-life when compared to other therapeutic agents and has little toxicity. Should the protective antigens be more fully identified and hyperimmune serum globulin prepared, this material should be even more effective.

References

1. Alexander, J. W., Fisher, M. W., and MacMillian, B. G. Immunological control of *Pseudomonas* infection in burn patients: A clinical evaluation. *Arch. Surg.* 102:31, 1971.
2. Alexander, J. W., et al. Prevention of invasive *Pseudomonas* infection in burns with a new vaccine. *Arch. Surg.* 99:249, 1969.
3. Allison, A. C. Interactions of antibodies, complement components and various cell types in immunity against viruses and pyogenic bacteria. *Transplant. Rev.* 19:3, 1974.
4. Bjornson, A. B., and Michael, J. G. Factors in human serum promoting phagocytosis of *Pseudomonas aeruginosa*. I. Interaction of opsonins with the bacterium. *J. Infect. Dis.* 130:119, 1974.
5. Bjornson, A. B., and Michael, J. G. Factors in human serum promoting phagocytosis of *Pseudomonas aeruginosa*. II. Interaction of opsonins with the phagocytic cell. *J. Infect. Dis.* 130:127, 1974.
6. Bohigian, G., Okumoto, M., and Valenton, M. Experimental *Pseudomonas* keratitis. *Arch. Ophthalmol.* 86:432, 1971.
7. Bryant, R. E., et al. Factors affecting mortality of gram-negative rod bacteremia. *Arch. Intern. Med.* 127:120, 1971.
8. Burdon, K. L. *Textbook of Microbiology* (3rd ed.). New York: Macmillan, 1949.
9. Davis, S. D. Efficacy of modified human immune serum globulin in the treatment of experimental murine infections with seven immunotypes of *Pseudomonas aeruginosa*. *J. Infect. Dis.* 134:717, 1975.
10. Fisher, M. W. Gamma globulin. *Pediatr. Clin. North Am.* 8:1105, 1961.
11. Fisher, M. W., Devlin, H. B., and Gnabasik, F. J. New immunotype schema for *Pseudomonas aeruginosa* based on protective antigens. *J. Bacteriol.* 98:835, 1969.
12. Fisher, M. W., and Manning, M. C. The specific antibody nature of the therapeutic action of gamma globulin in experimental bacterial infections in mice. *Antibiotics Annual,* 1957/1958, p. 572.
13. Fisher, M. W., and Manning, M. C. Studies on the immunotherapy of bacterial infections. I. The comparative effectiveness of human γ-globulin against various bacterial species in mice. *J. Immunol.* 81:29, 1958.
14. Fisher, M. W., and Manning, M. C. The influence of certain experimental variables on the antibacterial activity of human gamma-globulin in mice. *J. Pathol.* 82:293, 1961.
15. Fishman, L. S., and Armstrong, D. *Pseudomonas aeruginosa* bacteremia in patients with neoplastic disease. *Cancer* 30:764, 1972.
16. Freid, M. A., and Vosti, K. L. The importance of underlying disease in patients with gram-negative bacteremia. *Arch. Intern. Med.* 121:418, 1968.
17. Haghbin, M., Armstrong, D., and Murphy, M. L. Controlled prospective trial of *Pseudomonas aeruginosa* vaccine in children with acute leukemia. *Cancer* 32:761, 1973.
18. Hanessian, S., et al. Isolation and characterization of antigenic components of a new heptavalent *Pseudomonas* vaccine. *Nature* 229:209, 1971.
19. Hirsch, J. G., and Strauss, B. Studies on heat-labile opsonin in rabbit serum. *J. Immunol.* 92:145, 1964.
20. Homma, J. Y. Serological typing of *Pseudomonas aeruginosa* and several points to be considered. *Jpn. J. Exp. Med.* 44:1, 1974.
21. Hughes, W. T., Feldman, S., and Cox, F. Infectious diseases in children with cancer. *Pediatr. Clin. North Am.* 21:583, 1974.
22. Johnston, R. B., Jr., et al. The enhancement of bacterial phagocytosis by serum. *J. Exp. Med.* 129:1275, 1969.

23. Kefalides, N. A., et al. Role of infection in mortality from severe burns. Evaluation of plasma, gamma globulin, albumin and saline-solution therapy in a group of Peruvian children. *N. Engl. J. Med.* 267:317, 1962.

24. Liu, P. V., and Hsieh, H. Exotoxins of *Pseudomonas aeruginosa.* III. Characteristics of antitoxin A. *J. Infect. Dis.* 128:520, 1973.

25. Markley, K., and Smallman, E. Protection by vaccination against *Pseudomonas* infection after thermal injury. *J. Bacteriol.* 96:867, 1968.

26. Mates, A., and Zand, P. Specificity of the protective response induced by the slime layer of *Pseudomonas aeruginosa. J. Hyg.* (Camb.), p. 75, 1974.

27. Osler, A. G., and Sandberg, A. L. Alternate complement pathways. *Prog. Allergy* 17:51, 1973.

28. Osler, W., and McCrae, T. *Modern Medicine: Its Theory and Practice,* Vol 1. Philadelphia: Lea and Febiger, 1913.

29. Reynolds, H. Y., Kazmierowski, J. A., and Newball, H. H. Specificity of opsonic antibodies to enhance phagocytosis of *Pseudomonas aeruginosa* by human alveolar macrophages. *J. Clin. Invest.* 56:376, 1975.

30. Reynolds, H. Y., et al. *Pseudomonas aeruginosa* infections: Persisting problems and current research to find new therapies. *Ann. Intern. Med.* 83:819, 1975.

31. Root, R. K., Ellman, L., and Frank, M. M. Bactericidal and opsonic properties of C4-deficient guinea pig serum. *J. Immunol.* 109:477, 1972.

32. Ruddy, S., and Austen, K. F. Activation of the complement system in rheumatoid synovitis. *Fed. Proc.* 32:134, 1971.

33. Sadoff, J. C. Cell-wall structures of *Pseudomonas aeruginosa* with immunologic significance: A brief review. *J. Infect. Dis.* 130:61, 1974.

34. Sensakovic, J. W., and Bartell, P. F. The slime of *Pseudomonas aeruginosa:* biological characterization and possible role in experimental infection. *J. Infect. Dis.* 129:101, 1974.

35. Schless, A. P., and Harell, G. S. Human gamma globulin in the treatment of bacterial infections. *Am. J. Med.* 44:325, 1968.

36. Speirs, C. F., Selwyn, S., and Nicholson, D. N. Hypogammaglobulinemia presenting as *Pseudomonas* septicemia. *Lancet* I:710, 1963.

37. Stewart, G. T. Limitations of the germ theory. *Lancet* 1:1077, 1968.

38. Stone, H. H., et al. Evaluation of gamma globulin for prophylaxis against burn sepsis. *Surgery* 58:810, 1965.

39. Stossel, T. P., et al. The opsonic fragment of the third component of human complement. *J. Exp. Med.* 141:1329, 1975.

40. Winkelstein, J. A., Shin, H. S., and Wood, W. N., Jr. Heat labile opsonins to pneumococcus. III. The participation of immunoglobulin and of the alternate pathway of C3 activation. *J. Immunol.* 108:1681, 1972.

41. Wollman, M. R., et al. Anti-*Pseudomonas* heat-stable opsonins in acute lymphoblastic leukemia of childhood. *J. Pediatr.* 86:376, 1975.

42. Young, L. S. Role of antibody in infections due to *Pseudomonas aeruginosa. J. Infect. Dis.* 130:111, 1974.

43. Young, L. S., Stevens, P., and Ingram, J. Functional role of antibody against "core" glycolipid of Enterobacteriaceae. *J. Clin. Invest.* 56:850, 1975.

44. Young, L. S., Meyer, R. D., and Armstrong, D. *Pseudomonas aeruginosa* vaccine in cancer patients. *Ann. Intern. Med.* 79:518, 1973.

5. Biochemical Properties of Human "Transfer Factor"

A. Arthur Gottlieb

Since the pioneering experiments of Merrill Chase, it has been clear that leukocytes obtained from an immunologically sensitive individual can confer that sensitivity on a nonsensitive recipient, as measured by the ability of the recipient to exhibit a positive skin test to an intradermal injection of antigen [5]. In general, these skin reactions arise within 24 to 48 hours, appearing as an indurated area covered by an erythematous patch. The histology of such a reaction generally reveals the presence of infiltrating mononuclear cells, and it is this cellular infiltrate that is characteristic of this type of "delayed" hypersensitivity.

In the early 1950s, Dr. H. Sherwood Lawrence in New York demonstrated that this type of skin reaction could be transferred to a previously nonsensitive individual by an extract of leukocytes obtained from antigen-sensitive individuals and, more remarkably, by the dialyzable materials present in this cellular extract, that is, the materials that passed through a membrane filter having a molecular weight cutoff of 12,000 [10].

Lawrence referred to the active principle in the crude dialysate as transfer factor. Other investigators have applied this term to the entire crude extract without regard to the obvious fact that the dialysate is a crude mixture of many molecular components, some of which are certainly immunologically active (perhaps in concert with each other), some of which may be suppressive, and the balance of which are immunologically inert.

The general transfer factor phenomenon can be described as follows: Consider an individual who is sensitive to tuberculin (having had tuberculosis or received BCG vaccination). If his leukocytes are repeatedly freeze-thawed and the extract is treated with DNAse and dialyzed, the dialysate will confer sensitivity to tuberculin on a tuberculin-negative donor, as shown by the ability of this previously nonsensitive individual to react to an intradermal injection of tuberculin. If lymphocytes are obtained from an individual who has received transfer factor from a sensitive donor, these lymphocytes will now respond by proliferation in vitro on addition of tuberculin. This raises a critical point. There is a real question as to whether administration of the crude leukocyte dialysate, as described above, does indeed confer a new sensitivity on the recipient's lymphocytes or simply augments a previously acquired weak immune response to tuberculin. Since no one is truly immunologically virgin, it seems reasonable to suppose that a very small number of T cells that are indeed sensitive to an antigen such as tuberculin reside in each individual and that the difference between one who is skin-test positive and one who is skin-test negative is the absolute

Supported by Grants AI 12090 and AI 13386 from NIH and grants from the Research Corporation and the E. G. Schleider Foundation.

number of circulating T cells present. One can argue that the transfer factor simply causes a heightened proliferation of previously sensitized T cells in response to antigen. This points up one of the critical issues in the interpretation of studies of transfer factor, namely the issue of specificity.

Lawrence's original description of the transfer factor stated that such transfers were highly specific, in the sense that if a donor were not skin-test positive to a given antigen (which implies a relatively strong sensitivity to the antigen), then transfer of sensitivity to that antigen did not occur. Indeed, Lawrence indicated that in order to observe transfer, one had to use donors that have very strong sensitivities to antigen. Moreover, in a series of experiments using crude leukocyte extracts from donors who were negative to coccidioidin, weak skin reactions (which unfortunately were not biopsied) were seen in nonsensitive recipients [12]. Additionally, more recent evidence accumulating from several laboratories appears to show that the response of peripheral lymphocytes in vitro to crude leukocyte extracts and PPD is determined by the number of T cells present in the culture that are already sensitive to PPD.

Notwithstanding the controversy regarding the issue of specificity, the crude dialysates appear to have some remarkable properties in regard to the treatment of certain infectious diseases and, as I will indicate, the ability to reverse the anergic state. However, our interpretation of the presently available data, including those from our own laboratory, is that the majority of the active molecules in crude leukocyte dialysates appear to exert their action in a nonspecific fashion. I believe that there is a need to reexamine those studies that claim to demonstrate the immunologic specificity of transfer factor preparations to determine whether true delayed hypersensitivity is observed histologically.

The properties of crude transfer factor have been extensively reviewed by Lawrence [11]. Some of the more interesting properties of crude transfer factor are the ease with which systemic sensitization can be achieved and the persistence of sensitivity once transfer is accomplished. The active material in the crude extract is small (as indicated by its ability to pass a dialysis membrane), free of immunoglobulin, and probably free of antigenic fragments, although the latter have not been rigorously excluded [4]. It is clear that the crude extracts contain substantial amounts of polypeptide, orcinol reactive material, and traces of deoxyribose. In my judgment, there is no evidence that double-stranded RNA exists in preparations of crude transfer factor or that such a moiety is responsible for the observed effects of the crude preparations. Reports [7, 13] suggesting that the effects of transfer factor are due to double-stranded RNA have apparently been retracted [6].

While local intradermal transfers can be performed with as few as 10^7 cells, systemic transfers require at least 2×10^8 cells. Unfortunately, quantitation in this area is poor, and since the immunologically active moieties cannot be assayed directly, it is common to refer to units of transfer factor: the amount of crude dialysate containing active transfer factor derived from one unit, or approximately 500 ml of blood (equivalent to 5 to 8×10^8 leukocytes). Another major difficulty in the study of transfer factor is the difficulty of finding suitable animal or in vitro assays for this material, although recent studies in guinea pigs suggest progress in this area [3].

With respect to in vitro assays, progress seems to have been made in the use of ^3H thymidine uptake into DNA, as described by Ascher et al. [1]. However, it is not clear what this molecular parameter is measuring, and it may well be that it simply reflects augmented DNA synthesis by cells having prior sensitivity to one or another antigen. Other in vitro assays that have been employed to measure transfer factor activity include MIF production and chemotaxis, but these have not found wide applicability. It is important to recognize, however, that these assays may measure activities of molecules in the crude dialysate that are not related to the ability of the crude dialysate to induce a positive skin test in a previously unresponsive recipient.

One of the obvious approaches to an understanding of the nature of transfer factor is fractionation by appropriate biochemical means and recovery of the immunologically active components. In doing this, one needs to be sure that the components recovered are truly active in the transfer of delayed hypersensitivity, both morphologically and histologically. One simple method of fractionation is gel filtration of the crude dialysate. We have previously reported that crude leukocyte extracts gave three major ultraviolet absorbance peaks on Sephadex G-10 gel filtration, and the immunologically active component appeared to be part of the second fraction [8]. It was of interest to note that this fraction did display a degree of nonspecificity in transfer of delayed hypersensitivity responses. Following these initial studies, we employed fluorescamine [Fluram (Roche), a nonfluorescent compound that becomes fluorescent when complexed with molecules containing primary amines, such as polypeptides or amino acids] to determine the location of the major polypeptide fraction of the crude dialysate eluting from Sephadex G-10. Figure 5-1A displays the polypeptide peak as measured by this technique as well as the orcinol reactive and deoxynucleotide material present in these fractions.

The fractions eluting from Sephadex G-10 were grouped, lyophilized, and tested by intradermal injection into the skin of normal recipients and patients with Hodgkin's disease who were immunologically anergic. These fractions were tested in separate arms with and without antigen. The results are shown in Figures 5-1 and 5-2. It is apparent that in both cases, the normal individual and the anergic Hodgkin's recipient, the only fractions that evoked skin reactions were those containing fluorescamine-reactive material. These reactions were of comparable size and intensity and, in the normal subject, were the same whether antigen was injected with the fractions or not. Moreover, both morphologically and histologically, an im-

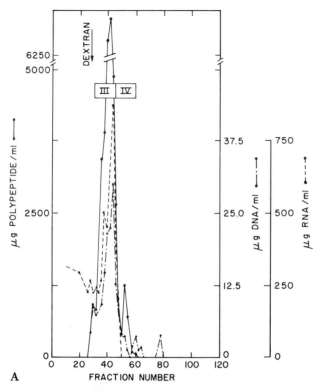

A

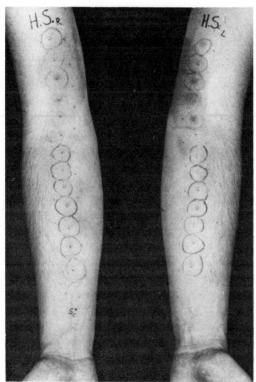

B

mediate inflammatory response was observed shortly after injection, and this subsequently developed into reactions that are characteristic of delayed hypersensitivity. Similar types of immediate hypersensitivity have been observed with crude, unfractionated leukocyte dialysates.

Two patients with Hodgkin's disease, who were clearly anergic before receiving the fluorescamine-reactive component of transfer factor, became capable of responding to an intradermal injection of PPD after receiving these fractions. In brief, their anergy was reversed, and this reversal was sustained for several weeks.

These studies demonstrate the utility of fluorescamine in the analysis of immunologically active components of transfer factor. The components of the crude dialysate that react with fluorescamine and appear to be polypeptide in nature are capable of inducing mixed immediate and delayed hypersensitivity reactions in vivo and can reverse the state of immunologic anergy seen in Hodgkin's disease.

In addition, the fluorescamine-reactive peak from Sephadex G-10 can be dialyzed against a membrane that excludes molecules having molecular weights greater than 3,500. This procedure yields two fractions: one smaller than 3,500, the other larger than 3,500. In preliminary studies, it appears that the small fraction, which represents 85% of the polypeptide in the preparation, is responsible for some nonspecific effects of the fluorescamine-reactive material [9]. The small fraction has been subjected to two-dimen-

---

Figure 5-1. Induction of delayed hypersensitivity by chromatographically prepared fractions of crude leukocyte extract, response in a normal recipient. The crude leukocyte extract prepared from 4×10^8 leukocytes of a donor sensitive to *Candida* was dialyzed against a membrane having a molecular weight cutoff of 12,000. The dialysate was subjected to gel filtration on a 1×80 cm column of Sephadex G-10 using 5 mM ammonium bicarbonate as eluent. 0.8 ml fractions were assayed for polypeptide using the fluorescamine technique [2]; the results are shown in the graph (A). Groups of 15 fractions were pooled, lyophilized, and dissolved in 0.6 ml of normal saline. 0.08 ml of each fraction was injected intradermally in the right arm, while 0.08 ml of each fraction was injected intradermally in the left arm. The earliest eluting fraction (fraction I) was placed at the top, and fractions II through XIII were placed sequentially toward the wrist. One hour later, the sites on the left arm were challenged with saline, while the sites on the right arm were challenged with 0.1 ml of Bencard Candida Antigen. The photo (B) displays the results at 24 hours. A control of 0.1 ml normal saline (Sc) was injected close to the right wrist. Note the erythema evident in reaction to fractions II through V. Induration was found to be comparable to the extent of the erythematous reaction induced by these fractions; little reaction was observed to fractions VI through XII. The reactions to fractions II through V in the presence of *Candida* antigen were, in this instance, comparable to the reactions induced by the fractions alone. (From Gottlieb, A. A., et al. Use of Fluorescamine to Identify a Nonspecific Component of Human Transfer Factor. In M. S. Ascher, A. A. Gottlieb, and C. H. Kirkpatrick [Eds.], *Transfer Factor*. New York: Academic Press, 1976.)

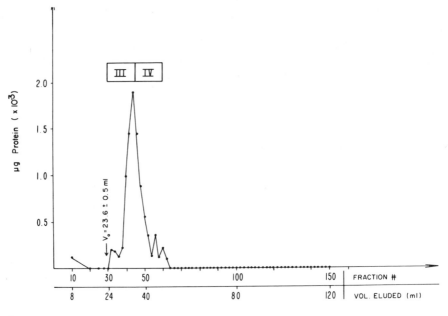

A

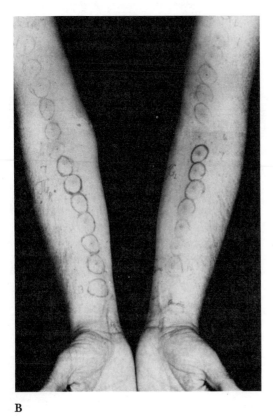

B

sional thin layer chromatography and appears to contain 14 polypeptide components. Studies are currently under way to determine which of these components is immunologically active, and if these active components are capable of reversing immunologic anergy.

Summary

Crude leukocyte dialysates contain a collection of heterogeneous molecules, only some of which are responsible for the transfer factor phenomenon. The term *transfer factor* should properly be applied only to this molecule or molecules.

Over 85% of the polypeptides present in crude leukocyte dialysates pass through a dialysis membrane having a molecular weight cutoff of 3,500. This fraction appears to act nonspecifically, and it appears from our studies that this fraction is capable of reversing the state of immunologic anergy seen in Hodgkin's disease.

These studies have reached a point at which the identification and sequence analysis of these components is achievable. Such small molecules are likely to be readily synthesized and would have interesting pharmacologic properties.

References

1. Ascher, M. S., et al. *In vitro* properties of leukocyte dialysates containing transfer factor. *Proc. Natl. Acad. Sci. U.S.A.* 71:1178, 1974.
2. Bohlen, P., et al. Fluorometric assay of proteins in the nanogram range. *Arch. Biochem. Biophys.* 155:213, 1973.
3. Burger, D. R., and Jeter, W. S. Cell-free passive transfer of delayed hypersensitivity to chemicals in guinea pigs. *Infect. Immun.* 4:575, 1971.

Figure 5-2. Induction of delayed hypersensitivity by chromatographically prepared fractions of crude leukocyte extract, response in an anergic recipient. The crude leukocyte dialysate derived from 4×10^8 leukocytes of a donor sensitive to *Candida* and streptokinase-streptodornase (SK/SD) were subjected to gel filtration on Sephadex G-10 using the same conditions outlined in Figure 5-1A. 0.8 ml fractions were collected and assayed for polypeptide by the fluorescamine technique [2]; the results are shown in the graph (A). Groups of 15 fractions were pooled, lyophilized, and taken up in 0.6 ml of normal saline. 0.08 ml of each fraction was injected intradermally in both arms of an anergic recipient having Hodgkin's disease (photo, B). The sites on the left arm were challenged with 0.1 ml of a 1 : 100 dilution of *Candida* antigen. Saline and *Candida* antigen alone were injected near the left wrist. As in the case of the normal recipient (Fig. 5-1B), erythema and induration are noted in response to fractions II through V, while little reaction was noted in response to other fractions. The photograph was taken at 24 hours. (From Gottlieb, A. A., et al. Biochemical analysis of dialyzable leukocyte extracts. *J. Reticuloendothel. Soc.* 21:407, 1977.)

4. Burger, D. R., Vetto, R. M., and Malley, A.   Transfer factor from guinea pigs sensitive to dinitrochlorobenzene: Absence of super antigen properties. *Science* 175:1473, 1972.
5. Chase, M. W.   The cellular transfer of cutaneous hypersensitivity to tuberculin. *Proc. Soc. Exp. Biol. Med.* 59:134, 1943.
6. Dressler, D., and Potter, H.   Author's statement. *Proc. Natl. Acad. Sci. U.S.A.* 72:409, 1974.
7. Dressler, D., and Rosenfeld, S.   On the chemical nature of transfer factor. *Proc. Natl. Acad. Sci. U.S.A.* 71:4429, 1974.
8. Gottlieb, A. A., et al.   What is transfer factor? *Lancet* 2:822, 1973.
9. Gottlieb, A. A., et al.   Biochemical analysis of dialyzable leukocyte extracts. *J. Reticuloendothel. Soc.* 21:403, 1977.
10. Lawrence, H. S.   The transfer in humans of delayed skin sensitivity to strepto-coccal M substance and to tuberculin with disrupted leukocytes. *J. Clin. Invest.* 34:219, 1955.
11. Lawrence, H. S.   Transfer factor in cellular immunity. *The Harvey Lectures* 68:239, 1974.
12. Rapaport, F. T., et al.   Transfer of delayed hypersensitivity to coccidioidin in man. *J. Immunol.* 84:358, 1960.
13. Rosenfeld, S., and Dressler, D.   Transfer factor: A subcellular component that transmits information for specific immune responses. *Proc. Natl. Acad. Sci. U.S.A.* 71:2473, 1974.

6. Detection of Defects in Host Defense Mechanisms and Their Repair in the Infection-Prone Patient

J. Wesley Alexander, Renzo Dionigi,
and J. Dwight Stinnett

Immunologic reactions have been known to play a role in resistance to bacterial infection for three-quarters of a century, but it was not until 1952, when Bruton discovered hypogammaglobulinemia [16], that defects in immune defense were proved to be associated with an increased susceptibility to infection in man. Since that time, a large variety of inherited abnormalities of the immune processes have been studied, which has led to a better understanding of their precise role in antimicrobial defense. These studies, in turn, have generated interest in documenting acquired defects of immunity associated with physiologic changes, disease, or the treatment of disease. Acquired defects are now known to be numerous, and they frequently contribute to the development of infections in the hospitalized patient. In fact, most if not all patients considered to be infection-prone can now be assumed to have abnormalities of host defense.

Identification and characterization of such abnormalities, however, remains difficult because of the incompletely understood, complex interactions within the immune system and the uncertainty of the clinical relevance of many immune system components. In addition, many of the tests now available do not measure what clinicians would really like to know. An attempt will be made to identify the utility of certain tests for detecting defects in immunity, and data will be presented which indicate that many defects can be corrected by appropriate therapy. Since the inherited diseases of immunity will be discussed in another chapter, primary emphasis here will be given to acquired defects.

Methods for Detecting Defects and Assessing Their Relevance to Infection

Antibody and Immunoglobulin Production

Levels of circulating immunoglobulins in the serum of patients can be measured by standard radioimmunodiffusion tests [35]. Low levels of IgM and IgG have been associated with an increased susceptibility to infection in inherited diseases, but depressions of IgA, IgE, or IgD have not in themselves been associated with decreased resistance [5, 30]. In our experience with

Part of the research described herein was supported by USPHS Grant No. 5-PO1-GM15428-08 and the Paul I. Hoxworth Blood Center of the University of Cincinnati.

surgical patients, acquired low immunoglobulin levels are rarely the underlying cause for infection except when interacting with other factors. Munster, Hoagland, and Pruitt [39] have reported that persistently low IgG levels in the sera of burn patients are associated with a higher mortality than when normal or increased levels are present.

Poor response to a specific antigen may be an inherited characteristic, a result of disease, or a result of its treatment, such as with immunosuppressive agents. However, poor antibody formation associated with other disease appears to be less important than other variables of host immunity.

Delayed Hypersensitivity and Cutaneous Responses
T cell activity can be tested both in vitro and in vivo. The in vitro measurements [46] consist primarily of measuring the responsiveness of lymphocytes in culture to a mitogenic stimulus, such as phytohemagglutinin, pokeweed mitogen, concanavallin, or allogeneic cells. Responsiveness is measured by the uptake of tritiated thymidine by the responding cells. In other tests, sensitization of T cells can be measured by the production of migration inhibitory factor (MIF) in vitro in the presence of specific antigen. Also, a variety of cell-mediated cytotoxicity tests can be performed, but their usefulness has not been evaluated in measurement of resistance to infection. In vivo assessment of delayed hypersensitivity can be made by decreasing the primary immune response to sensitization and challenge with an antigen such as dinitrochlorobenzene (DNCB) [22] or by recall responses of delayed hypersensitivity to a battery of available antigens, including tuberculin, histoplasmin, *Trichophyton*, mumps, streptokinase, *Candida*, and others [43]. For this purpose, antigens having a high frequency of response in the general population are usually used. The delayed hypersensitivity response in vivo probably measures both T cell reactivity and nonspecific factors.

T cell function as determined by response to mitogens or allogeneic cells has been shown to be abnormal in patients with severe sepsis, following trauma, and following major burn injury [18, 34]. However, there has not been a good correlation with susceptibility to infection. On the other hand, lack of reaction to delayed hypersensitivity antigens and challenge with DNCB (anergy) has been associated with death from sepsis in seriously ill individuals [34, 43]. MacLean and his coworkers found that anergy in patients preoperatively was predictive of septic complications in patients undergoing surgical operation [34].

Along this line, it may be that lymphokine production by T cells, rather than a blastogenic response, is a more realistic indication of their in vivo role in host resistance. The exact role of T cell function in typical bacterial infections needs to be further clarified.

Neutrophil Function
The function of neutrophils can be assessed by a wide variety of tests, including measurement of intracellular enzymes, the metabolic responses to

stimulation, chemotaxis, and the ingestion and killing of microorganisms. Metabolic tests, including oxygen consumption, are interesting but do not seem to have predictive value for the development of sepsis [27]. Likewise, the nitroblue tetrazolium (NBT) test statistically has a predictive value for the development of sepsis in the burn patient, but individual determinations have little benefit [33]. Chemotactic studies with neutrophils using the Boyden chamber technique are only now being performed in prospective studies, and while abnormalities have been clearly associated with infections [59], they have not yet been shown to be responsible for them. On the other hand, patients have been reported to have inherited defects of chemotaxis that have been responsible for recurrent infections [37, 48].

More importantly, acquired abnormalities of the antibacterial function of human neutrophils have been clearly shown to be associated with susceptibility to infection in a variety of diseases, including patients with leukemia, protein-calorie malnutrition, sepsis, and, following transplantation, severe traumatic injury, or major burn injury [7]. The studies in burn injury have been particularly valuable in determining that abnormalities of neutrophil function can predispose to infection. Early studies in our laboratory in seriously burned patients showed that defects in the ability of neutrophils to kill *Staphylococcus aureus* occurred frequently [6]. Burned patients who did not develop sepsis had an average neutrophil bactericidal index (NBI) of almost 6, meaning that six times as many bacteria survived in an in vitro test using the patient's neutrophils compared to a test in which neutrophils from normal persons were used. When patients who developed sepsis at some time during their burn course were examined, the neutrophil function was significantly worse than in those without sepsis. Immediately preceding the onset of sepsis, the abnormalities were still worse. When the degree of abnormality was plotted against the incidence of positive blood cultures within 48 hours subsequent to the time individual tests were performed, an extremely good correlation was obtained (Figure 6-1). Normal or better-than-normal neutrophil function characterized by NBI values of less than 1 were not associated with positive blood cultures, but 25% of the time in which the NBIs were greater than 8, there was a positive blood culture within the next 48 hours. A series of tests on a patient with a typical course is shown in Figure 6-2. Neutrophil function was markedly abnormal throughout this patient's course, but, in addition, there was a superimposed cyclic variation of the ability of his neutrophils to kill bacteria, and associated with this cyclic variation was the development of systemic sepsis as evidenced by positive blood cultures. As neutrophil function got better, the septic course improved. More often, such patients converted positive blood cultures to negative ones with this improvement. When the kinetics of bacterial killing by neutrophils from burned patients was examined, killing appeared to be normal or even better than normal for the first few minutes because of an increased phagocytosis. Later, how-

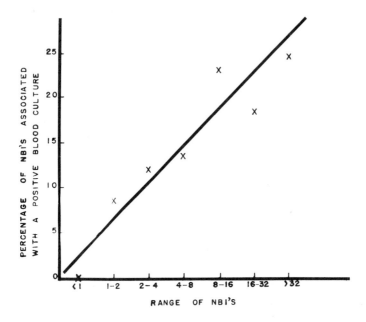

Figure 6-1. Relations of neutrophil function to the development of bacterial infection in patients with serious burn injuries. NBI = neutrophil bactericidal index. Increasing values for NBI reflect diminishing ability of blood neutrophils to kill bacteria. (From Alexander, J. W., and Meakins, J. L. A physiological basis for the development of opportunistic infection. *Ann. Surg.* 176:273, 1972.)

ever, not only was there a lack of killing, but in many instances growth of bacteria occurred within the ineffective cells.

The defect in burn neutrophils was therefore basically similar to that found in patients with chronic granulomatous disease of childhood inasmuch as phagocytosis was normal or increased, intracellular killing was decreased, and their response to NBT in both nonstimulated and stimulated tests was markedly deficient and correlated with the inability to kill bacteria, implying reduction in NADH and NADPH activity.

During sequential studies of neutrophil function in burn patients, it was noted that a cyclic variation occurred with a periodicity of approximately 14 days. Sequential studies of neutrophil function and quantitative wound bacteriology showed that the cyclical changes in antibacterial function influenced the numbers of bacteria in the burn wound by as much as 10,000 times (Figure 6-3). This cyclical variation also occurs in normal individuals and may well have an important role in resistance to infection [8]. We have hypothesized that patients exposed to brief periods of bacterial contamination may be more or less resistant to infection because of these cyclical changes [1]. Unfortunately, numerous experiments to examine a precise relation to endocrinologic function have been fruitless [8].

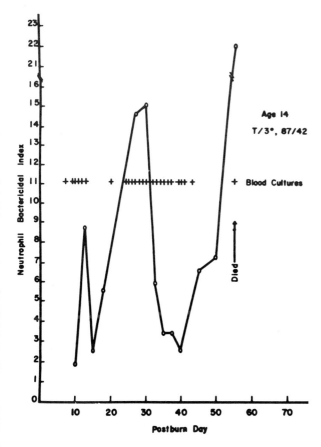

Figure 6-2. Example of serial neutrophil function tests in a seriously burned patient. Note the cyclical variation in neutrophil function and the association of positive blood cultures with increased abnormalities of neutrophil function. (From Alexander, J. W., and Meakins, J. L. A physiological basis for the development of opportunistic infection. *Ann. Surg.* 176:273, 1972.)

The ability of neutrophils to ingest and kill *Escherichia coli,* interestingly enough, does not correlate with the ability to kill *S. aureus,* nor does it seem to be significantly correlated with the development of infection (unpublished data).

Complement System Activity
The complement system has been shown to be of crucial importance for resistance to bacterial infection in man. Both the classic pathway and the alternative pathway may play a role but, of the two, the alternative pathway appears to be more important in resistance to infection. The classic pathway is composed of 11 serum proteins (nine components), the first com-

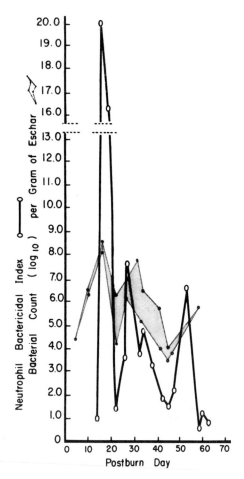

Figure 6-3. Influence of cyclical neutrophil function on quantitative cultures of the burn wound eschar. Serial measurements of each were made in this patient. The shaded area represents the range of bacterial counts in different areas. (From Alexander, J. W. Immunological Considerations of Burn Injury and the Role of Vaccination. In H. C. Polk, Jr., and H. H. Stone, *Contemporary Burn Management.* Boston: Little, Brown, 1971.)

ponent being comprised of three proteins bound together in the presence of calcium. Specific IgM antibody and three of the four subclasses of IgG antibody complexed with antigen can activate these components sequentially, although not in direct numerical order (C1, 4, 2, 3, 5, 6, 7, 8, 9) (Figure 6-4). Full expression of this pathway results in the formation of opsonins (C3b), chemotoxins (C3a, C5a, and C567), anaphylatoxins (C3a and C5a), and hemolytic activity. The distal components of the complement sequence, beginning with C3, can also be activated by a different set of mechanisms

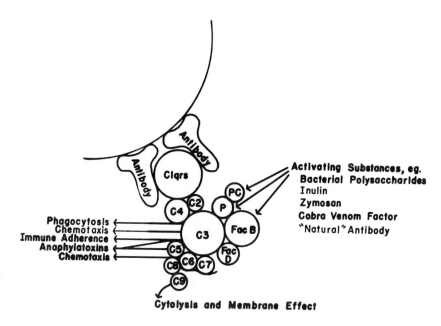

Figure 6-4. Schematic representation of the classic and alternative pathways of the complement sequence. C1, C4, etc. = classic components. P = properdin. PC = properdin convertase. Fac B = factor B or C3 proactivator. Fac D = factor D or C3 proactivator convertase. (From Altemeier, W. A., and Alexander, J. W. Surgical infections and choice of antibiotics. In D. C. Sabiston, Jr. [Ed.], *Textbook of Surgery* [11th ed.]. Philadelphia: Saunders, 1977.)

now known as the alternative, or properdin, pathway, first discovered by Pillemer et al. in 1954 [44]. The present concept of activation of the alternative pathway involves several proteins, including C3, factor B, factor D, and others that are less well defined [42]. An amplification feedback mechanism is initiated by C3b acting on factor D, which in turn acts on factor B to generate C3 activator. The amplification loop is regulated by an enzyme known as C3b inactivator (KAF). Absence of C3b inactivation can result in unregulated activation of the alternative pathway by C3b and an increased susceptibility to infection because of consumption of these components. C3 is the most important of the opsonic proteins of the alternative pathway, and a reduction in C3 levels or activity is clearly associated with an increased susceptibility to infection [61]. These conditions include inherited homozygous deficiency of C3, hypercatabolism of C3, systemic lupus erythematosus, premature infants, and patients with severe bacterial infections [24]. In addition, patients with severe burn injury have transiently low levels of C3 [13], and patients with severe malnutrition characteristically have low levels of C3 and complement activity [20, 32, 52]. The pivotal role of C3 activation via the alternative pathway in resistance to bacterial infection has been made remarkably clear by the good health of humans and animals with genetic defects in C4, C2, and C5, C6, and C7 [24]. Also, sera made deficient in factor B or properdin have diminished opsonic activity against a variety of organisms.

There is now clear evidence that severe infection can result in the consumption of opsonic proteins, a condition that can lead to both progression of the existing infection and increased susceptibility to infection by other organisms. We have called this condition a consumptive opsoninopathy [9]. Fearon et al. [23] showed that the components of the alternative pathway of complement were remarkedly depleted in patients with gram-negative bacteremia and hypotension. Bokisch et al. [15] also showed low complement levels in patients with dengue hemorrhagic shock syndrome, and Neva et al. [40] showed periodic consumption of complement in malaria. Bach et al. [10] described patients in whom gram-negative bacteremia developed following transuretheral resection. In two of these, C3 dropped remarkably. We have studied 10 patients with life-threatening infections, five of which were fatal, and these patients had marked decreases in C3 levels related to severity of the infection [9]. Three of the seven patients in whom properdin was measured also had levels lower than 50% of normal values. In vitro, restoration of C3, properdin, and factor B restored opsonic activity.

The effects of low levels of C3 and C5 on chemotactic activity in vivo is not known at this time. However, at least one patient has been described in whom repeated infections occurred associated with a functional defect in C5 that could be restored by the transfusion of normal plasma [37].

The complement system can be investigated with a large number of tests. Perhaps the most common of these is the standard assay to measure hemolytic complement activity. Individual components can also be measured by radioimmunodiffusion, but the method has the disadvantage of not measuring functional activity. Functional activity of the classic components can be measured using specifically deficient sera and purified components that are available commercially. Commercial antisera to C3 are currently available only as antibody to βlc/βla. In our laboratory more consistent and meaningful results have been obtained when C3 is measured using antisera that are specific for the B antigen, which is lost when the molecule is converted to its active fragments, C3a and C3b [38]. Functional integrity of the alternative pathway can be measured by the addition of activators of this pathway (e.g., endotoxin, inulin, or zymosan) and measuring the disappearance of the C3B antigen [2]. This technique may be useful for examining the sera from patients treated with large doses of antibiotics that must otherwise be removed by dialysis. Activity of the alternative pathway can also be measured by opsonophagocytic tests, using organisms that require participation of the alternative pathway for opsonization. Two organisms frequently used are *E. coli* 075 and *Pseudomonas aeruginosa* immunotype 1. The ability of a patient's serum to generate chemotactic activity for normal neutrophils can also be studied by the Boyden chamber technique.

Other opsonic proteins have been described that do not seem to be related to specific antibody or to proteins of the complement system. However, their role in resistance to bacterial infection in man must still be defined.

Immunologic Surveillance in the Susceptible Patient
Literally hundreds of tests can be used to survey immunologic competence in infection-prone patients. Those we consider to be of practical value are listed in Table 6-1 with references for details of their performance. These tests are tedious and time-consuming and require a laboratory dedicated to excellence. However, there is no reason why they cannot be performed routinely in most major hospitals dealing with infection-prone patients.

Repair of Defects of Host Defense
In an effort to restore defects of host defense to normal, first consideration should be given to the discontinuation of any therapy that may contribute to the abnormality. For this, considerable clinical judgment must often be exercised, but the degree of severity of defects as measured by in vitro testing can aid as guidance in these important decisions. One of many examples in this regard is a patient receiving immunosuppressive therapy for a renal transplant, who is admitted with a pulmonary infection caused by *Pneumocystis carinii* (Figure 6-5). Assessment of the immunologic competence of such patients may aid greatly in the decision to stop or continue immunosuppressive therapy. In the susceptible patient, antibiotic therapy should be

Table 6-1. Suggested Tests for Surveillance of Immune Competence in the Infection-Prone Patient

---

T Cell Function

Sensitization to DNCB [22]
Battery of skin tests (**PPD**, *Trichophyton*, **SKSD**, *Candida*)
Response of lymphocytes *in vitro* to mitogens [46, 57]

B Cell Function

Serum levels of IgG and IgM [35]

Neutrophil Function

Test for ingestion and killing of *Staphylococcus aureus* 502 A [6]
Chemotactic response [37, 59]

Complement System Activity

Serum levels of C3 (B antigenic determinant) and properdin [35, 38]
Measurement of the ability of serum to opsonize *Escherichia coli* 075 [9, 28]
Measurement of the ability of serum to support chemotaxis

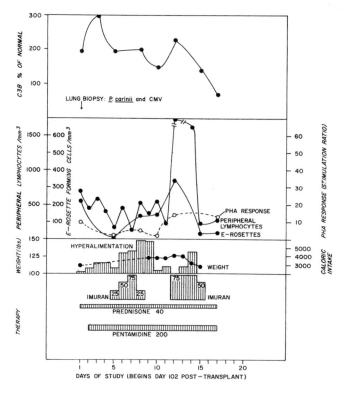

Figure 6-5. Serial measurements of immune function in an immunosuppressed patient with pneumonia caused by *Pneumocystis carinii.* Measurement of T cell function was abnormal in this patient, whereas tests of neutrophil function and complement activity (not shown) were normal.

limited as much as possible, since many of the antibiotics interfere with complement activity [2].

There are four means by which clinicians can currently repair immunologic defects. These are (1) nutritional support, (2) hemotherapy, (3) immunization, and (4) the use of immunoadjuvants.

Nutritional Support

Gordon and Scrimshaw [25] have estimated that problems involving interaction between nutrition and infection affect three-quarters of the world's population. Often ignored as a contributing problem in medical practice in the United States, there are still many diseases associated with a high frequency of relative or overt malnutrition. These include patients undergoing chemotherapy for malignancy, patients with advanced stages of malignancy, intestinal fistulas, abscesses, septicemia, extensive trauma or burn injury, cirrhosis, inflammatory bowel disease, intestinal obstruction, prolonged ileus, central nervous system disease requiring respiratory therapy, and numerous chronic illnesses [3]. In many of these diseases there is an increased requirement for nutritional substances, and diseases such as severe burn injury or severe sepsis can almost double the metabolic requirements for calories and other nutrients. Infection can also result in an increased requirement for certain nutrients as well as a decreased intake, decreased absorption, or an alteration of metabolism. Infection can precipitate acute clinical manifestations of vitamin deficiency in many individuals with marginal vitamin intake.

Protein-calorie malnutrition has long been recognized as having adverse effects on infection. As early as 1936, Studley [55] recognized that postoperative fatality rates could be correlated with the extent of preoperative weight loss. Cannon and his colleagues in 1944 [17] demonstrated that protein malnutrition resulted in a striking impairment in antibody synthesis. Two years later Guggenheim and Buechler [26] showed that protein and calorie malnutrition inhibited bactericidal factors and phagocytic properties of peritoneal fluid in rats. Scrimshaw, Taylor, and Gordon [49] extensively reviewed the relation of nutritional deficiencies to infection and found they were regularly associated in man as well as in experimental animals. Perhaps the best studied forms of protein-calorie malnutrition in man have been kwashiorkor and marasmus, long known to be associated with an increased incidence of infection. These deficiencies also are associated with multiple deficiencies of vitamins and minerals. Selverage and Bhat [50] have shown that patients with kwashiorkor have a decreased phagocytic capability, a defect in the glycolytic pathway, and a defect in the intracellular killing of bacteria by neutrophils. Their findings have recently been confirmed and extended by Schopfer and Douglas [47]. Smythe et al. [53] showed that the lymphocytes from patients with protein-calorie malnutrition respond poorly to phytomitogens, and those patients who died had a high proportion of chronic atrophy of the thymus and wasting of peripheral lymphoid tissues both in T cell and B cell dependent areas. Sirisinha et al. [52] showed that factor B of the properdin pathway and all the classic complement components except C4 were markedly lowered in malnourished children. Protein deficiency has been shown to markedly affect the cellular composition of acute inflammatory exudates in experimental animals, possibly via reduction in the generation of the polypeptide mediators of the acute immune response.

Of the very greatest importance is that immune defects related to nutritional deficiencies can be corrected by nutritional repletion. Selverage and Bhat [50] showed that the defect in killing of bacteria by neutrophils in patients with kwashiorkor could be corrected by dietary protein and caloric intake. The quantity of dietary protein and caloric intake was also reported to markedly influence the repair of deficiencies of the complement system in the study of Sirisinha and his colleagues [52]. Law, Dudrick, and Abdou [32] demonstrated that immune competence, as measured by delayed skin reactivity to primary or secondary antigens or in vitro lymphocyte responses to phytohemagglutinin, could be improved by intravenous hyperalimentation in man, and they showed that primary antibody response and the response of lymphocytes to phytomitogens could be restored in markedly depleted animals given protein repletion, beginning 48 hours before an immunologic challenge [31]. In fact, the response was often better than normal. Partial restoration of the immune response could be obtained in animals where repletion was begun 48 hours after an immunologic challenge. Dionigi and his colleagues [20] have studied the effect of total parenteral hyperalimentation in malnourished surgical patients, and they demonstrated improvement in lymphocyte counts, response to phytohemagglutinin, immunoglobulin concentration, neutrophil migration, chemotactic responses, and serum levels of C3. They have further shown that subacute starvation in animals affects C3, IgG, and IgM levels, and chemotaxis more than any other variables and that this can be restored to normal levels in a relatively short period of time [19].

Vitamin deficiencies have a variable effect on host resistance. Among the more important are vitamin B deficiencies. The effect of most mineral deficiencies on infection is still poorly understood, but it is important to remember that administration of excess iron during a bacterial infection may potentiate the infection [60].

From this discussion, it is evident that nutritional deficiencies may influence a wide variety of immunologic processes that may contribute to the development of infection or its progression. Studies from our unit have shown that the institution of oral hyperalimentation regimens in seriously burned children has resulted in a dramatic reduction in death from sepsis and that this reduction in death was accompanied by an improvement in neutrophil function. However, not all the benefit may have come from the improvement in neutrophil function alone, since hyperalimentation in the malnourished individual can also improve complement function and activities, delayed hypersensitivity response, and the responsiveness of T cells, antibody synthesis to specific antigenic stimuli, skin reactivity, and chemotaxis. We have recently had the opportunity to study patients who developed moderately severe weight loss from anorexia nervosa following a renal transplant. Restoration of immunologic competence in a post-transplant patient with dietary supplementation is shown in Figure 6-6.

Nutritional support of the malnourished patient is perhaps the most important and easily accomplished clinical mechanism for repair of acquired defects of host defense. Our current recommendations for nutritional therapy to prevent infection or supplement the treatment of infections is as follows:

1. Hyperalimentation should be instituted in anyone who is expected to be unable to take oral nourishment for periods longer than 5 to 7 days.
2. Patients with preexisting malnutrition should have correction of the

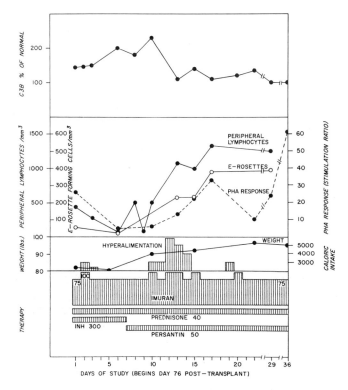

Figure 6-6. Serial measurements of immune function in a post-transplant patient. Pre-transplant weight was 106 pounds. The patient progressively lost weight in the post-transplant period and was admitted for parenteral hyperalimentation on the 76th post-transplant day. She refused such treatment, and associated with this was a progressive worsening of T cell immune responsiveness and a febrile illness believed to be caused by viral infection. A 5-day course of hyperalimentation significantly improved lymphocyte function. Caloric intake on this chart represents intake by both oral and intravenous routes in excess of the patient's normal diet.

nutritional deficits by either oral supplementation or intravenous hyperalimentation before any planned elective surgical intervention or the institution of therapy that may aggravate the nutritional problem.

3. Patients with severe infections who do not respond promptly to therapy should have supplemental hyperalimentation by the oral or intravenous route.

4. Supplemental oral hyperalimentation is best administered by continuous or intermittent drip via a nasogastric tube. Intravenous hyperalimentation using a central venous catheter should be reserved for those patients who are not able to take nourishment orally.

5. The hyperalimentation form may be varied with the condition being treated, but it should ensure adequate caloric intake for the basal meta-

bolic needs plus the estimated needs required by conditions associated with hypercatabolism, such as burn injury. Amino acid and caloric composition should take into consideration basal metabolic needs, increased catabolism, increased urinary loss, or loss from any wounds or fistulas.

6. Supplementation with vitamins for individuals not previously vitamin deficient should be in the range of 2 to 3 times the minimum daily requirement. It is doubtful whether doses of vitamin C more than 500 mg per day will be of any benefit, and pronounced excesses of many of the other vitamins may actually cause harm.

7. The requirements for metals during infection have not been determined, although they are apparently important. Oral hyperalimentation programs probably contain enough trace metals to ensure against deficiencies, but they must be added to hyperalimentation regimens. Iron therapy may aggravate acute infection and should rarely be given during an acute infection.

Component Therapy

In patients with low levels of complement components related to the properdin pathway, including C3, it may be of value to administer blood products containing these components. There are many anecdotal examples of the benefit of plasma or blood therapy in chronic or severe infections, but we know of no well controlled clinical studies at this time. Serum from patients with diminished opsonic activity, however, can be restored functionally by the addition of either normal serum or purified components of the alternative pathway. Studies in our laboratory have shown that cryoextracted plasma retains full opsonic capability, and there is only slight reduction in opsonic capacity in the plasma of blood stored at 4°C in plastic bags when CPD is used as an anticoagulant [36]. At the present time, our recommendation for patients with severe infections, who are not responding adequately to antibiotic therapy and in whom we suspect there may be a defect in opsonic proteins, is to administer whole blood, cryoextracted blood, or cryoextracted plasma daily. In these patients, the use of packed or washed red cells, albumin, or solutions of plasma protein derivative is discouraged.

Transfusion therapy with peripheral neutrophils has apparent benefit in patients who are severely leukopenic with evidence of infection [14, 58]. However, the benefit of this technique in patients with peripheral neutrophil counts greater than 1,000 per milliliter is much more questionable. Transfusion with blood lymphocytes to correct specific abnormalities of immune function has not proved beneficial at the present time with the exception of a few highly selected conditions, such as mucocutaneous candidiasis. Our current recommendation for leukocyte transfusion therapy is limited to neutrophil transfusion obtained by leukophoresis, preferably from histocompatible donors, and administered to patients with evidence of bacterial infection who have peripheral neutrophil counts lower than 500.

Immunization

Resistance to infection by selected pathogens can be increased by active programs of immunization. Prominent among infections occurring in hospitalized patients are those caused by *P. aeruginosa.* A heptavalent vaccine against this organism has been evaluated in clinical trials at our center and the results are summarized in Table 6-2. In these patients, active immunization resulted in an approximate 80% reduction in the incidence of death from burn wound sepsis or septicemia caused by this organism. In the last group, a hyperimmune polyvalent gamma globulin preparation was available for the treatment of patients who developed bacteremia or signs of invasive burn wound sepsis caused by *Pseudomonas.* The combined use of these modalities has resulted in virtual elimination of *Pseudomonas* infections in our burn population as a cause of death. We have demonstrated that a selective consumption of specific antibody may occur during heavy colonization by a particular immunotype and that when low levels of the specific antibody are reached, systemic invasion may occur [1, 4]. Specific anti-*Pseudomonas* IgG antibody generated by active immunization may not require participation of the alternative pathway to function as an opsonin, but complement activity improves the opsonic defect. On the other hand, natural antibody for *P. aeruginosa* requires participation of the alternative pathway for some strains, although not for others. Therefore the administration of hyperimmune anti-*Pseudomonas* gammaglobulin may be especially effective in patients who have *Pseudomonas* infections accompanied by abnormalities involving the alternative pathway of the complement system. Recent experiments in our laboratory have shown that it is possible to extract specific immune antibody from crude gammaglobulin, plasma, or serum by the technique of immune affinity chromatography with greater than 90% yield of the specific functionally active antibody molecules against

Table 6-2. Effect of Immunotherapy on Infection with *Pseudomonas aeruginosa* in Patients with 20% Burns or More

	Number of Patients	Percent Positive Blood Cultures (*Pseudomonas*)	Percent Septic Deaths (*Pseudomonas*)
Antecedent control	75	18.7	14.7
Vaccination only	96	8.3	3.1
Vaccination plus hyperimmune globulin for *Pseudomonas* bacteremia	186	5.9	0.0

Source: Adapted from Alexander, J. W., and Fisher, M. W. Immunization against *Pseudomonas* infection after thermal injury. *J. Infect. Dis.* 130(Suppl.):152, 1974.

the corresponding immunotype [41]. Experiments are currently under way to use this technique for extraction of antibody to other immunotypes. It may become possible to prepare specific immunoglobulin preparations for a large number of the problematic pathogens that now respond poorly to antibiotic therapy.

Unfortunately, at the present time, neither are effective bacterial vaccines against the common pathogens available, nor are the hyperimmune globulin preparations available commercially. If the *Pseudomonas* hyperimmune globulin preparation is approved for commercial distribution, we can highly recommend its use in patients with *Pseudomonas* infections.

Immunoadjuvants

Historically, immunoadjuvants have generally been conceded to be anything that, when administered with an antigen, results in a greater antibody response against that antigen. With our growing awareness of the complexity of host defense mechanisms, it has become obvious that such agents could enhance the cell-mediated arm of immunity as well as the humoral factors; thus the more general term, *immunopotentiator,* has come into vogue. These agents include biological and synthetic products (see Table 6-3 for a representative list).

It has been known for some time that animals treated with BCG (or other mycobacterial products) were highly resistant to a wide variety of infectious agents [21]. This effect seems to be true for most of the agents listed in Table 6-3 [29, 45, 51, 56]. However, interest in these agents waned with the advent of effective antibiotic therapy, only to be rekindled when their antitumor activity began to be exploited [11, 12].

Table 6-3. A Brief List of Selected Immunoadjuvants

Biological Products
Bacille Calmette-Guerin (BCG) and a variety of cell wall products
Bordetella pertussis
Corynebacterium parvum
Double-stranded RNA
Lipopolysaccharides

Synthetic Products
Pyran
Tilorone
Triton WR
Styrene-maleic anhydride copolymers
Poly-rI:rC
DMAE-fluorenone
DBAP-anthraquinone
Levamisole

A clear mode of action has not been delineated for any of the immuno-potentiators. Indeed, as one might suspect on examining the list of such agents, there is considerable diversity in their modes of action. Some agents seem to depress T cell function almost totally, while enhancing the activity of B cells and macrophages (e.g., pyran and *Corynebacterium parvum*). Others seem to enhance T cell responsiveness (e.g., levamisole). The combination of effects on T cells, B cells, macrophages, or serum factors seems endless, but one function seems common to all these agents — the activation of macrophages. Thus we return to the body's basic defense mechanism against infection, phagocytosis.

Macrophages from animals treated with a variety of immunopotentiators have been shown to have antitumor activity [12, 45], enhanced bactericidal activity [21, 29], greater activity against parasites [56], and more effective killing of fungi [51]. The number of animal studies is increasing every day, but the majority of human studies with immunopotentiators are cancer studies. These studies can provide useful information for designing effective therapy in infection-prone patients and for determining the appropriateness of a particular agent.

For example, adverse reactions to BCG have been clearly documented [54] and include hepatic dysfunction, fever, and ulcers. Consequently, the physician would be justifiably wary of using a live vaccine, such as BCG, in an already seriously immunocompromised patient. However, killed vaccines, such as *C. parvum,* and synthetic agents, such as levamisole and pyran, may be seriously considered. Pyran and *C. parvum* offer the advantage of functioning in spite of T cell depletion and do not enhance allograft rejection. Thus their use in the highly susceptible transplant recipient may be justified when other therapeutic modalities fail (e.g., *P. carinii* infection). Where a general T cell depression is being experienced and graft rejection is not an issue, levamisole may be appropriate.

Unfortunately, no clear suggestions in this area can be made until solid clinical trials, designed after extensive animal investigations, have been conducted. Clearly this is an area of active research and one that holds promise for the transiently immunocompromised patient.

Summary

Acquired defects in host-resistance mechanisms occur, frequently related to a variety of causes, and specific infections are associated with specific defects. These abnormalities can be detected by relatively simple tests and followed sequentially. At the present time, malnutrition, which is usually easily correctable, appears to be a major contributing factor to acquired defects of host defense, predisposing to infection. Other contributing factors are the disease process itself and therapy for the disease. Some of the defects can be corrected by replacement therapy, and specific immunization or passive treatment with immune IgG antibody shows significant promise as a therapeutic modality. Immunoadjuvants also show promise, but their use is largely speculative at the present time.

References

1. Alexander, J. W. Emerging concepts in the control of surgical infections. *Surgery* 75:934, 1974.
2. Alexander, J. W. Antibiotic agents and the immune mechanisms of defense. *Bull. N.Y. Acad. Med.* 51:1039, 1975.
3. Alexander, J. W. Nutrition and surgical infections. In W. Ballinger (Ed.), *American College of Surgeons Manual of Surgical Nutrition*. Philadelphia: Saunders, 1975.
4. Alexander, J. W., and Fisher, M. W. Immunization against *Pseudomonas* infection after thermal injury. *J. Infect. Dis.* 130(Suppl):S152, 1974.
5. Alexander, J. W., and Good, R. A. *Immunobiology for Surgeons*. Philadelphia: Saunders, 1970.
6. Alexander, J. W., and Meakins, J. L. A physiological basis for the development of opportunistic infections in man. *Ann. Surg.* 176:273, 1972.
7. Alexander, J. W., and Meakins, J. L. Acquired abnormalities of the antibacterial function of neutrophils. *Int. Med. Dig.* 8:38, 1973.
8. Alexander, J. W., et al. Lack of pituitary, adrenal, thyroid, gonadal, and pineal endocrine control of cyclic changes in the antibacterial function of neutrophils. *J. Reticuloendothel. Soc.* 14:266, 1973.
9. Alexander, J. W., et al. Consumptive opsoninopathy. Possible pathogenesis in lethal and opportunistic infections. *Ann. Surg.* 184:672, 1976.
10. Bach, G., et al. Biologic role of rheumatoid factor. Relationship between antiglobulin consumption and complement system activation during bacteremia in man. *Acta Biol. Med. Ger.* 31:311, 1973.
11. Bartlett, G. L., and Zbar, B. Tumor-specific vaccine containing *Mycobacterium bovis* and tumor cells: Safety and efficacy. *J. Natl. Cancer Inst.* 48:1709, 1972.
12. Bast, R. C., Jr., et al. BCG and cancer. *N. Engl. J. Med.* 290:1458, 1974.
13. Bjornson, A. B., and Alexander, J. W. Alterations of serum opsonins in patients with severe thermal injury. *J. Lab. Clin. Med.* 83:372, 1974.
14. Boggs, D. R. Transfusion of neutrophils as prevention or treatment of infection in patients with neutropenia. *N. Engl. J. Med.* 290:1055, 1974.
15. Bokisch, V. A., et al. The potential pathogenic role of complement in dengue hemorrhagic shock syndrome. *N. Engl. J. Med.* 289:996, 1973.
16. Bruton, O. C. Agammaglobulinemia. *Pediatrics* 9:722, 1952.
17. Cannon, P. R., et al. The relationship of protein deficiency to surgical infection. *Ann. Surg.* 120:514, 1944.
18. Daniels, J. C., Sakai, H., and Ritzmann, S. E. Lymphoid response of the burn patient. *South. Med. J.* 68:865, 1975.
19. Dionigi, R., et al. The effects of total parenteral nutrition on immunodepression due to malnutrition. *Ann. Surg.* 185:467, 1977.
20. Dionigi, R., et al. Antibody formation and phagocytic function in patients undergoing parenteral nutrition. Proceedings of the International Congress of Parenteral Nutrition, Montpellier, 1974. In press.
21. Dubos, R. J., and Schaedler, R. W. Effects of cellular constituents of mycobacteria on the resistance of mice to heterologous infections. I. Protective effects. *J. Exp. Med.* 106:703, 1957.
22. Eilber, F. R., and Morton, D. L. Impaired immunologic reactivity and recurrence following cancer surgery. *Cancer* 25:362, 1970.
23. Fearon, D. T., Ruddy, S., Schur, P. H., and McCabe, W. R. Activation of the

properdin pathway of complement in patients with gram-negative bacteremia. *N. Engl. J. Med.* 292:937, 1975.

24. Frank, M. M., and Atkinson, J. P. Complement in clinical medicine. *DM* 1:000, 1975.
25. Gordon, J. E., and Scrimshaw, N. S. Infectious disease in the malnourished. *Med. Clin. North Am.* 54:1495, 1970.
26. Guggenheim, K., and Buechler, E. Nutrition and resistance to infection. Bactericidal properties and phagocytic activity of peritoneal fluid of rats in various states of nutritional deficiency. *J. Immunol.* 54:349, 1946.
27. Heck, E. L., et al. Evaluation of leukocyte function in burned individuals by *in vitro* oxygen consumption. *J. Trauma.* 15:486, 1975.
28. Hirsch, J. G., and Strauss, B. Studies on heat-labile opsonin in rabbit serum. *J. Immunol.* 92:145, 1964.
29. Irwin, M. R., and Knight, H. D. Enhanced resistance to *Corynebacterium pseudotuberculosis* infections associated with reduced serum immunoglobulin levels in levamisole-treated mice. *Infect. Immun.* 12:1098, 1975.
30. Johnston, R. B., Jr., Lawton, A. R., and Cooper, M. D. Disorders of host defense against infection. Pathophysiologic and diagnostic considerations. *Med. Clin. North Am.* 57:421, 1973.
31. Law, D. K., Dudrick, S. J., and Abdou, N. I. The effect of dietary protein depletion on immunocompetence: The importance of nutritional repletion prior to immunologic induction. *Ann. Surg.* 179:168, 1973.
32. Law, D. K., Dudrick, S. J., and Abdou, N. I. The effects of protein calorie malnutrition on immune competence of the surgical patient. *Surg. Gynecol. Obstet.* 139:257, 1974.
33. Lennard, E. S., et al. An immunologic and nutritional evaluation of burn neutrophil function. *J. Surg. Res.* 16:286, 1974.
34. MacLean, L. D., et al. Host resistance in sepsis and trauma. *Ann. Surg.* 182:207, 1975.
35. Mancini, G., Carbonara, A. O., and Heremans, J. F. Immunochemical quantitation of antigens by single radial immunodiffusion. *Immunochemistry* 2:235, 1965.
36. McClellan, M. A., and Alexander, J. W. The opsonic activity of stored blood. *Transfusion* 17:227, 1977.
37. Miller, M. E. Pathology of chemotaxis and random reaction. *Semin. Hematol.* 12:59, 1975.
38. Molenaar, J. L., et al. Changes in antigenic properties of human C3 upon activation and conversion by trypsin. *J. Immunol.* 112:1444, 1974.
39. Munster, A. M., Hoagland, H. C., and Pruitt, B. A., Jr. The effect of thermal injury on serum immunoglobulins. *Ann. Surg.* 172:965, 1970.
40. Neva, F. A., et al. Relationship of serum complement levels to events of the malarial paroxysm. *J. Clin. Invest.* 54:451, 1974.
41. Ogle, J. D., Stace, P., and Alexander, J. W. Extraction and purification of specific antibody against *Pseudomonas aeruginosa* by immune affinity chromatography. *J. Lab. Clin. Med.* 89:433, 1977.
42. Osler, A. G., and Sandberg, A. L. Alternate complement pathways. *Prog. Allergy* 17:51, 1973.
43. Palmer, D. L., and Reed, W. P. Delayed hypersensitivity skin testing. II. Clinical correlates and anergy. *J. Infect. Dis.* 130:138, 1974.
44. Pillemer, L., et al. The properdin system and immunity. I. Demonstration and isolation of a new serum protein, properdin, and its role in immune phenomena. *Science* 120:279, 1954.
45. Regelson, W. Host modulation of resistance to infection and neoplasia. *Annu. Reports Med. Chem.* 8:160, 1973.

46. Rocklin, R. E.   Clinical applications of *in vitro* lymphocyte tests. *Prog. Clin. Immunol.* 2:21, 1974.
47. Schopfer, K., and Douglas, S. D.   Neutrophil function in children with kwashiorkor. *J. Lab. Clin. Med.* 88:450, 1976.
48. Scott, H., et al.   Familial opsonization defect associated with fatal infantile dermatitis, infections, and histiocytosis. *Arch. Dis. Child.* 50:311, 1975.
49. Scrimshaw, N. S., Taylor, C. E., and Gordon, J. E.   *Interactions of nutrition and infection.* Monograph Series, No. 57. Geneva: World Health Organization, 1968.
50. Selvaraj, R. J., and Bhat, K. S.   Metabolic and bactericidal activities of leukocytes in protein-calorie malnutrition. *Am. J. Clin. Nutr.* 25:166, 1972.
51. Sher, N. A., et al.   Effects of BCG, *Corynebacterium parvum*, and methanol-extraction residue in the reduction of mortality from *Staphylococcus aureus* and *Candida albicans* infections in immunosuppressed mice. *Infect. Immun.* 12:1325, 1975.
52. Sirisinha, S., et al.   Complement and C3-proactivator levels in children with protein-calorie malnutrition and effect of dietary treatment. *Lancet* I:1016, 1973.
53. Smythe, P. M., et al.   Thymolymphatic deficiency and depression of cell-mediated immunity in protein-calorie malnutrition. *Lancet* II:939, 1971.
54. Sparks, F. C., et al.   Complications of BCG immunotherapy in patients with cancer. *N. Engl. J. Med.* 289:827, 1973.
55. Studley, H. O.   Percentage of weight loss. A basic indicator of surgical risk in patients with chronic peptic ulcer. *J.A.M.A.* 106:458, 1936.
56. Swartzberg, J. E., Krahenbuhl, J. L., and Remington, J. S.   Dichotomy between macrophage activation and degree of protection against *Listeria monocytogenes* and *Toxoplasma gondii* in mice stimulated with *Corynebacterium parvum*. *Infect. Immun.* 12:1037, 1975.
57. Thurman, G. B., et al.   Human mixed lymphocyte cultures. Evaluation of a microculture technique utilizing the multiple automated sample harvester (MASH). *Clin. Exp. Immunol.* 15:289, 1973.
58. Vallejos, C., et al.   White blood cell transfusions for control of infections in neutropenic patients. *Transfusion* 15:28, 1975.
59. Warden, G. D., Mason, A. D., Jr., and Pruitt, B. A., Jr.   Evaluation of leukocyte chemotaxis *in vitro* in thermally injured patients. *J. Clin. Invest.* 54:1001, 1974.
60. Weinberg, E. D.   Iron and susceptibility to infectious disease. In the resolution of the contest between invader and host, iron may be the critical determinant. *Science* 184:952, 1974.
61. Winkelstein, J. A., Smith, M. R., and Shin, H. S.   The role of C3 as an opsonin in the early stages of infection. *Proc. Soc. Exp. Biol. Med.* 149:397, 1975.

7. Host Defense Mechanism Defects in Neonates

Michael A. Medici and Richard A. Gatti

Protection against infection requires the successful interaction of a number of nonspecific and specific host defense systems. These mechanisms include the inflammatory response, the complement cascade, phagocytosis, and the immune response. Whereas most of these functions are only marginally compromised in the normal term infant, in infants who are small for gestational age and in premature neonates, they are sufficiently inadequate to predispose to infections.

Normal Host Mechanisms

Confinement of an invading organism to the portal of entry requires the activation of a series of host factors that result in the inflammatory response. Hageman factor (XII) is activated by (1) the presence of endotoxin, (2) disruption of mucosal surfaces of the endothelial lining of blood vessels with the resultant exposure of the collagen fibrils of the basement membrane, or (3) foreign substances with negative surface charges (e.g., glass) (Figure 7-1). Factor XII, a β or λ globulin with a molecular weight of 80,000 daltons, is then converted to its active form, a proteolytic enzyme designated as factor XII_A. Directly or indirectly, XII_A activates coagulation and the inflammatory response, as mediated by the kinin and complement systems. The fibrin clot for hemostasis is produced through the intrinsic coagulation cascade, leading to the production of thrombin. Factor XII_A via plasminogen proactivator also initiates the production of plasmin in the fibrinolytic system.

Kinin formation is initiated by factor XII_A and plasmin via prekallikrein activators (PKA). These plasma proteases hydrolyze prekallikrein to kallikrein with subsequent activation of kininogen, a plasma α globulin, to release the nonapeptide, bradykinin. In addition to causing pain, the kinins also have pronounced vascular effects. The resultant dilatation of peripheral arterioles and increased capillary permeability cause the exudation of plasma proteins, such as antibody and complement, into the perivascular tissues. These hemodynamic changes also reverse the normal laminar flow of blood in the vessels, with resultant margination of leukocytes. Marginated cells then adhere to the vascular endothelium and migrate into the extravascular tissue spaces by diapedesis. In addition, the kinins have chemotaxic effects on leukocytes, attracting them to the area of injury [33].

Complement is a series of distinct serum proteins that react sequentially with one another, forming biologically active inflammatory and opsonic products, in addition to having lytic and cytotoxic effects on certain target

This work was partially supported by the Amie Karen Fund for Children with Cancer, Los Angeles, California.

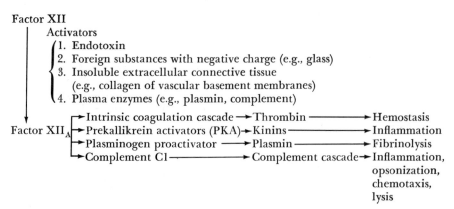

Figure 7-1. Activation of Hageman factor (XII) and subsequent reactions of factor XII$_A$.

cells. The first component of complement circulates in plasma as a trimolecular protein complex C1q, r, and s with Ca^{2+} as a ligand (Figure 7-2). Binding of C1q to the Fc portion of (1) immunoglobulin aggregates, (2) antibody-antigen complexes, or (3) specific antibody-target cell interaction converts C1s to an active proteolytic enzyme whose natural substrate is C4. Activated C4 interacts with C2, forming a new enzyme-active fragment $C\overline{42}$ or C3 convertase, which splits C3 into C3a and C3b. The C3b fragment is bound in a complex ($C\overline{142a3b}$) and can attach to specific receptors on red blood cells and neutrophils, causing the phenomenon of immune adherence and enhanced phagocytosis. The soluble factor C3a, released into the fluid phase, is an anaphylatoxin that causes significant vasomotor responses as well as exhibiting chemotaxis for neutrophils. Further amplification of the binding of C1 is mediated through the subsequent reaction of C3b with C5. This causes (1) the release of C5a, a vasoactive and chemotactic fragment, into the fluid phase and (2) the binding of C5b to the complex. C5b can then interact with C6 and C7 and stabilize as the complex $C\overline{142a3b5b67}$ or can release the trimolecular fragment $C\overline{567}$ to promote further neutrophil chemotaxis. Binding and activation of C8 and C9 results, finally, in the enzymatic production of membrane defects and osmotic lysis of the target cell.

An alternate pathway for the activation of C3 by properdin (Figure 7-3) has recently been elucidated. This allows activation of the complement cascade without the prerequisite specific immunoglobulin. This system is activated by complex polysaccharides and lipopolysaccharides of fungal and bacterial cell walls (e.g., endotoxin). These activating substances interact with properdin, factor D, and other plasma factors to generate activated properdin and factor D. These two activated factors and C3 activate factor B, resulting in the conversion of C3 into the two active fragments described above, C3a and C3b, thus initiating the remaining complement cascade. This alternate, or properdin, pathway provides the major defense to gram-

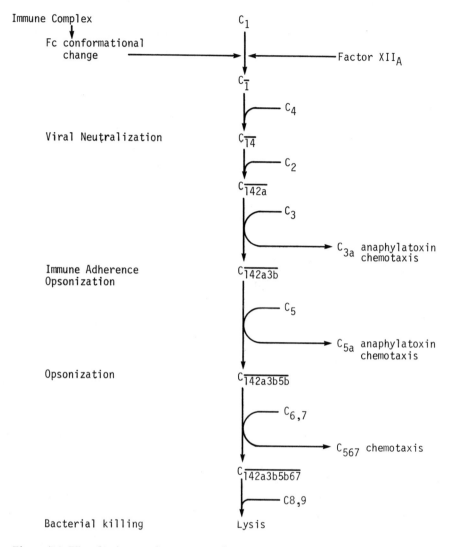

Figure 7-2. The classic complement cascade.

negative organisms. As would be expected, the levels of properdin, factor B, and C3 are depressed in patients with gram-negative shock, while C1, C4, and C2 remain at normal levels [47].

Defects in the classic and alternate complement pathway have led to recurrent infections that appear to be secondary to deficiencies in phagocytosis and the inflammatory response. Inability to activate complement secondary to C1r deficiency has been responsible for recurrent infections [36]. Several patients with significantly increased susceptibility to infection were found

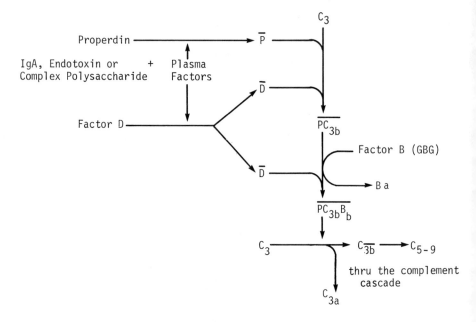

Figure 7-3. The alternate, or properdin, pathway of complement activation. (GBG = Factor B.)

to have abnormalities in C3 metabolism. Degradation by an aberrant serum enzyme was found, splitting C3 into an inactive conversion product C3c. In addition, hyposynthesis and hypercatabolism contribute to low serum C3 levels in other patients [5, 6, 8]. Complete absence of C3 in man has recently been reported [7, 16] and is associated with recurrent infections with encapsulated and gram-negative organisms. Given the pivotal importance of C3 in both the classic and alternate activation of complement, the increased susceptibility of these patients to infection is not unexpected. The fifth component of complement is another important generator of chemotactic and vasoactive factors; it also amplifies the activation of C3. Familial deficiencies of C5 have also been described [112, 127]. These patients have deficient phagocytosis and are particularly susceptible to gram-negative bacteria and coagulase-positive staphylococci. In addition, some patients may have a lupus-like syndrome. The phagocytic-enhancing activity of their serum can be restored by the addition of C5. Clinically, several kindreds manifest a syndrome similar to Leiner's disease [91]. Along similar lines, patients with sickle cell disease have deficient opsonization of pneumococci and inability to utilize the alternate, or properdin, pathway [93].

Neutrophils are the first phagocytic cells to respond to the inflammatory stimulus. With the generation of chemotactic factors, neutrophils migrate along the concentration gradient and accumulate in the area of inflammation within 4 to 6 hours. Mononuclear cells begin to accumulate at 6 hours and are the predominant cell type by 12 hours. The ability to respond to chemotactic stimuli depends in part on the mobility and deformability of the cell. Leukocytes can also generate chemotactic factors from serum and lysosomal granules.

The phagocytic efficiency of a leukocyte is strongly influenced by the surface character of the foreign material to be ingested. Opsonins condition the surface, thereby enhancing phagocytosis. Both antibody and complement may function as opsonins, since neutrophils and macrophages have membrane receptors for complement components and for the Fc portion of antibody molecules. By an ATP-dependent anaerobic glycolytic process, phagocytosis results in the formation of a phagocytic vacuole. Following fusion with intracellular lysosomes, intracellular killing occurs during a metabolic burst, characterized by increased O_2 consumption and the production of peroxide and O_2^-. The microorganism is killed as myeloperoxidase and peroxide fix halide. This mechanism and the resultant increase in O_2 utilization through the hexosemonophosphate (HMP) shunt can be evaluated by the nitroblue tetrazolium (NBT) reduction test.

Patients with chronic granulomatous disease have recurrent infections. The NBT test is negative and the neutrophils of these patients ingest but fail to kill microorganisms. They also lack the characteristic metabolic burst of the hexosemonophosphate shunt or the concurrent increased oxygen consumption following phagocytosis. Recent studies [35] have demonstrated that the production of superoxide (O_2^-) is also defective in these patients. The intracellular killing defect therefore appears to be directly related to deficient oxygen metabolism, with resultant inadequate peroxide and superoxide production. This disorder is discussed at length elsewhere in this volume.

Absence of myeloperoxidase is associated with decreased intracellular *Candida albicans* killing capacity. Patients with Chediak-Higashi syndrome have lysosomes that do not release their contents and therefore cannot assist in intracellular killing. In these patients there is a delayed intracellular killing of microorganisms, and recurrent infections are common. Defective leukocyte migration has been demonstrated to be associated with recurrent staphylococcal disease in Job's syndrome and has been found in male patients with markedly elevated IgE levels [81, 82, 132]. In Miller's "lazy leukocyte" syndrome, decreased neutrophil mobility and impaired marrow release of granulocytes have been associated with recurrent upper respiratory infections as well as with other local infections [113]. Leukotactic defects have also been described in juvenile diabetes mellitus [83].

Foreign substances are also phagocytosed and processed by macrophages. Normally, macrophages do not possess the extensive lysosomal system of the neutrophil. After activation by lymphocyte mediators or certain microbial substances, there is significantly increased intracellular killing and processing of antigenic material. The uptake and surface trapping of antigen by macrophages in the highly organized microenvironment of the lymph node and spleen further amplifies the immunogenicity of the antigen [131]. Here, macrophage-focused antigens stimulate lymphocytes and initiate a specific immune response.

The specific immune response encompasses two main types of lymphocytes: T, or thymus-dependent, and B, or bursa-dependent, lymphocytes. B lymphocytes arise from the bone marrow and, after maturation to an immunocompetent cell, produce specific antibody. The exact mode of induction of the immune response is not known, but antibody production seems to involve the interaction of macrophage-processed antigen, a T lymphocyte in a "helper" function, and an immunocompetent B cell. Recent in vitro studies by Rosenthal, Lipsky, and Shevach [128] indicate several sequential steps. After an antigen-independent, rapidly reversible interaction between macrophage and lymphocyte, a second, nonreversible, antigen-dependent binding occurs. This second step only occurs if the macrophage has a surface antigen to which the lymphocyte has a receptor. Following interaction of this complex with antigen receptors on B cells, antibody production is initiated. This antibody has the capacity to react specifically with the antigen that caused its production. After antibody-antigen combination, a conformational change in the Fc portion of IgM and in certain subclasses of IgG occurs, resulting in the activation of complement via the classic pathway. In addition, if the antibody is directed to the surface coat of a particulate antigen, it serves as a heat-stable opsonin, allowing augmented phagocytosis of this foreign material.

Thymic dependent or T lymphocytes originate in the bone marrow, mature in the thymus, and mediate cellular immunity. These lymphocytes are the primary defense against intracellular residing organisms (viruses, fungi, and mycobacterium) as well as against foreign tissue cells. The mediators, or lymphokines produced by T cells can kill foreign cells directly (lymphotoxin), prevent viral spread (interferon), recruit other lymphocytes to respond to the antigen (transfer factor), localize macrophages to an area (migration inhibitory factor), and stimulate the intracellular metabolic and phagocytic processes of macrophages. The action of these mediators is therefore to improve intracellular killing. In the peripheral blood, T cells comprise 60 to 80% of the circulating lymphocyte population, with B cells accounting for another 20 to 30%.

Patients with congenital hypoimmunoglobulinemia (Bruton type) lack the capacity to produce specific antibody and have recurrent bacterial infections caused predominately by encapsulated organisms. Although their cell-mediated immunity (CMI) is grossly intact, they have difficulty with hepatitis and polio as well. Occasionally these patients also develop a chronic panencephalitis associated with rubeola, herpes, ECHO-30, and adenovirus [29, 137, 138]. Patients with congenital thymic hypoplasia lack an intact T cell system and have severe defects in cell-mediated immunity. These individuals suffer from infections caused by intracellularly residing organisms. In the neonatal period, these patients may present with hypocalcemic tetany, misshapen ears, mild hypertelorism, shortened philtrum, and micrognathia (DiGeorge's syndrome). However, not all infants who manifest this syndrome have an immunologic deficiency [61].

The most devastating form of immunodeficiency is the severe combined immunodeficiency. These infants manifest defects of both humoral and cell-mediated immunity. There are at least four well-defined forms of SCID: autosomal recessive [85], X-linked recessive [67], that associated with short-limbed dwarfism [62], and infants who are adenosine deaminase deficient [66]. These infants rarely survive beyond 1 year of age without treatment, usually succumbing to sepsis with bacterial, viral, fungal, or protozoan organisms, such as *Pneumocystis carinii*. Vaccinia gangrenosa, following smallpox vaccination, and graft-versus-host disease, following administration of fresh blood products, are common iatrogenic causes of death in this group of patients. We have limited our discussion of the primary immunodeficiency disorders in this review because this subject will be presented at length by others and has been extensively reviewed elsewhere in the literature [17, 60].

Neonatal Deficiencies

Clinical studies indicate that the newborn has widespread impairments of both nonspecific and specific defense mechanisms (Table 7-1). The inflammatory response that is critical in localizing the insulting organism is decreased in the newborn, a deficiency that is exaggerated further with increasing prematurity. Factor XII, an important nonspecific activator of the inflammatory response, is present at 50% of adult levels in term infants and only 30% in 32 to 36-week-old premature infants [80]. It is likely that serum levels would be even lower in 26 to 32-week-old premature infants. Factor XII and other physiologically low clotting factors reach normal adult levels after several weeks of age [99]. There is also evidence that factor XII is activated at birth by changes in temperature and P_{AO_2}. With kinin activation, vasoconstriction of the umbilical cord vessels and the ductus arteriosis occurs. Kinins may also be responsible for vasodilatation of the pulmonary vasculature [33, 106]. Recent studies have demonstrated further reduction in factor XII levels in debilitated newborns. Significant deficiencies are found in debilitated prematures (20% of adult levels), particularly in those infants with severe RDS. These low levels of factor XII were independent of other problems in coagulation, such as disseminated intravascular coagulation [34].

The major nonspecific humoral defense mechanism is the complement system. The cytotoxic and bactericidal reactions are dependent on the entire sequence. Generation of chemotactic and vasoactive factors, as well as opsonization of bacteria and fungi, are dependent on C3 and C5. Although C5 production is detected as early as 8 weeks gestational age, and C3 and C5 production are consistently found by 11 weeks [98], the term infant has only 50% of adult serum activity for C3 and C5 [50, 122]. Since complement

Table 7-1. Comparison of Neonatal and Adult Defense Factors

Factor	32–36 weeks	Term	Comments
XII	30%	50%	Proportional to gestational age
C3, C5	?	50%	Proportional to gestational age
Properdin	?	?	
Factor B	?	< 50%	In 15% of cord bloods
Alpha$_2$ globulin	?	65%	Needed for RES phagocytosis
PMN function			
Migration	▼	▼	Rebuck skin window; high eosinophil count, days 1–21 in 34-week and older neonates
Membrane rigidity	?	▲	
Chemotaxis	▼	▼	(?) secondary to rigidity of membrane
Killing	▼	▼	Abnormal to *Candida*, abnormal to *S. aureus*, during first 12 hr in 36% of term cord blood studied
Opsonization	?	▼	
Macrophage	?	?	Decreased in animal models
IgM	▼	▼	▲ with intrauterine antigen stimulation
IgG	Normal or ▼	▲	Proportional to gestational age
T cell function			
Lymphotoxin	?	▼	40% of adult level
T cell rosettes	▼	Normal	▼ in SGA
DNCB	▼	Normal	▼ in SGA
PHA	▼	Normal	▼ in SGA

components do not cross the placenta [122], levels are dependent on fetal production, and the degree of deficiency is usually proportionate to the prematurity of the infant [50].

The alternate, or properdin, activated pathway is found to be markedly deficient in factor B in 15% of cord sera. This correlates with defective opsonic activity in such sera [130]. The premature infant is particularly compromised in effective protection against gram-negative organisms, since the predominant defense against these infections involves complement activation, either through the alternate pathway or through specific IgM. The substantial deficiency of factor XII in debilitated premature infants also precludes activation of complement by gram-negative organisms through Hageman factor and plasmin.

In vitro studies on the response and function of neonatal neutrophils by Miller demonstrate decreased chemotactic response [109], somewhat decreased random mobility [107], and a more rigid membrane as measured by cell deformability [111]. It is possible that this increased membrane rigidity accounts for some of the decreased chemotaxic response, demonstrated by the Boyden chamber technique, since neonatal cells would have greater difficulty passing through the 3-micron pores in the filter. Phagocytosis by term and premature neonatal cells is normal [51] under usual test conditions. When limiting amounts of adult sera are used (2.5%), neonatal neutrophils phagocytose significantly fewer yeast particles as compared to adult cells [109]. Cord blood does not support phagocytosis as well as adult serum, although this deficiency can be restored by the addition of C5 [108]. No differences have been noted in complement-dependent immune adherence [109].

The metabolic burst leading to intracellar killing of ingested organisms has also been shown to be decreased in the neonatal leukocyte [32, 77, 92], although the resting level as indicated by the NBT test is significantly higher than normal adult levels [89]. Intracellular bactericidal function of neutrophils was decreased in 36% of full-term infants within the first 12 hours of life. This was related to failure of the normal stimulation of the hexosemonophosphate shunt during phagocytosis [32]. Other studies have revealed metabolic differences in all specimens taken from cord blood leukocytes [92]. Intracellular killing by neutrophils from term and premature infants has been evaluated in vitro using a variety of microorganisms. C. albicans was killed to a significantly lower degree by neutrophils from newborns when compared to cells from adults in autologous serum [140]. There was no difference between the intracellular killing capacity between neutrophils from term and premature infants. The addition of adult serum to the test system did not improve the ability of neonatal cells to kill ingested Candida. Using Pseudomonas aeruginosa as a test organism, Cocchi and Marianelli [30] demonstrated comparable killing in the first 1½ hours of incubation in term and premature newborn infants and the cells of older children. By 3½ hours, however, the premature infants' cells demonstrated significantly impaired killing. In addition, after 3 hours incubation, the premature infants' neutrophils demonstrated cytopathic lesions, including rupture of the cell membrane with loss of cytoplasm and ingested organisms. This cellular disruption was not demonstrable in the term neonate or control cell suspensions. Neutrophils from septic neonates show further decreases in bactericidal capacity [139].

In vivo, the kinetics of the inflammatory response in the newborn are significantly different from those of adults, both in the dermal response to irritants, such as topical croton oil, and in the leukocyte response, as observed by the Rebuck skin window. In adults, neutrophils appear rapidly in the Rebuck window, accounting for 85 to 95% of the cells at 4 hours. The proportion of mononuclear cells increases steadily, becoming the predominant cell at 10 to 12 hours. These cells also become larger with pale-staining vacuolated cytoplasm during that time. Significant numbers of eosinophils are not found in the adult at any time during the 12-hour observation period. In the full-term neonate, from 1 to 21 days of age, an early eosinophil response in excess of 2% of the cells is observed. For example, at 2 hours eosinophils may represent an average of 19% of the cells (1 to 93% range). Comparable eosinophilia is not demonstrated in infants under 24 hours of age or older than 21 days [121]. Although infants with high circulating eosinophil counts have a higher percentage of eosinophils in the exudate, the proportion of eosinophils in the skin lesion is significantly higher than in the peripheral circulation. Another consistent difference is the slower appearance of mononuclear cells in the neonate; these cells never predominate [45]. Infants of less than 34 weeks gestational age demonstrate a similarly delayed response by neutrophils and mononuclear cells but without the eosinophilia that is prevalent in term infants [24].

Phagocytosis by the reticuloendothelial system (RES) also represents an important host defense mechanism. This appears to be dependent on a specific α_2 globulin for optimal activity. Quantitation of this circulatory factor in term newborns reveals levels that are only 65% of adult norms [74]. To date, there has been no evaluation of this factor in preterm infants. However, this impaired RES clearance may correlate with the ease that bacteremia and septicemia can develop. Although human neonatal macrophage function has not been evaluated, studies in animals have shown that some in vitro and in vivo defects of immune reactivity can be corrected by the addition of adult macrophages [21, 76].

The specific immune response develops from the cells of the blood islands and yolk sac, which then migrate into the developing embryo to become the lymphoid and hematopoietic precursors. Later, the fetal liver is the major source of stem cells and, finally, the bone marrow assumes this function, as in the adult [121]. Lymphocytes bearing membrane immunoglobulins (mIg) can be identified by 12 weeks of gestation. In vitro synthesis of IgM can be detected at $10\frac{1}{2}$ weeks, IgG, and IgE are detectable at 11 weeks, and IgA at 30 weeks. Passive transfer of maternal IgG produces detectable serum levels by 38 days. A linear relationship between the log of IgG concentration and gestational age was found for infants 24 to 42 weeks of gestational age [116] but did not correlate with birth weight [18]. In the last trimester, immunoglobulins are actively transported so that fetal levels are generally higher than maternal serum levels. In infants born prior to 33 weeks' gestation, immunoglobulin levels below 100 mg per 100 ml may occur within the first 6 months of life. It has been suggested that administering exogenous gamma globulin to these infants may provide some protection against infection [86].

In the neonate, passively transferred IgG affords protection against infection only if adequate titers of specific antibodies existed in the mother. Infections with rubeola, rubella, group A beta-hemolytic streptococci, and *Hemophilus influenzae* produce persistent circulating IgG long after the infection has resolved. It is this antibody that will be transmitted to the newborn and will provide protection during the neonatal period. As the maternal antibody titer declines, proportional to a half-life of approximately 3 weeks, the infant once again becomes susceptible to these infections. It is perhaps worth stressing that with rapid treatment and prolific use of antibiotics, the levels of these specific antibodies are decreasing in the general population, thus placing neonates at a higher risk to infection from these organisms. For example, the significant rise in neonatal susceptibility to *H. influenzae* in recent years has been attributed to a deficiency of bactericidal antibody in the mother [73]. Only 10% of neonates and 25% of mothers currently have bactericidal antibodies to *H. influenzae*, while over 90% of newborns that were born in past years were protected. Further, antibodies of the IgM class appear to have a major protective role against gram-negative infections. Since these antibodies do not cross the placenta, the infant is vulnerable to such pathogens as *Escherichia coli* and *Klebsiella*. This specific opsonic defect, coupled with the above-mentioned nonspecific opsonic defects in the complement system, greatly increase the infectious risk of the term and, more so, the premature infant.

Specific antibody acquired transplacentally also has a modulating effect on fetal and neonatal immune responses. With antigenic stimulation in utero, such as with congenital infections by *Treponema pallidum*, rubella, cytomegalovirus, and *Toxoplasma gondii*, the fetus does respond with both IgM and IgA production [3, 4], and elevated specific antibody levels of these classes are indications of congenital infection. Fetal production of IgG is limited, however, by a regulatory feedback inhibition involving maternal transplacental antibody. This is one of the reasons for withholding immunization early in life. Studies have revealed that immunizations given within 24 hours of birth not only fail to produce the desired serologic response [25, 123] but may result in a period of temporary immunoparalysis [123]. Colostral antibody has also been shown to limit neonatal responses to oral polio vaccine [102].

Cell-mediated immunity is detectable by in vitro responsiveness of thymic cells to PHA at 12 weeks of gestation [12, 95]. This is temporally related to the development of the demarcation of thymic cortex and medulla [95]. Several weeks later PHA responsive cells can be demonstrated in the spleen concurrent with the development of the small lymphocyte periarteriolar cuffs, known to be thymic dependent areas [12]. Delayed hypersensitivity skin testing is more difficult to evaluate because of the impaired inflammatory responsiveness of the neonates. In vitro studies, however, have revealed that neonates respond normally to PHA, pokeweed mitogen, staphylococcal filtrate, and mixed leukocyte cultures [101]. The percentage of lymphocytes forming spontaneous (E) rosettes with sheep erythrocytes (T cells) is also comparable to adult levels [44]. Lymphotoxin production, however, is only 40% that of the adult response [28]. In infants who are small for their gestational ages, T cell levels, PHA response, and 2,4-dinitrochlorobenzene (DNCB) sensitivity are deficient. These impairments were noted to be present 9 to 20 months after birth, especially in those children who remained lower than the third percentile on the growth chart [28].

Evaluation of the Neonate for Sepsis

The initial indications of sepsis in a newborn are usually so subtle that it is difficult to be certain if the change is due to sepsis or related to other etiologies. Increasing jaundice, apnea, poor feeding, abdominal distention with or without gastric residuals, lethargy, hypoglycemia, or difficulty with temperature regulation may herald life-threatening infection. Increasing respiratory distress, acidosis, a fullness of the fontanelle, thrombocytopenia, disseminated intravascular coagulation (DIC), hypotension, and vasomotor instability are common in progressive sepsis but can also be seen in premature neonates with respiratory distress syndrome or other disorders. Signs of shock or severe toxicity occur late in the course. (This could be only 6 to 12 hours later in a fulminant infection [72].) Therefore it is often impossible to reliably differentiate bacterial sepsis from other pathologic processes. If an alternate explanation for even subtle changes cannot be found, the patient should be properly cultured and appropriate antibiotics instituted without further delay.

The perinatal history can be of great clinical significance, especially in premature infants and those who are small for their gestational ages. Flora of the vaginal vault, e.g., *E. coli, S. aureus,* and group B beta-hemolytic streptococci, may ascend and induce inflammation and infection of the fetal membranes, placenta, and umbilical cord [42]. Aspiration of infected amniotic fluid is a major source of neonatal septicemia [22], with pneumonia the most commonly associated infection [114]. Maternal events predisposing to ascending infection include premature rupture of the fetal membranes, lengthy labor, peripartum infection, extensive manipulation, bleeding, and eclampsia. It is important to note therefore whether there was a history of maternal fever, whether the amniotic fluid was turbid or foul smelling, or whether the placental membranes were cloudy. Histologic examination of the placenta for chorioamnionitis and of the umbilical cord for funisitis can be of significant assistance in this regard [20].

The reliability of gastric aspirate analysis as a correlate of sepsis is controversial. Neutrophils found in the gastric aspirate are predominantly of maternal origin, since cytogenetically these cells are female, irrespective of the sex of the infant [133]; they do not represent a fetal response to infection. If the aspirate is collected within the first hour of life, the risk of sepsis does correlate with the number of neutrophils in the gastric aspirate [70, 120]. This correlation decreases rapidly with specimens collected later than 1 hour after birth. Using a system to score perinatal risk factors (maternal pyrexia, rupture of membranes longer than 24 hours before delivery), fetal risk factors (prematurity, 1 min APGAR scores less than 7), and whether the gastric aspirate contains more than five neutrophils per high-powered field; there is good correlation with the risk of sepsis [70]. In addition, since most infections are the result of aspirating contaminated amniotic fluid, the gastric aspirate usually provides a reliable, easily available source for culturing and identifying potential pathogens.

Acute phase reactants in the serum are nonspecific indicators of infection and may be useful in evaluation of a newborn for sepsis. The C-reactive protein (CRP) is an acute phase reactant. In vitro it is a phagocytosis-promoting factor [90, 96] and thus may be an indirect sign of bacteremia

[129]. The time of appearance and the amount of CRP in the serum are related to the onset and degree of the inciting stimulus [49]. The normal CRP is negative, but may rise to 2 mm at 2 to 3 days of life. This may be secondary to necrosis of the umbilical cord stump [115]. Thus a reaction of 2 mm or greater during the first week of life and any reaction in older neonates should be considered significant. The CRP becomes positive within 12 hours after the onset of infection or inflammation, and the return to normal is usually complete several days after successful treatment. Therefore it is valuable in establishing an initial diagnosis of sepsis as well as for evaluating the efficacy of treatment. The CRP is maximally elevated with *E. coli* infections and correlates best of several parameters with impending relapse. It is also noted to be as reliable as the CSF culture for following the remission or relapse in *E. coli* meningitis, where it is more consistent than the CSF cell count, protein or glucose, and the peripheral blood leukocyte count. In meningitis caused by *H. influenzae,* the CRP is as reliable as the CSF culture, pleocytosis, and protein elevation for following the clinical course [129]. For these reasons, the recent introduction of a rapid, semi-quantitative agglutination method and the quantitative "rocket" (EIQ) technique for measuring CRP are of interest and should prove to have great value as aids in the rapid evaluation of the newborn for possible sepsis.

Another acute phase reactant, the erythrocyte sedimentation rate (ESR), is dependent on fibrinogen levels and is known to be elevated in collagen diseases, cancer, tissue necrosis, and infection. Recent clinical studies using a modified mini-ESR method have defined the normal values in neonates. During the first day of life the ESR is 1 mm/hr or less. From 3 to 14 days of age, this value gradually rises to a maximum of 17 mm/hr. This probably reflects improved liver function and fibrinogen formation. In most septic neonates, the ESR is elevated within 24 hours of the onset of sepsis and is not influenced by antibiotics. With remission there is a slow return to normal. Patients with DIC give falsely low values, while false-positive results are obtained in infants with Coombs-positive hemolytic disease. Significantly, the ESR is not elevated in uncomplicated hyaline membrane disease [1].

The leukocyte count is normally elevated in the newborn and there is a marked lymphocytosis. Peripheral blood leukocyte counts are significantly lower in premature infants and those who are small for gestational age [103]. Therefore the total leukocyte count is not a reliable indication of sepsis in the neonate. The absolute band count, however, is significantly increased beyond the normal range in newborns with proven bacterial infection, even when leukocyte counts are within normal limits [2].

Another indication of phagocytosis of bacteria in the blood is the NBT test. The ability of neutrophils to reduce the nitroblue tetrazolium dye to formazan is dependent on the stimulation of the hexosemonophosphate (HMP) shunt. This occurs after the ingestion of particulate matter, e.g., bacteria, but not with pinocytosis of fluid or viruses [117]. In normal adults, the level of NBT positive cells is usually below 10%, and both the percentage and absolute number of NBT positive cells increase with bacteremia [48]. In term newborns, NBT reduction, oxygen consumption, and HMP activity are significantly elevated [89, 118]. These values return to resting adult levels after the fourth week of life [69]. In premature infants, the absolute NBT count is significantly depressed, although the percentages of NBT positive cells and HMP shunt activity are similar to those found in term infants [69]. Several studies have shown that these values change with infection. However, these changes are not consistent and there is significant overlap with normal newborn values [9, 31, 79, 94]. Serial evaluation of the NBT test in the infected neonate might be useful in evaluating response to therapy.

Unfortunately, there is no one best laboratory test to select initially for the diagnosis of bacterial sepsis. Although each of the above laboratory procedures has its own usefulness and reliability, the most reasonable approach to the neonate with possible sepsis appears to be the concurrent evaluation of several parameters. Serial evaluation of the patient also offers the best method for following improvements and relapses, especially if baseline values are available.

Neonatal Infections with E. coli, Group B Streptococcus, and S. aureus

E. coli is the predominant gram-negative organism causing sepsis in the newborn and is the most common cause of neonatal purulent meningitis. Even with the current advances in antibiotic therapy and ancillary medical support, the combined mortality and morbidity of E. coli sepsis remains high [125]. The most likely time of acquiring this organism is at parturition, since bacterial organisms do not usually cross the placental barrier. Approximately 50% of all women harbor K_1 antigen positive E. coli at delivery, as demonstrated by rectal culture. Two-thirds of their offspring have subsequent colonization by the same strain. Another source is probably nosocomial, since the same intestinal colonization rate is probably true of the population in general.

The Neonatal Meningitis Cooperative Study has reported that 38% of all cases of meningitis in the newborn are caused by E. coli [88]. Of the 100 possible K antigens associated with E. coli, K_1 is responsible for nearly 85% of neonatal E. coli meningitis and 43% of neonatal E. coli sepsis. The K_1 antigen therefore is associated with virulence, especially in the newborn infant. Recent studies have demonstrated that the prognosis in E. coli meningitis is directly related to the amount of K_1 antigen in the CSF and the length of time that it is detectable [105]. Similar correlations have been shown for prognosis in H. influenzae and Neisseria meningiditis meningitis. The exact mechanism by which K_1 antigen predisposes to meningitis is not known; however, it is of interest that this antigen is immunochemically identical to the group B polysaccharide of N. meningiditis [125]. Since IgM does not cross the placenta, opsonization of E. coli is dependent on complement activation by properdin and factor XII [53, 54].

Group B beta-hemolytic *Streptococcus* (GBS) was demonstrated to cause 31% of meningitis by the Neonatal Meningitis Cooperative Study [88]. Recently, it has become the major cause of purulent meningitis in some neonatal centers and is responsible for up to 70% of neonatal meningitis [141]. The infection is acquired by the ascending route: 2 to 33% asymptomatic vaginal carrier rates have been reported [10, 14, 19, 43, 57]. Isolation of the organism from the male urethra indicates that there is a venereal mode of transmission [57]. Infant colonization rates vary from 1.2 to 37% and, in a recent study, up to 60% of infants from carrier mothers were colonized with maternal serotypes within the first week of life [10]. The actual disease attack rate was significantly lower, ranging from 0.5 to 2% with a mortality rate of 1 per 1,000 [87, 124].

Clinically, there are two distinct presentations of GBS infections in the neonate. The first has an acute onset of disease within the first few days of life, characterized by increasing respiratory distress and fulminant pneumonia. Infants predominantly have low birth weights and are characterized by a high incidence of maternal obstetric complications, particularly premature labor and prolonged rupture of fetal membranes [14]. The course deteriorates rapidly with mortality rates between 58 and 100% [13, 57]. Maternal colonization with serotypically identical organisms is found in up to 75% of the cases. Infection with type B_{Ia} organisms has the worst prognosis, with up to 100% mortality reported [57]. Since the organism is acquired from the vaginal vault in the perinatal period, the serotype of the infecting organism should correspond with the local carrier rates. In studies where B_I infection predominates, 48.9% of mothers had group B_I organisms on culture [57]. These infants usually present with fulminant pneumonia. In other infections, where mothers harbor predominantly group B_{III} organisms, those infants with early onset of disease have a high incidence of group B_{III} organisms, and meningitis constitutes a significant part of the clinical course [13, 14, 15].

The second presentation is characterized by infants with late onset of symptoms and is seldom associated with maternal obstetric complications. These patients have a purulent leptomeningitis and show B_{III} organisms almost exclusively on culture. The clinical course is much less progressive and the mortality rate is significantly lower. The maternal colonization rate is low (about 25%), and the possibility of nosocomial acquisition must be considered [57].

A recent study evaluated host defenses against group B streptococci [97]. Protection to group B_{Ia} organisms correlates with three factors: (1) a B_{Ia} plasma factor, (2) phagocytic capacity, and (3) type-specific agglutinins. Most newborn infants are deficient in all three of these components, and these deficiencies correlate with the poor prognosis with B_{Ia} infections. Group B_{Ia} organisms have extremely long fimbriae projecting from their surfaces, and it is postulated that these fimbriae interfere with phagocytosis. The heat-labile B_{Ia} plasma factor (not associated with the complement system) enhances neutrophil phagocytosis by interacting with these fimbriae.

Normal neutrophils rarely have the capacity to phagocytose group B_{Ia} organisms. In contrast, more than 85% of maternal and cord blood neutrophils have good phagocytic ability toward other types of group B streptococci. When maternal neutrophils can phagocytose B_{Ia} organisms, this ability is conferred to the fetus. The third factor correlating with protection is a type-specific agglutinin. Agglutinins for group B_{III} and B_{Ia} have been detected in maternal serum; however, the type B_{III} agglutinins do not cross the placenta.

S. aureus is another important epidemic cause of neonatal infection. It is ubiquitous and is the first organism to colonize the skin of the normal newborn. Pyogenic skin infections are commonly caused by staphylococci, although pneumonia and osteomyelitis also occur. The umbilicus is an important reservoir and omphalitis can seed organisms to the liver with resultant hepatic abscesses. Before the introduction of penicillin, *S. aureus* was the predominant neonatal pathogen. The capsule and cell wall, as well as certain extracellular protein products, are responsible for virulence. These products include: coagulase; hemolysin, which causes tissue necrosis; leukocidin, which damages leukocytes and inhibits phagocytosis; and catalase, which destroys the peroxide needed for intracellular killing. In addition, protein A and aggressin significantly interfere with the initiation of the inflammatory response.

Efficient opsonization of *S. aureus* requires both antibody and complement, since there is no activation of the alternate pathway [136]. Type-specific antibody does cross the placenta and can provide some protection during the first months of life. *S. aureus,* however, has a factor, protein A, that causes nonspecific aggregation of IgG [56] and IgM [75] by interaction with the Fc portion of the molecule. Protein A is widely distributed among coagulase-positive strains of *S. aureus* [52] and can be secreted into the surrounding microenvironment. A correlation has been shown between protein A concentration and resistance of that strain of *S. aureus* to phagocytosis [38]. By combining with the immunoglobulin Fc portion, this area is no longer available to interact with membrane receptors of neutrophils and macrophages and thus could decrease phagocytosis. In addition, the Fc portion of the molecule might not be able to activate complement due to steric hindrance of the Cl_q binding site in the same region. In fact, it has been demonstrated that low concentrations of protein A inactivate the classic complement pathway [55].

Aggressin is another cell wall mucopeptide associated with the virulence of *S. aureus* [84]. It inhibits the migration of neutrophils toward a chemotactic stimulus and markedly inhibits early edema formation. Treatment of this factor with lysozyme destroys the lesion-potentiating and edema-inhibiting effects, but the capacity to inhibit chemotaxis is unaffected or even enhanced [135]. This antichemotactic factor apparently interacts directly with the neutrophil, since it cannot be removed by washing and does not directly neutralize the chemotactic generating factors. The effects of aggressin are not due to cytotoxicity since 90% of the neutrophils remain viable by excluding trypan blue dye when it is present. The mechanism of the anti-inflammatory property of this factor has recently been investigated. From the time sequence of interaction and the use of bioassays, it was determined that both histamine and kinin action are in some way affected, although there is no direct antagonism. It has been hypothesized that activation of Hageman factor may be inhibited [41].

Treatment and Prognosis

Once the potentially septic neonate has been identified, appropriate laboratory tests drawn, and adequate cultures taken, antibiotics should be initiated. Currently, the combination of ampicillin with an aminoglycoside to which *E. coli* is sensitive seems to be the best clinical approach. If *S. aureus* is suspected, a penicillinase-resistant penicillin should be instituted. Because of decreased renal excretion during the first weeks of life, dosages must be modified to minimize toxic side effects. Several excellent sources may be consulted for specific recommendations [64, 104].

It is the practice in our neonatal unit to monitor coagulation in debilitated premature neonates by serial prothrombin time (PT) and partial thromboplastin time (PTT) evaluation. If the PTT is prolonged beyond 100 to 120 sec, cryoprecipitate or fresh frozen plasma is administered to correct this coagulation defect. The administration of fresh frozen plasma has potentially many other important effects on neonatal defense mechanisms. Factor XII or Hageman factor is given at the full adult level, and since levels of this critical initiator of inflammation are significantly depressed in septic neonates, this could be of substantial benefit. Properdin, factor B, and complement components C3, and C5 are likewise depressed in premature infants, and these are also present in both cryoprecipitate and fresh frozen plasma. Finally, since IgM does not cross the placenta, these important opsonins for gram-negative organisms are also provided.

The deficiency of specific plasma factors and antibody could also be corrected if the donor of the fresh frozen plasma were previously immunized against important pathogens. Thus in *E. coli* septicemia and meningitis, not only would the broad spectrum of IgM and alternate pathway components be provided, but it would be possible to administer specific K_1 antibody. In animal studies, specific antibody to this capsular polysaccharide protected mice from lethal infections [105].

The possible use of immunotherapy to alter the course of group B *Streptococcus* infections is even more promising. Since the ability to phagocytose GBS is comparable in the mother and the fetus, it seems reasonable to evaluate these functions prenatally in the population at risk. Mothers with prolonged rupture of the fetal membranes, who are delivering before the 37th week of gestation, should be cultured for GBS. Newer culture techniques [46] allow rapid recognition of group B organisms. If these organisms are found, serotyping should follow. Recently developed immunofluorescent techniques allow GBS identification directly on the swab specimen [126]. Evaluation of maternal phagocytosis and specific plasma factors could then proceed. If the mother is deficient in phagocytosis, the amniotic fluid and tracheal aspirate should also be cultured. Specific B_{Ia} plasma factor as well as type-specific agglutinins could be administered to the neonate at risk in fresh frozen plasma as a prophylactic modality or could be used at the first sign of respiratory distress. If type B_{III} organisms are identified, the proper antibodies could be provided in an attempt to prevent or treat the meningitis. Recently, Lancefield, McCarty, and Everly have shown that antibody to either the type-specific polysaccharide or the protein antigens can afford protection to infection in an animal model [100]. It is theoretically possible to predict the efficacy of serotherapy using maternal neutrophils and specific bacterial suspension in vitro before the infant has been delivered.

Breast-feeding also provides specific and nonspecific factors to the neonate. Breast milk per se is high in lactose and low in protein, phosphate, and residual bulk. It has less buffering capacity and a higher pH than cow's milk. This difference in pH and buffering capacity seems to be directly responsible for the high lactobacillus count in stools of breast-fed infants and may selectively inhibit E. coli from growing in the digestive tract [23, 78]. In addition, there is higher resistance to gastroenteritis and respiratory infections. Where breast- versus bottle-feeding has been compared in underdeveloped areas, a significantly decreased neonatal mortality has been observed with the former [65]. It is of interest that whereas some of the beneficial effects of breast milk can be achieved by correcting the pH of bottled milk, many of the protective effects of breast milk are abrogated by boiling.

The immunologic properties of breast milk and colostrum were not well appreciated until recently and now appear to be substantial. Colostrum has a higher content of IgA than serum [68]. Another factor found in human, animal, and soy milk preparations has some of the functional activities of C5 [59]. Although this C5-like factor could reconstitute opsonic activity in C5 deficient sera, it is not functional in hemolytic assays [59]. In addition, breast milk has a lysozyme that cleaves bacterial cell peptidoglycans and is found in concentrations 3,000 times greater than in cow's milk [27].

Cells are also present in colostrum. Total cell counts range from 1,600 to 2,400 cells per milliliter. These cells are predominantly macrophages (85%) and lymphocytes (13%). Approximately 35% of the lymphocytes are T cells, as measured by E rosette formation. B cells average 35% and half show IgA by membrane fluorescence [37]. In an animal model, the macrophages are effective in in vitro killing assays against Klebsiella. Although freezing destroys this ability, it can be reconstituted by adding peritoneal cells [119]. It is of interest that Klebsiella is present in significantly higher numbers of infants with necrotizing enterocolitis than in normal neonates

[58]. The presence of macrophages, lysozyme, and antibody may be an important part of the protective effect to necrotizing enterocolitis attributed to breast milk.

The specific protective function of colostrum was demonstrated by Goldblum et al. [71] in an in vitro assay. Lactating women were fed a strain of *E. coli* that was not present in their gastrointestinal tract and produced IgA antibodies specific against that strain. These antibodies were synthesized in vitro by breast milk lymphocytes within 1 week of ingestion of the bacteria by the donor. There was no concurrent elevation of serum antibody titers so a generalized bacteremia was unlikely. It was postulated that cells sensitized in the gastrointestinal tract migrate to the mammary glands, where specific IgA is produced [71]. This locally produced IgA has a direct protective effect on the gastrointestinal tract. It is therefore conceivable that specific breast milk antibody could be provided to infants at risk from *E. coli* or *Klebsiella* by feeding antigens from these strains beforehand to lactating breast milk donors. This may provide the local mucosal protection necessary to prevent both gastroenteritis and necrotizing enterocolitis with the transmural invasion of hydrogen-gas producing organisms.

Several animal studies have shown other immunologic properties of breast milk. In the immunologically deficient pituitary dwarf mouse, Duquesnoy, Kalpaktsoglou, and Good demonstrated a protective effect by nursing. In these Snell-Bagg dwarf mice, severe lymphopenia and death normally occur soon after weaning. This was prevented by prolonged nursing. Histologically, the lymphoid tissue of nursed mice had increased cellularity, particularly in the thymic dependent areas [40]. In addition to the cellular reconstitution of these T cell areas, antibody responses to sheep erythrocytes that require T cell helper function were normal. Significantly increased spleen weight compared to body weight was also consistently demonstrated, suggesting the presence of a specific lymphopoietic influence rather than better nutrition alone [39].

Specific immunologic unresponsiveness can also be transmitted to newborn mice from tolerant nursing mothers. Transfer experiments in the mothers demonstrated that the inhibition resided in the serum and could not be attributed to tolerant or suppressor cells. Tolerance was transmitted to the newborn mice through breast milk. Animals born to tolerant mothers but nursed by normal mice were responsive, while normal newborns nursed by tolerant mothers were tolerant. The authors suggested that a circulating antibody-antigen complex might be responsible for this tolerogenic effect [11]. This transmission of specific unresponsiveness must be evaluated in newborns of infected mothers, where transmission of infection is likely.

Beyond Koch's Postulates

It now appears clear that although certain microorganisms are crucial to the development of specific infections, there are equally important underlying factors that predispose the host to infectious diseases. Despite Koch's postulates, it has long been apparent that most healthy individuals do not develop tuberculosis even when exposed to patients with this disease over a period of many years. The protective influence of "good health" has, in modern terminology, been transliterated as "intact host responses." The latter would include all the mechanisms discussed in this review as well as many others that have not been mentioned. Perhaps the most striking recent example of infection-prone persons has been that of patients with primary immunodeficiency disorders. Within this group of patients, infectious diseases, such as vaccina gangrenosa, candidiasis, *P. carinii* pneumonitis, and bacterial sepsis have been rampant. Now we must nurture a new level of consciousness in the physician dealing with infectious diseases, for it appears that even among apparently healthy persons, there exists a spectrum of rather individualistic immune responses to a variety of, and perhaps all, infectious agents that is dependent on the inheritance of immune response genes. These genes appear to be located primarily, if not entirely, on chromosome 6 in man. They cannot truly be called abnormal, since we each have our own share of these immune response genes that render us somewhat less adequate in combating a specific infectious agent than other individuals in the general population. Genes controlling at least four of the complement components are also located in this chromosome area.

Evidence is rapidly accumulating which suggests that persons with HLA-D w2, for example, are especially prone to the slow virus effects of measles virus. Similar evidence suggests that persons carrying HLA-B 27 develop various types of arthritis (i.e., ankylosing spondylitis, Reiter's disease, and juvenile rheumatoid arthritis) and that this arthritic problem may follow infections with *Shigella, Salmonella,* or *Yersinia,* but only (or primarily) in persons who carry a specific gene; this gene appears to be similar to or identical with B27. Perhaps the most striking demonstration of these interrelated factors is the report of Calin and Fries [26], recounting a celebration banquet aboard a U.S. naval cruiser in which two infected cooks apparently transmitted shigellosis to 602 of the 1,276 men. Of these, nine developed Reiter's disease. In followup histocompatibility typing studies of five of these men with Reiter's disease, all but one were B27 and the fifth one was HLA-7. Other histocompatibility studies indicate that B27 and B7 are linked with Dw1 and Dw2, respectively [63]. Recent reports of a genetic propensity for juvenile diabetes mellitus associated with HLA-D w3 and the observation of virus particles in the pancreas of diabetic animal models further suggests that diabetic patients do not handle a particular infectious agent as effectively as the rest of the general population. These observations would also explain the inconsistent hereditary pattern of this disease. Many other examples of this orientation to infectious disease are appearing.

One must conclude that it is no longer compatible with modern concepts of infectious disease to simply identify and eradicate a specific organism in an infected patient. We must be ready to examine the relation between the patient and that organism more closely if the infection proves difficult to eradicate or if it recurs. We should further begin to ask ourselves why only certain infants develop severe or fatal infections with *E. coli, S. aureus,* or beta-hemolytic *Streptococcus.* Obviously, many neonates come into contact with these organisms, yet only a few develop clinical problems. Rather than set our priorities on the development of a larger armamentarium of antibiotic agents, perhaps we should be analyzing more closely the host mechanisms that prevent the infections we have discussed from developing in healthy neonates.

References

1. Adler, S. M., and Denton, R. L. The erythrocyte sedimentation rate in the newborn period. *J. Pediatr.* 86:942, 1975.
2. Akenzua, G. I., et al. Neutrophil and band counts in the diagnosis of neonate infections. *Pediatrics* 54:38, 1974.
3. Alford, C. A. Immunoglobulin determinations in the diagnosis of fetal infection. *Pediatr. Clin. North Am.* 18:99, 1971.
4. Alford, C. A., et al. A correlative immunologic, microbiologic and clinical approach to the diagnosis of acute and chronic infections in newborn infants. *N. Engl. J. Med.* 277:437, 1967.
5. Alper, C. A., et al. Increased susceptibility to infection associated with abnormalities of complement-mediated functions and of the third component of complement (C_3). *N. Engl. J. Med.* 282:349, 1970.
6. Alper, C. A., Block, K. J., and Rosen, F. S. Increased susceptibility to infection in a patient with type II essential hypercatabolism of C_3. *N. Engl. J. Med.* 288:601, 1973.
7. Alper, C. A., et al. Homozygous deficiency of C_3 in a patient with repeated infections. *Lancet* II:1179, 1972.
8. Alper, C. A., and Rosen, F. S. Increased susceptibility to infection in patients with defects affecting C_3. In D. Bergsma, et al. (Eds.), *Immunodeficiencies in Man and Animals.* Birth Defects: Original Article Series, No. XI. Sunderland, Mass.: Sinauer Associates, 1975.
9. Anderson, D. C., Pickering, L. K., and Feigin, R. D. Leukocyte function in normal and infected neonates. *J. Pediatr.* 85:420, 1974.
10. Anthony, B. F., Okada, D., and Hobel, C. J. Group B streptococci (GBS) in perinatal infections: Natural history of maternal and neonatal colonization. *Pediatr. Res.* 9:296, 1975.
11. Auerback, R., and Clark, S. Immunological tolerance: Transmission from mother to offspring. *Science* 189:811, 1975.
12. August, C. S., et al. Onset of lymphocyte function in the developing human fetus. *Pediatr. Res.* 5:539, 1971.
13. Baker, C. J., et al. Suppurative meningitis due to streptococci of Lancefield group B: A study of 33 infants. *J. Pediatr.* 82:724, 1973.
14. Baker, C. J., and Barrett, F. F. Transmission of group B streptococci among parturient women and their neonates. *J. Pediatr.* 83:919, 1973.
15. Baker, C. J., and Barrett, F. F. Group B streptococcal infection in infants. The importance of the various serotypes. *J.A.M.A.* 230:1158, 1974.
16. Ballow, M., et al. Complete absence of the third component of complement in man. *J. Clin. Invest.* 56:703, 1975.

17. Belohradsky, B. H., et al. Meeting report of the second international workshop on primary immunodeficiency diseases in man. *Clin. Immunol. Immunopathol.* 2:281, 1974.
18. Berg, T. Immunoglobulin levels in infants with low birth weight. *Acta Paediatr. Scand.* 57:369, 1968.
19. Bevanger, L. Carrier rate of group B streptococci with relevance to neonatal infections. *Infection* 2:123, 1974.
20. Bisberg, D. S., Schidlow, D. V., and Dweck, H. S. Prolonged rupture of membranes (PROM): Value of laboratory studies in assessment of infection. *Pediatr. Res.* 9:338, 1975.
21. Blaese, R. M. Macrophages and the development of immunocompetence. *Pediatr. Res.* 7:363, 1973.
22. Blanc, W. A. Pathways of fetal and early neonatal infection. *J. Pediatr.* 59:473, 1961.
23. Bullen, C. L., and Willis, A. T. Resistance of the breast-fed infant to gastroenteritis. *Br. Med. J.* 3:338, 1971.
24. Bullock, J. D., et al. Inflammatory response in the neonate re-examined. *Pediatrics* 44:58, 1969.
25. Butler, N. R., Barr, M., and Glenny, A. T. Immunization of young babies against diphtheria. *Br. Med. J.* 1:476, 1954.
26. Calin, A., and Fries, J. F. Epidemic Reiter's syndrome, genetics and environment. *Arthritis Rheum.* 18:390, 1975.
27. Chandan, R. C., Shahani, K. M., and Holly, R. G. Lysozyme content of human milk. *Nature* 204:76, 1964.
28. Chandra, R. K. T lymphocytes and cell-mediated immunity (CMI) in low birth weight (LBW) infants. *Pediatr. Res.* 9:328, 1975.
29. Chang, T. W., Weinstein, L., and MacMahon, H. E. Paralytic poliomyelitis in a child with hypogammaglobulinemia: Probable implication of type 1 vaccine strain. *Pediatrics* 37:630, 1966.
30. Cocchi, P., and Marianelli, L. Phagocytosis and intracellular killing of *Pseudomonas aeruginosa* in premature infants. *Helv. Paediatr. Acta* 1:110, 1967.
31. Cocchi, P., Mori, S., and Betcattini, A. N.B.T. tests in premature infants. *Lancet* II:1426, 1969.
32. Coen, R., Grush, O., and Kauder, E. Studies of bactericidal activity and metabolism of the leukocyte in full-term neonates. *J. Pediatr.* 75:400, 1969.
33. Colman, R. W. Formation of human plasma kinin. *N. Engl. J. Med.* 291:509, 1974.
34. Corrigan, J. J., Sell, E. J., and Pagel, C. Level of coagulation factor XII in sick newborns. *Pediatr. Res.* 7:354, 1973.
35. Curnutte, J. T., Kipnes, R. S., and Babior, B. M. Defect in pyridine nucleotide dependent superoxide production by a particulate fraction from granulocytes of patients with chronic granulomatous disease. *N. Engl. J. Med.* 293:628, 1975.
36. Day, N. K., et al. C_{1r} deficiency: An inborn error associated with cutaneous and renal disease. *J. Clin. Invest.* 51:1102, 1972.
37. Diaz-Jouanen, E., and Williams, R. C. T and B lymphocytes in human colostrum. *Clin. Immunol. Immunopathol.* 3:248, 1974.
38. Dossett, J. H., et al. Antiphagocytic effects of staphylococcal protein A. *J. Immunol.* 103:1405, 1969.
39. Duquesnoy, R. J., and Good, R. A. Prevention of immunologic deficiency in pituitary dwarf mice by prolonged nursing. *J. Immunol.* 104:1553, 1970.
40. Duquesnoy, R. J., Kalpaktsoglou, P. K., and Good, R. A. Immunological

studies of the Snell-Bagg pituitary dwarf mouse. *Proc. Soc. Exp. Biol. Med.* 133:201, 1970.

41. Easmon, C. S. F., Hamilton, I., and Glynn, A. A. Mode of action of A staphylococcal anti-inflammatory factor. *Br. J. Exp. Pathol.* 54:638, 1973.

42. Eickhoff, T. C., et al. Neonatal sepsis and other infections due to group B beta-hemolytic streptococci. *N. Engl. J. Med.* 271:1221, 1964.

43. Eidelman, A. I., and Szilagi, G. Group B beta strep (GBS) colonization of mothers and infants. *Pediatr. Res.* 9:296, 1975.

44. Eife, R., et al. Dissociated lymphocyte function in newborn infants. *Pediatr. Res.* 8:412, 1974.

45. Eitzman, D. V., and Smith, R. T. The nonspecific inflammatory cycle in the neonatal infant. *Am. J. Dis. Child.* 97:326, 1959.

46. Fallon, R. J. The rapid recognition of Lancefield group B haemolytic streptococci. *J. Clin. Pathol.* 27:902, 1974.

47. Fearon, D. T., et al. Activation of the properdin pathway of complement in patients with gram-negative bacteremia. *N. Engl. J. Med.* 292:937, 1975.

48. Feigin, R. D., et al. Nitroblue tetrazolium dye test as an aid in the differential diagnosis of febrile disorders. *J. Pediatr.* 78:230, 1971.

49. Felix, N. S., Nakajima, H., and Kagan, B. M. Serum C-reactive protein in infections during the first six months of life. *Pediatrics* 37:270, 1966.

50. Fireman, P., Zuchowski, D. A., and Taylor, P. M. Development of human complement system. *J. Immunol.* 103:25, 1969.

51. Forman, M. L., and Stiehm, E. R. Impaired opsonic activity but normal phagocytosis in low-birth-weight infants. *N. Engl. J. Med.* 281:926, 1969.

52. Forsgren, A. Significance of protein A production by staphylococci. *Infect. Immun.* 2:672, 1970.

53. Forsgren, A., and Quie, P. G. Influence of the alternate complement pathway on opsonization of several bacterial species. *Infect. Immun.* 10:402, 1974.

54. Forsgren, A., and Quie, P. G. Opsonic activity of human serum chelated with ethylene glycoltetra-acetic acid. *Immunology* 26:1251, 1974.

55. Forsgren, A., and Quie, P. G. Effects of staphylococcal protein A on heat labile opsonins. *J. Immunol.* 112:1177, 1974.

56. Forsgren, A., and Sjöquist, J. "Protein A" from *S. aureus.* I. Pseudo-immune reaction with human γ globulin. *J. Immunol.* 97:822, 1966.

57. Francoisi, R. A., Knostman, J. D., and Zimmerman, R. A. Group B streptococcal neonatal and infant infections. *J. Pediatr.* 82:707, 1973.

58. Frantz, I. D., et al. Necrotizing enterocolitis. *J. Pediatr.* 86:259, 1975.

59. Ganges, R. G., and Miller, M. E. Studies on the fifth component of complement (C_5) comparison of hemolytic and opsonic activity in bovine milk and human plasma. *Pediatr. Res.* 9:329, 1975.

60. Gatti, R. A., and Seligmann, M. The primary immunodeficiency diseases: Classification, pathogenesis, and treatment. *Turk. J. Pediatr.* 15:195, 1973.

61. Gatti, R. A., et al. Combined system immunodeficiency with DiGeorge syndrome and dissociation of PHA/MLC responses. *Adv. Exp. Med. Biol.* 29:327, 1972.

62. Gatti, R. A., et al. Hereditary lymphopenic agammaglobulinemia associated with a distinctive form of short-limbed dwarfism and ectodermal dysplasia. *J. Pediatr.* 75:675, 1969.

63. Gatti, R. A. Unpublished data, 1975.

64. Gellis, S. S., and Kagan, B. M. *Current Pediatric Therapy* (6th ed.). Philadelphia: Saunders, 1973.

65. Gerrard, J. W. Breast feeding: Second thoughts. *Pediatrics* 54:757, 1974.

66. Giblett, E. R., et al. Adenosine-deaminase deficiency in two patients with severely impaired cellular immunity. *Lancet* II:1067, 1972.

67. Gitlin, D., and Craig, J. M.   The thymus and other lymphoid tissues in congenital agammaglobulinemia. I. Thymic alymphoplasia and lymphocyte hypoplasia and their relation to infection. *Pediatrics* 32:517, 1963.

68. Gitlin, J. D., and Gitlin, D.   The selective transport of maternal plasma proteins across the mammary gland. *Pediatr. Res.* 8:413, 1974.

69. Goel, K. M., and Vowels, M. R.   Leukocyte function in normal and pre-term infants. *Acta Paediatr. Scand.* 63:122, 1974.

70. Goldberg, B., Siegel, N. J., and Campbell, A. G. M.   Risk of neonatal sepsis following rupture of membranes (ROM). *Pediatr. Res.* 7:402, 1973.

71. Goldblum, R. M., et al.   Antibody production by human colostrum cells. *Pediatr. Res.* 9:330, 1975.

72. Gotoff, S. P., and Behrman, R. E.   Neonatal septicemia. *J. Pediatr.* 76:142, 1970.

73. Graber, C. D., et al.   Changing patterns of neonatal susceptibility to *Hemophilus influenzae*. *J. Pediatr.* 78:948, 1971.

74. Graham, C. W., et al.   Deficient serum opsonic activity for macrophage function in newborn infants. *Proc. Soc. Exp. Biol. Med.* 143:991, 1973.

75. Grov, A.   Human IgM interacting with staphylococcal protein A. *Acta Pathol. Microbiol. Scand.* [C] 83:173, 1975.

76. Hardy, B., Globerson, A., and Danon, D.   Ontogenic development of the reactivity of macrophages to antigenic stimulation. *Cell. Immunol.* 9:282, 1973.

77. Harris, M. B., and Root, R. K.   Metabolic and functional defects in neonatal granulocytes (PMN). *Pediatr. Res.* 8:413, 1974.

78. Harrison, V. C., and Peat, G.   Significance of milk pH in newborn infants. *Br. Med. J.* 4:515, 1972.

79. Hartley, P. S., Malan, A. F., and Heese, H. de V.   The histochemical nitroblue tetrazolium reduction test in newborn infants. *S. Afr. Med. J.* 49:1263, 1975.

80. Hathaway, W. E.   The bleeding newborn. *Semin. Hematol.* 12:175, 1975.

81. Hill, H. R., and Quie, P. G.   Raised serum-IgE levels and defective neutrophil chemotaxis in three children with eczema and recurrent bacterial infections. *Lancet* I: 183, 1974.

82. Hill, H. R., et al.   Defects in neutrophil granulocyte chemotaxis in Job's syndrome of recurrent "cold" staphylococcal abscesses. *Lancet* II:617, 1974.

83. Hill, H. R., et al.   Impaired leukotactic responsiveness in patients with juvenile diabetes mellitus. *Clin. Immunol. Immunopathol.* 2:395, 1974.

84. Hill, M. J.   A staphylococcal aggressin. *J. Med. Microbiol.* 1:33, 1968.

85. Hitzig, W. H., Kay, H. E. M., and Cottier, H.   Familial lymphopenia and agammaglobulinemia. An attempt at treatment by implantation of foetal thymus. *Lancet* II:151, 1965.

86. Hobbs, J. R., and Davis, J. A.   Serum γG-globulin levels and gestational age in premature babies. *Lancet* I:757, 1967.

87. Horn, K. A., et al.   Group B streptococcal neonatal infection. *J.A.M.A.* 230: 1165, 1974.

88. Howard, J. B., and McCracken, G. H.   The spectrum of group B streptococcal infections in infancy. *Am. J. Dis. Child.* 128:815, 1974.

89. Humbert, J. R., Kurtz, M. L., and Hathaway, W. E.   Increased reduction of nitroblue tetrazolium by neutrophil of newborn infants. *J. Pediatr.* 45:125, 1970.

90. Iwaszko-Krawczuk, W.   Stimulating effect of C-reactive protein on phagocytosis in the newborn. *Acta Paediatr. Acad. Sci. Hung.* 15:115, 1974.

91. Jacobs, J. C., and Miller, M. E.   Fatal familial Leiner's disease: A deficiency of opsonic activity of serum complement. *Pediatrics* 49:225, 1972.

92. Jemelin, M., et al. Impaired phagocytosis in leukocytes from newborn infants. *Enzyme* 12:642, 1971.
93. Johnston, R. B., Newman, S. L., and Struth, A. G. An abnormality of the alternate pathway of complement activation in sickle-cell disease. *N. Engl. J. Med.* 288:803, 1973.
94. Kalpaktsoglou, P. K., et al. Evaluation of nitroblue-tetrazolium test in low-birth-weight infants. *J. Pediatr.* 84:441, 1974.
95. Kay, H. E. M., Doe, J., and Hockley, A. Response of human foetal thymocytes to phytohaemagglutinin (PHA). *Immunology* 18:393, 1970.
96. Kindmark, C. O. Stimulating effect of C-reactive protein on phagocytosis of various species of pathogenic bacteria. *Clin. Exp. Immunol.* 8:941, 1971.
97. Klesius, P. H., et al. Cellular and humoral immune response to group B streptococci. *J. Pediatr.* 83:926, 1973.
98. Kohler, P. F. Maturation of the human complement system. I. Onset time and sites of fetal C_{1q}, C_4, C_3 and C_5 synthesis. *J. Clin. Invest.* 52:671, 1973.
99. Kurkcuoglu, M., and McElfresh, A. E. The Hageman factor: Determinations of its concentration during the neonatal period and presentation of a case of Hageman factor deficiency. *J. Pediatr.* 57:61, 1960.
100. Lancefield, R. C., McCarty, M., and Everly, W. N. Multiple mouse-protective antibodies directed against group B streptococci. Special reference to antibodies effective against protein antigens. *J. Exp. Med.* 142:165, 1975.
101. Leikin, S., Mochir-Fatemi, F., and Park, K. Blast transformation of lymphocytes from newborn human infants. *J. Pediatr.* 72:510, 1968.
102. Lepow, M. L., et al. Effect of Sabin type I poliomyelitis vaccine administered by mouth to newborn infants. *N. Engl. J. Med.* 264:1071, 1961.
103. Martinez, G., et al. Influence of gestational age (GA) and birth weight (BW) on the white blood cell count (WBC) in the neonate. *Pediatr. Res.* 8:405, 1974.
104. McCracken, G. H., and Eichenwald, H. F. Antimicrobial therapy: Therapeutic recommendations and a review of newer drugs. Part I. Therapy of infectious conditions. *J. Pediatr.* 85:297, 1974.
105. McCracken, G. H., et al. Relationship between *Escherichia coli* K_1 capsular polysaccharide antigen and clinical outcome of neonatal meningitis. *Lancet* II:246, 1974.
106. Melmon, K. L., et al. Kinins: Possible mediators of neonatal circulatory changes in man. *J. Clin. Invest.* 47:1295, 1968.
107. Miller, M. E. Phagocytosis in the newborn infant: Humoral and cellular factors. *J. Pediatr.* 74:255, 1969.
108. Miller, M. E. Demonstration and replacement of a functional defect of the fifth component of complement in newborn serum. A major tool in the therapy of neonatal septicemia. *Pediatr. Res.* 5:379, 1971.
109. Miller, M. E. Chemotactic function in the human neonate: Humoral and cellular aspects. *Pediatr. Res.* 5:487, 1971.
110. Miller, M. E. Functional activity of the fifth component of complement (C_5) in human, animal, proprietary and soy milks. Therapeutic and biological implications. *Pediatr. Res.* 8:415, 1974.
111. Miller, M. E., and Myers, K. Decreased membrane deformability of neonatal leukocytes and its relationship to neutrophil movement. *Pediatr. Res.* 8:406, 1974.
112. Miller, M. E., and Nilsson, U. R. A familial deficiency of the phagocytosis-enhancing activity of serum related to a dysfunction of the fifth component of complement (C_5). *N. Engl. J. Med.* 282:354, 1970.
113. Miller, M. E., Oski, F. A., and Harris, M. B. Lazy leukocyte syndrome. A new disorder of neutrophil function. *Lancet* 1:665, 1971.

114. Naeye, R. L., Dellinger, W. S., and Blank, W. A.   Fetal and maternal features of antenatal bacterial infections. *J. Pediatr.* 79:733, 1971.
115. Nemir, R. L., Roberts, P. H., and Barry-LeDeaux, S.   Observations of anti-streptolysin-O, C-reactive protein and electrophoretic protein patterns in maternal and neonatal sera. *J. Pediatr.* 51:493, 1957.
116. Papadatos, C., et al.   Immunoglobulin levels and gestational age. *Biol. Neonate* 14:365, 1969.
117. Park, B. H., Fikrig, S. M., and Smithwick, E. M.   Infection and nitroblue-tetrazolium reduction by neutrophils, a diagnostic aid. *Lancet* II:532, 1968.
118. Park, B. H., Holmes, B., and Good, R. A.   Metabolic activities in leukocytes of newborn infants. *J. Pediatr.* 76:237, 1970.
119. Pitt, J., et al.   Macrophages and the protective action of breast milk in necrotizing enterocolitis. *Pediatr. Res.* 8:384, 1974.
120. Pole, J. R. G., and McAllister, T. A.   Gastric aspirate analysis in the newborn. *Acta Paediatr. Scand.* 64:109, 1975.
121. Prindull, G.   Maturation of cellular and humoral immunity during human embryonic development. *Acta Paediatr. Scand.* 63:607, 1974.
122. Propp, R. P., and Alper, C. A. C_3 synthesis in the human fetus and lack of transplacental passage. *Science* 162:672, 1968.
123. Provenzano, R. W., Wetterlow, L. H., and Sullivan, C. L.   Immunization and antibody response in the newborn infant. I. Pertussis inoculation within twenty-four hours of birth. *N. Engl. J. Med.* 273:959, 1965.
124. Reid, T. M. S.   Emergence of group B streptococci in obstetric and perinatal infections. *Br. Med. J.* 2:533, 1975.
125. Robbins, J. B., et al.   *Escherichia coli* K_1 capsular polysaccharide associated with neonatal meningitis. *N. Engl. J. Med.* 290:1216, 1974.
126. Romero, R., and Wilkinson, H. W.   Identification of group B streptococci by immunofluorescence staining. *Appl. Microbiol.* 28:199, 1974.
127. Rosenfeld, S. I., and Leddy, J. P.   Hereditary deficiency of fifth component of complement (C_5) in man. *J. Clin. Invest.* 53:67a, 1974.
128. Rosenthal, A. S., Lipsky, P. E., and Shevach, E. M.   Macrophage-lymphocyte interaction and antigen recognition. *Fed. Proc.* 34:1743, 1975.
129. Sabel, K. G., and Hanson, L. A.   The clinical usefulness of C-reactive protein (CRP) determinations in bacterial meningitis and septicemia in infancy. *Acta Paediatr. Scand.* 63:381, 1974.
130. Stossel, T. P., Alper, C. A., and Rosen, F. S.   Opsonic activity in the newborn: Role of properdin. *Pediatrics* 52:134, 1973.
131. Unanue, E. R., and Calderon, J.   Evaluation of the role of macrophages in immune induction. *Fed. Proc.* 34:1737, 1975.
132. Van Scoy, R. E., et al.   Familial neutrophil chemotaxis defect, recurrent bacterial infections, mucocutaneous candidiasis and hyperimmunoglobulinemia E. *Ann. Intern. Med.* 82:766, 1975.
133. Vasan, U., et al.   The origin of gastric polymorphonuclear leukocytes. *Pediatr. Res.* 9:346, 1975.
134. Verhaart, W. J. C.   Polio-encephalopathy or masked encephalitis in familial hypogammaglobulinaemia. *J. Neuropathol. Exp. Neurol.* 20:380, 1961.
135. Weksler, B. B., and Hill, M. J.   Inhibition of leukocyte migration by a staphylococcal factor. *J. Bacteriol.* 98:1030, 1969.
136. Wheat, L. J., Humphreys, D. W., and White, A.   Opsonization of staphylococci by normal human sera: The role of antibody and heat-labile factors. *J. Lab. Clin. Med.* 83:73, 1974.
137. Whisnant, J. K., et al.   Prolonged CNS viral infection with ECHO-30 in an agammaglobulinemic child with intact cell-mediated immunity. *Pediatr. Res.* 9:336, 1975.

138. White, H. H., et al. Subacute encephalitis and congenital hypogammaglobu-linemia. *Arch. Neurol.* 26:359, 1972.
139. Wright, W. C., et al. Impaired antibacterial activity of leukocytes of sick newborns. *Pediatr. Res.* 7:380, 1973.
140. Xanthou, M., et al. Phagocytosis and killing ability of *Candida albicans* by blood leukocytes of healthy term and pre-term babies. *Arch. Dis. Child.* 50:72, 1975.
141. Yow, M. D. Epidemiology of group B streptococcal infections, 1975. In S. Krugman, and A. A. Gershon (Eds.), *Progress in Clinical and Biological Research,* Vol. 3. New York: Alan R. Liss, 1975.

8. Infections in Children with Congenital Defects in Host Defense Mechanisms

Vincent A. Fulginiti

The hallmark of most immunodeficient states is susceptibility to infection. Manifest as clinical disease or colonization by unusual organisms, such susceptibility is predicated on the specific immune dysfunctions. For most congenital defects in host defense mechanisms, a clearly defined spectrum of infectious susceptibility has been described. Such susceptibility is potential; clinical expression is dependent on exposure to the organism(s) and lack of preventive or therapeutic interference.

This chapter deals with the specific infectious susceptibility associated with each of a variety of congenital defects in host immune mechanisms. Factors in the genesis of potential susceptibility and means of prevention are also discussed.

Throughout this chapter, standardized nomenclature will be used as suggested by an expert committee of the World Health Organization [19]. Major categories of immunodeficiencies will be discussed in terms of overall infectious susceptibility. Deviations from the general pattern for specific defects will be indicated when they occur. The major defects to be discussed are (1) antibody immunodeficiency, (2) cellular immunodeficiency, (3) combined immunodeficiency, (4) phagocytic immunodeficiency, and (5) complement immunodeficiency.

Antibody Immunodeficiency: Specific Infectious Susceptibility

The Infectious Agents
The most frequently encountered infectious agents in children with antibody immunodeficiency are bacteria [7, 12, 14, 21, 25]. Varying in onset, severity, and extent among specific types of antibody immunodeficiencies, bacterial infections account overwhelmingly for clinical disease in these infants and children. A few viruses, a parasite, and a presumed protozoan have also caused infections on occasion.

The most frequently encountered bacteria are the pyogenic cocci and *Hemophilus influenzae.* Occasionally, enteric bacilli, particularly *Pseudomonas aeruginosa,* are encountered. Most infections are due to *Diplococcus pneumoniae,* the pneumococcus. Second in importance is *H. influenzae.* Occasionally streptococci produce clinical infections. Curiously, staphylococci and other gram-positive cocci are not encountered. With the employment of antimicrobial agents, gram-negative bacilli become more prominent, particularly *Pseudomonas* species.

Types of Infection

Infections due to bacteria are generally of five types: (1) severe, systemic infections, (2) respiratory tract infections, (3) skin infections, (4) infectious conjunctivitis, and (5) gastrointestinal infections.

Severe, systemic infection usually takes the form of bacteremia or bacterial meningitis. As many as 10 to 15 separate episodes of these severe infections have been recorded prior to diagnosis and treatment of the underlying immunodeficiency. On occasion a single episode may be lethal, but more often recovery follows institution of appropriate antibacterial therapy. Individual episodes do not differ from those occurring in healthy children; it is the recurrence and repetitiveness that are unique.

Infections of the respiratory tract include otitis media, sinusitis, chronic tracheobronchitis, pneumonia, lung abscess, and bronchiectasis. Otitis media is common in infancy and early childhood; repetitive single episodes evolve into chronic otitis media. The initial infectious agents are the pneumococci and *H. influenzae;* with the use of antimicrobial agents, *Pseudomonas* species become predominant.

Chronicity characterizes the pulmonary infections. Isolated, repetitive episodes of pneumonia are superseded by chronic tracheobronchial and pulmonary disease. Chronic cough, sputum production, and reduced pulmonary function form the background in later childhood and adolescence. Pulmonary abscesses and bronchiectasis produce persistent disability and diminishing pulmonary reserves. There is considerable variation among individuals and among types of antibody immunodeficiency in the rate of progression of pulmonary disease. Most patients with sex-linked, recessive antibody immunodeficiency will develop some degree of chronic pulmonary infection, usually the life-limiting factor in this congenital defect. Less severe forms of congenital antibody immunodeficiency may be associated with little or no pulmonary disability.

Skin infections may be present early in life or develop as a late manifestation, probably related to individual hygienic and epidemiologic factors. Many of these infections are identical to pyoderma and impetigo encountered in healthy children. A few unusual chronic skin infections have been described, including eczematous forms and verrucous disease, which may be viral.

Conjunctivitis is a common early manifestation of antibody immunodeficiency, usually caused by the pneumococci. Profuse, purulent discharge is present. Therapy is effective but the lesion recurs in a repetitive fashion. For some patients, conjunctivitis is the major early hallmark of their disease; diminished gamma globulin effect is heralded by the appearance of conjunctivitis.

Gastrointestinal disease, usually in the form of chronic diarrhea or malabsorptive syndromes, occurs frequently [16]. Only rarely is a specific bacterial etiology identified. It is unclear whether this type of disease is related to susceptibility to members of the normal flora or due to another infectious agent such as *Giardia lamblia.* A third possible explanation is a coinherited defect in disaccharidase deficiency. Present information does not permit separation of these potential causes. The diarrhea can be severe, but most often it is mild or moderate.

In general, viral disease is not unusual in patients with antibody immunodeficiency [21, 25]. Measles, varicella, smallpox vaccination, and the common respiratory and enteric viruses all produce diseases that do not differ significantly from those observed among healthy children. In a few instances polio virus (wild or vaccine-type) results in paralytic disease, and hepatitis virus may cause severe liver disease [25]. There is no explanation for the occurrence of these viral diseases in light of current immunologic knowledge.

In patients with isolated, deficient IgM synthesis, generalized vaccinia has been described [8]. This is not the progressive form of vaccinia infection; rather, repeated crops of vaccinia vesicles develop after primary vaccination with ultimate healing (in 1 month). The primary lesion is slightly more severe than normal and heals slowly over a 3-month period.

Verrucous lesions of the skin have been described in several congenital antibody deficiencies [47]. Insufficient data are available to implicate viruses.

G. lamblia, an intestinal parasite, has been implicated in a malabsorptive syndrome that is associated with antibody immunodeficiency [41]. It does not appear to be different from disease observed among healthy individuals and it is responsive to appropriate therapy.

A few instances of infection with *Pneumocystis carinii,* a presumed protozoan, have been described in individuals with antibody immunodeficiency [44]. Most often this parasite produces pulmonary disease in patients with cell-mediated immune deficient states. *Pneumocystis* causes an interstitial pneumonia that results in an interference in oxygen transport. It is a progressive disease that is lethal if untreated. Pentamidine isethionate and trimethoprim-sulfa have been effectively utilized in treatment and have resulted in cures.

Onset and Course of Infections

Congenital defects in antibody function generally are not manifest by infection until 5 to 6 months of age or later [7, 12, 14, 21, 25]. Transplacental transmission of maternal IgG appears to protect the young infant. Sex-linked, recessive antibody deficiency is usually manifest in the second half of the first year of life, when antibody is degraded. Occasionally, onset may be delayed until 4 to 5 years of age in less severe congenital antibody deficiencies. Some adolescents and adults have been described with presumably congenital defects in antibody synthesis, whose disease was not manifest until much later in life.

Any type of infection may occur first, but otitis media, conjunctivitis, and bacteremia are most common. The first evidence of disease can also be the appearance of diarrhea. Most often, the initial episodes do not suggest immunodeficiency and are responsive to antimicrobial therapy. Only with repetitive episodes is the condition recognized and diagnosis established.

The course of infections in congenital antibody deficiency states varies with the degree and specificity of the defect. Also, administration of passive antibody can alter the natural course. In severe deficiencies, infection is the most persistent and important clinical event. In milder deficiencies, infection may be infrequent. Thus further discussion of the factors operative in these varying courses is presented.

The prognosis of infections in antibody deficiency is dependent on the specific defect present. In severe defects, any of the systemic infections can be lethal. However, with recognition of the defect and the employment of immunologic therapy, the major problem becomes the persistent and progressive topical infections of the respiratory tract. Thus pulmonary function can be gradually and progressively reduced. Death occurs in pulmonary failure in adolescence or young adulthood. In less severe antibody immunodeficiency, a relatively normal life span is predictable, punctuated with episodes of infection or complicated by persistent, chronic respiratory disease, such as otitis media or sinusitis.

Immunologic Factors in Infectious Susceptibility Secondary to Antibody Deficiency

Current theory explains antibody function on the basis of a configurational match between a limited, but extensive, array of immunoglobulin molecules and certain antigens [26]. Thus diphtheria toxin is "matched" by a variety of immunoglobulin molecules that fit a portion of its structure. These immunoglobulin molecules, in the aggregate, are measured by their ability to interact with diphtheria toxin and are labeled *antitoxin,* or antibody to diphtheria toxin.

Absence of antibody synthesizing capacity will result in susceptibility to those agents that are completely inactivated by antibody. If the immunoglobulin-antibody system is solely responsible for limitation, inactivation, and elimination of the infectious agent, then recovery cannot occur in its absence. Even if other factors provide ancillary assistance in immunity, susceptibility will still occur if antibody is the principal mode of defense. Pneumococci can be captured and destroyed by phagocytes, but in the absence of antibody this modality can only function at a primitive and inefficient level. Interaction with specific antibody is necessary for effective removal of pneumococci by phagocytic cells. The interaction between specific antibody and the infectious agent can act as a primer for a variety of immune functions. Inability to interact either fails to trigger these functions or only permits minimal expression. Phagocytic cells, complement, the kinin system, properdin, and other nonspecific immune mechanisms fail to function effectively in the absence of the specific antibody-antigen complexes.

A separate problem is encountered in the topical immune system. Interaction between specific secretory IgA and infectious agents is believed to be the major line of defense at the mucosal level [48]. However, inability to synthesize secretory IgA limits the individual's ability to respond to certain agents. Pneumococci produce uncontrolled local disease in the absence of local immune mechanisms, principally IgA. In congenital deficiencies of antibody synthesis, the ability to manufacture secretory IgA permits such uncontrolled infections [7, 12, 14, 21, 25]. This defect is further accentuated by the inability to substitute IgG or IgM into the secretions produced by the infection, since these molecules are not being synthesized by the individual. These defects lead to chronic, local infections with agents against which antibody is the principal mode of defense. Antimicrobial therapy can only exert a partial controlling effect, since the underlying immunodeficiency remains present. Penicillin can kill pneumococci in the respiratory tract but other organisms will fill the void, since no effective local immune control is present.

Prevention of Infection in Antibody Deficiencies
The most effective preventive measure available is the administration of passive antibody [14, 25, 46]. Either pooled adult gamma globulin or plasma from individual donors is used [46]. Administration of passive antibody converts the individual from an antibody-deficient host into one who behaves as if he had already experienced contact with the infectious agents. Preformed antibody from adults with diverse infectious experience provides systemic protection against agents that are responsive to immunoglobulin-antibody defense. Early recognition, specific diagnosis, and appropriate passive antibody administration results in relative freedom from severe, systemic bacterial infections. Not all episodes are prevented in every individual, but the frequency is greatly diminished, and for some persons complete freedom results. No effective therapy is available to replace local antibody (secretory IgA) and susceptibility remains to these forms of infection occurring in the respiratory and, perhaps, the gastrointestinal tracts [48]. Antimicrobial therapy alone, administered prior to actual infection, does not provide adequate protection. Contact with some infectious agents is avoided by this means of prevention (e.g., pneumococci by penicillin) but are replaced by others as the basic, underlying defect persists.

Isolation measures are unnecessary and impractical [46]. The indigenous flora are acquired early in life, usually during the period of transplacental antibody protection. Members of this flora include those agents to which the individual is subsequently susceptible, i.e., the pneumococci and *H. influenzae*. At the age of diagnosis (usually after 6 months of age) contact with the organisms and colonization has already occurred. In addition, the organisms are ubiquitous; most children and some adults harbor pneumococci and *H. influenzae* in their respiratory tracts. Isolation would mean unreasonable restriction from most human contact; and since there is no permanent immunologic replacement possible now or in the foreseeable future, such restriction is unwarranted.

Cellular Immunodeficiency (Cell-Mediated Immune Deficiency): Specific Infectious Susceptibility

This section will include only those congenital conditions in which cell-mediated immune (CMI) function is absent, but in which antibody capacity is wholly or partially intact. Conditions included are thymic hypoplasia (Di George's syndrome), autosomal recessive immunodeficiency with lymphopenia (Nezelof's syndrome), and isolated disorders affecting only the CMI function [1].

The Infecting Agents

Children with congenital defects in CMI function but intact immunoglobulin antibody synthesis are susceptible to a wide variety of infectious agents [15, 20, 21, 27, 29, 40]. Fungal, many viral, protozoal, and bacterial infections are all encountered.

Oral candidiasis due to *Candida albicans* is the most frequent fungal infection. Occurring early in life, the candidal infection tends to be refractory to antifungal therapy [21]. Often it is the only infection apparent for months or years. There is such variability among patients with congenital CMI defects that generalizations should be made, and taken, with caution. Some individuals have been described with an isolated CMI defect to *Candida;* otherwise they appear fully capable of mounting an effective CMI response against other agents and antigens [9].

Rarely, other fungi may produce disease among these children. In southwestern United States, individuals with an inability to mount a CMI response to *Coccidiodes immitis* may develop disseminated disease on contact with this agent. *Cryptococcus neoformans* and *Histoplasma capsulatum* have the potential to produce severe infections in patients with congenital defects in CMI function.

Viral infections of unusual character or severity have been noted. Persistent, recurrent varicella, measles of unusual severity, and progressive vaccinia following smallpox vaccination have all occurred in this group of children [15, 20, 22, 27, 29, 40]. Cytomegalovirus pneumonia and persistent respiratory infections caused by parainfluenza and respiratory syncytial viruses have also been described [20, 21, 27].

P. carinii, a presumed protozoan, produces a severe, progressive interstitial pneumonia [20, 27, 44]. This infection will be discussed more fully in the section, Combined Immunodeficiency.

Bacterial infections have also been encountered. In contrast to those associated with antibody deficiencies, *P. aeruginosa* and other gram-negative bacilli have been predominant [20, 40].

Onset of Infections
There is a great deal of variability in the age at which congenital defects in CMI become clinically apparent [15, 20, 21, 27, 29, 40]. Patients with thymic hypoplasia may become infected in the newborn period or shortly thereafter [15, 29]. Patients with the autosomal recessive condition associated with lymphopenia (Nezelof's syndrome) may not develop significant infections until 4 or 5 years of age [20, 40]. Few instances of each of these varieties of isolated CMI defect have been described, thereby limiting the validity of generalizations. Those that have been described have been sufficiently variable to warrant caution in predicting the onset and course of the infections.

In general, the infections encountered in this group of patients have been less severe than those seen in association with combined immunodeficiency. Individual infections have been just as severe or even lethal. Overall, the course of infection has been slower with fewer complications. For example, in a series of patients with progressive vaccinia, complicating combined immunodeficiency, none survived. In a series of patients with progressive vaccinia, complicating cellular immunodeficiency with intact antibody synthesis, three patients were "cured" of their progressive vaccinia [22]. The progressive vaccinia lesions were fewer and less extensive in the children with defects solely in CMI function.

The prognosis in this group of defects is dependent on the specific defect and its degree. Among children with thymic hypoplasia, the defect in CMI has proved to be extremely variable. Predictions as to outcome are speculative at best. Further complicating prognostic predictions are as follows: (1) The first of these defects was recognized in 1964; thus long-range observations among the survivors are limited. (2) Attempts at reconstitution of immunologic function have been made, some of which have been successful, but the period of observation afterwards is too short to allow prediction. Some reconstitution attempts have resulted in the occurrence of graft-versus-host disease, thereby obscuring the natural history of the disease [22].

*Immunologic Factors in Infectious Susceptibility of Children with
Congenital Cellular Immunodeficiency*
Most of the organisms encountered in infections among this group of children are opportunistic. Normal control of these organisms is vested in an intact cell-mediated immune (CMI) system [9, 22, 24]. This system is dependent on the presence of T lymphocytes, an intact thymus, and interaction between the two, probably occurring in fetal life. The lymphocytes that result from this immunologic development are capable of responding to certain antigens and becoming "sensitized." They are then capable of interacting directly with the infectious agent or indirectly with cells of the body that are infected with that agent. The usual result of this interaction is a limitation of replication of the infectious agent such that recovery from the acute infection occurs and permanent immunity results. Absence of

lymphocytes capable of responding in this interaction and/or defects in thymic development or function result in an inability to mount an effective CMI response. This inability, in turn, allows the infectious agents to multiply without restriction or with limited control. The clinical counterpart of this deficiency is unusual, prolonged, severe, or recurrent infections.

Prevention of Infections in Children with Cellular Immunodeficiency

The most effective way to prevent infections in children with cellular immunodeficiency is for them to avoid contact with the infectious agents. However, since most of these organisms are abundant in nature and are frequently found in healthy, asymptomatic human carriers, avoidance is difficult if not impossible. The only certain way to isolate a patient is by means of the various devices that reduce environmental contamination in the immediate vicinity of the patient. Before such measures are contemplated, certain factors must be considered and weighed. These factors include: (1) the chances for ultimate benefit accruing to the patient, (2) the impact on the patient's physical and mental well-being, (3) the efficiency of the method to be used, and (4) an estimate of the cost, inconvenience, necessity for special procedures, trained personnel, etc., in relation to the other factors. Full consideration of these factors and of the currently available methods will be given in the section, Prevention of Infections in Combined Immunodeficiency.

Administration of gamma globulin or plasma offers little to some of these patients because they are capable of immunoglobulin synthesis. However, many of these individuals have dysglobulinemia; they produce immunoglobulins, even in normal quantities, but have little or no antibody function. Because of this disparity between globulin production and antibody function, passive antibody may afford a degree of protection against some infectious agents (see the section Antibody Immunodeficiency).

Antimicrobials, including antifungal and antiviral agents, have no place in preventive therapy. Their employment prior to infection can only result in selection of the more resistant opportunists from among the indigenous flora and extrinsic agents. Drugs useful against *P. carinii* should only be employed with the diagnosis of infection by this agent. All the antimicrobials effective against viruses, fungi, and protozoa are associated with significant toxicity. These two factors, selection of resistant opportunists and intrinsic drug toxicity, prevent the consideration of their use prophylactically.

Combined Immunodeficiency: Specific Infectious Susceptibility

The Infectious Agents and Types of Infections

The variants of combined immunodeficiency are associated with the most severe infectious susceptibility [22, 27, 29]. Since both antibody and CMI functions are absent, or greatly reduced, these patients are susceptible to most pathogens and to many opportunists. Bacteria, viruses, fungi, protozoa, and parasites have all been responsible for significant infections in this group of children.

Bacterial infections include those caused by the major pathogens and also by organisms of relatively low virulence (in healthy persons). Pyogenic bacteria are seldom encountered, which is possibly related to two factors: the umbrella protection of maternal antibody and the early use of antimicrobial agents. These patients have such a severe immunologic defect that they become infected early in life, frequently in the first weeks after birth. At this time, circulating IgG of maternal origin protects them from the common pyogenic bacteria. Also, many of the infections they experience are accompanied by signs and symptoms of bacterial sepsis, whether or not bacteria are involved etiologically. As a result, potent antimicrobial therapy is employed, further reducing the incidence of pyogenic bacterial infections. The bacteria most frequently encountered are *P. aeruginosa,* other members of the *Pseudomonas* family, and a variety of opportunistic gram-negative bacilli, such as *Serratia marcescens, Enterobacter* species, etc.

Immunization with live, attenuated tuberculosis vaccine, BCG (bacille Calmette-Guerin), has resulted in a progressive, fatal infection in more than 12 children with definite, or presumed, combined immunodeficiency [28, 37].

Fungal infections are very common; the most frequent is oral candidiasis. Thrush is a hallmark of CMI defects. In these children it develops very early in life, is extensive, and is resistant to therapy. Extension from the mouth is common with *Candida esophagitis,* and gastrointestinal tract infection is frequent. The organism frequently invades the respiratory tract and, not uncommonly, is involved in pneumonia of mixed etiology. Invasion of the bloodstream occurs, with candidemia resulting in widespread dissemination; *Candida* meningitis, renal disease, osteomyelitis, and other organ infections follow. *C. albicans* is ubiquitous and has produced disease in these children throughout the world. Other species of *Candida* are occasionally involved. Other fungi are more restricted in their distribution but still remain potential pathogens for children with combined immunodeficiency. *C. immitis, H. capsulatum, C. neoformans,* and others are capable of producing significant disease.

Unusual, severe, complicated, or prolonged infections with a variety of viruses have been described in these children. Lethal, disseminated measles with Hecht's giant-cell pneumonia has occurred. Prolonged or complicated varicella has been reported. A necrotizing pneumonia, caused by adenoviruses, can be lethal in these children. Cytomegalovirus pneumonia is frequent and represents a severe threat in these children. Prolonged infection with parainfluenza and respiratory syncytial viruses occurs, in contrast to the briefer illnesses seen in immunologically healthy children. Progressive vaccinia occurs invariably following primary smallpox vaccination [22]. Implantation of vaccinia virus in the skin results in unrestricted multiplication. A slowly progressive primary lesion occurs that enlarges inexorably, leaving a necrotic center. The virus enters the bloodstream and viremic lesions occur at distant sites, each behaving like the primary vaccination. Multiple organ invasion is common. The disease may follow a prolonged and slowly progressive course, stretching over weeks or months. Bacterial superinfection of local lesions is common and may give rise to bacteremia.

Polioviruses may also produce extensive CNS infection and paralysis. A few instances of polio, arising from attenuated vaccine administration, have occurred [45]. Not uncommonly, viruses are involved in the multiple-causation pneumonias encountered in these children.

Onset and Course of the Infections in Combined Immunodeficiency

In contrast to most other immunodeficiencies, children with combined immunodeficiency experience infections very early in life. Oral candidiasis is common within the first few days or weeks of life and persists thereafter, often spreading to the rest of the gastrointestinal tract and systemically. Bacteremia is common early in life. Usually, pneumonia becomes evident in the first few months of life; in individual patients it may be impossible to identify the specific etiologic agents causing the pneumonia. Frequently, pneumonia is produced by the first of the many opportunists that the patient encounters. It may then progress as that single etiologic disease, or it may be complicated by the addition of one or more infectious agents, which contribute to the pneumonic process. In one of our patients, vaccinia virus, cytomegalovirus, and C. albicans were all isolated from the lung [22]. Histologic examination demonstrated evidence for active infection by each agent.

Usually, the first weeks or months of life are characterized by the continual presence of a significant infection. Additional disease is added as the initial one is treated, resulting in a pattern of severe infectious disease, constantly present and worsening with age. Pneumonia, almost always present, is seldom fulminant, often extending across weeks or even months. Despite antimicrobial therapy, the variety of infectious agents and the persistence of the severe immunologic defect results in continual illness and ultimate death, usually prior to the second year of life. The only alterations in this pattern are observed with various forms of immunologic reconstitution. A few patients have had complete restoration of immunologic function with disappearance of the infectious susceptibility. Many more have had partial, or temporary, reconstitution, leaving them with partial or complete susceptibility. A few have developed graft-versus-host disease, which apart from the pathologic effects of that process, has made the patients even more susceptible to infection. In most patients, reconstitution has failed, and the disease has followed its expected course.

Prevention of Infection in Combined Immunodeficiency

There are no effective means of avoiding the multiple opportunistic and pathogenic agents to which these infants are exposed, unless one resorts to isolation techniques with stringent safeguards. As discussed earlier, certain factors should be considered and weighed before institution of an isolation program: ultimate benefit and risk to the patient, efficiency and expectations of the method, and cost, effort, and requirements of employing the method in relation to the other factors [31]. A brief discussion of each of these factors is warranted here.

Before strict isolation is undertaken, the major question to be answered is the probability of reversal of the defect. If there is a reasonable chance that immunologic reconstitution can be afforded the patient in the future, then one can consider protective isolation. If the chances are nonexistent or slim, embarking on a protective isolation program may result in the difficult decision later to abandon it. This is a difficult decision because the child may appear, and be, healthy, and a variety of emotional contacts develop between parents and child and health workers and child. To then decide that isolation has no beneficial end, and to discontinue it, means that the child will be subject to the infectious susceptibilities associated with the underlying combined immunodeficiency. To retain the isolation in the face of inadequate or absent means of immunologic reconstitution means prolongation of an abnormal life in a sealed environment with no fixed plan for removal.

If attempts at immunologic reconstitution are possible, then the next assessment must be of the risks of isolation-confinement to the patient. Most of the effective methods employed include total lack of skin-to-skin physical contact between the patient and the caretakers. One of the potential risks involved is physical malnutrition, unless strict attention is given to adequate intake of calories, protein, vitamins, and other nutriments. This risk is easily overcome but requires recognition of the patient as a growing, developing individual, requiring constant reappraisal of nutritional needs. The effects of indirect feeding, with no human skin-to-skin contact, is more difficult to assess. There is an abundance of evidence that mothering is an important phenomenon in the physical, as well as emotional, well-being of young infants [18]. The ultimate effect of deprivation of maternal contact cannot be assessed with accuracy; inference from other human experience indicates that growth failure may occur, despite seemingly adequate nutrition. Emotional deprivation is even more difficult to assess. We have little experience with infants and children confined to a separate environment in which they can see, but not touch (without rubber gloves or some such device), their caretakers. One can anticipate severe emotional disturbances in an individual who is thus confined for a prolonged period of time. Such disturbance can possibly be minimized if the period of confinement is relatively short. However, most efforts at immunologic reconstitution require long periods of time for diagnosis, search for compatible donors, and observation of postreconstitution for evidence of successful immunologic function. Counterbalancing these physical and psychological risks is the knowledge that without isolation, the patient undertakes a substantial, and inevitable, risk to health and life. Most physicians and investigators, indeed most parents, in Western society have decided, in specific instances, that the risk ratio was overbalanced in favor of the isolation-reconstitution approach.

The availability and operation of an efficient system of isolation is critical to the success of the effort [4, 5, 36, 42, 49]. No isolation attempt should be undertaken by a team or institution unfamiliar with the prolonged, stringent requirements. Obviously, unavailability of equipment, personnel, or commitment to such a program should rule against its initiation. In the latter instances, arrangements could be made with an institution and team capable of undertaking the appropriate program. Under no circumstances should a decision be made to substitute an inferior approach if a better one is accessible for the patient.

The fourth factor to be considered is really one of feasibility. Given a positive approach to isolation in relation to all the above factors, the responsible parties must decide in advance the feasibility of undertaking the project and seeing it to its conclusion. Also, complete commitment should be assured the family if the project is undertaken at all. If circumstances indicate that such an undertaking cannot be sustained, it should not be begun, even if all the factors have been considered and the decision to undertake isolation is favorable. Alternatives should be sought and, if not available, the project abandoned rather than initiated, only to be aborted in the future.

The actual means of isolation are varied [4, 5, 36, 42, 49]. Data supporting their effectiveness are few, because experience with patients of such high susceptibility is limited. Under ideal circumstances, presumptive diagnosis is sought prior to delivery. Based on familial occurrence and occasionally supported by intrauterine sex determination (for sex-linked conditions) and enzyme evaluation (for some forms of combined immunodeficiencies), the diagnosis of combined immunodeficiency may be suspected. Delivery is arranged with cooperating obstetricians in the same institution, where the isolation facilities exist. With advance planning, cesarean section can be performed under as sterile conditions as possible. The infant is handled by a trained team that utilizes sterile techniques, instruments, and linens. Transfer to the protected environment is as rapid as the infants' condition and medical care needs permit. From that point on, protective isolation is maintained until the infant is released from quarantine.

The ideal circumstances, as described above, may not be achievable. For each necessary variation, the effectiveness of protective isolation can be correspondingly compromised. It may not be possible to identify the infant in advance; and diagnosis may only be established by recognition of the infectious pattern after birth. Protective isolation may be instituted at the point the diagnosis is suspected or confirmed, but the child and his or her organisms enter the unit together. Further contact with pathogens or opportunists may be avoided, or minimized, but those already present may be sufficient to produce significant infections, even lethal ones. Also, it may not be possible to perform a cesarean section, and vaginal delivery exposes the infant to a limited but definite array of microorganisms of potential pathogenicity. Immediate protective confinement reduces, or eliminates, further contact with microorganisms but leaves the infant with some of potential pathogenicity.

Other alterations from the ideal will similarly be met by some infectious risk to the patient. The best guidelines to follow are to employ protective isolation techniques as soon as the disease is recognized and to decide whether to follow the isolation-reconstitution approach.

There are several techniques for protective isolation. However, details as to their operation are beyond the scope of this report. The reader is referred to appropriate references. A brief description of each method follows:

1. "Reverse" isolation: The most primitive and, presumably, the least efficient method of isolation. The patient is placed in a separate environment with sterile clothing and bedding. Entry into the patient's environment is limited to those who need to minister to him or her. Each is gowned in sterile overclothing, wears a cap and mask, and dons sterile gloves. Refinements of this technique include separate ventilation for the patient's area and sterilization, to the extent feasible, of all instruments, equipment, and even food entering the patient's area.

2. The laminar-flow environment: Depending on the size of the patient, equipment can vary from a small cubicle to an entire room. The principle employed is that continuous, directed airflow moving over the patient and exiting into a filtering system, which recirculates again past the patient, prevents microorganisms from gaining entry into the patient's environment. Filtration of the recirculated air removes particulate antigens, even viruses. The constant organized laminar airflow provides a physical restraint to air entry; such environmental air from the area surrounding the laminar-flow environment contains microorganisms. There are several variants to this technique, but all depend on the above principle.

   Entry to the patient's environment is avoided by devices that permit care through a flexible wall, containing means of handling the patient and the equipment. Gloved plastic sleeves projecting into the laminar flow room, allow access to the patient.

   All equipment, food, and supplies can be sterilized before introducing them into the patient's environment.

3. The life-island concept: A variety of devices that completely enclose the patient in a controlled environment. By means of filtration and impermeable barriers, the internal environment of such devices can be made germ-free, or nearly germ-free. A large amount of animal experimentation has established the protective efficacy of such devices, and recent human experience also indicates that long-term residence in such units is possible and effective, even for infants.

There are variations on these themes, but these three main types of protective isolation constitute the available means of preventing contact between a susceptible patient and environmental microorganisms.

Gamma globulin should be administered to all individuals with combined immunodeficiency who are not provided a protective isolation environment. These individuals are antibody-deficient, and significant protection against infections with certain microorganisms can be provided by administration of gamma globulin (see the section Prevention of Infection in Antibody Deficiency).

Prophylactic use of antimicrobial agents is ineffective. Employment of such therapy, on occasion, will result in enhancement of the risk of growth of opportunistic organisms and subsequent infections. However, immunologic reconstitution, when feasible, provides corrective therapy for the basic defect. Hence the best prevention is to restore immunologic capacity.

Phagocytic Immunodeficiency: Specific Infectious Susceptibility

This category includes congenital neutropenias as well as a variety of congenital conditions that are characterized by inefficient leukocyte function, despite adequate numbers. Although varying somewhat in the specific nature of the infectious susceptibility observed, there are some basic similarities. This section deals largely with the classic syndrome of phagocytic immunodeficiency, chronic granulomatous disease [43]. This disorder is a sex-linked recessive condition associated with a metabolic defect in the polymorphonuclear leukocyte, the neutrophil. The defect appears to limit the cells' ability to manufacture hydrogen peroxide, an essential element in the bactericidal capacity of the neutrophil. The specific infectious susceptibilities observed clinically are a direct result of this defect.

The Infecting Agents and Types of Infection in Phagocytic Immunodeficiency

The principal organisms observed in infections among children with phagocytic immunodeficiency are *Staphylococcus aureus, Staphylococcus epidermidis, Serratia marcescens, Escherichia coli, Pseudomonas* species, *Proteus* species, *Enterobacter* species, *Salmonella* species, *Candida* species, and *Aspergillus* species [3, 6, 43]. These organisms are most frequently encountered, especially the staphylococci, but as additional instances are reported less commonly observed organisms are added to the list.

Infections of the skin, bone, lung, and lymph nodes predominate [3, 6, 43]. Conjunctivitis, stomatitis, rhinitis, perianal abscesses, and diarrhea also occur with moderate frequency. Unexplained fever or bacteremia punctuate the course of other infections.

The skin infections are characteristically eczematoid and range from superficial to deep, interlaced abscesses. The lesions are indolent; histologically they consist of purulent exudate surrounded by a granulomatous reaction. Regional lymphadenopathy with eventual suppuration is characteristic.

Osteomyelitis is common, often occurring early in life [50]. The lesion differs from osteomyelitis observed in otherwise healthy children in that it is low-grade and often confined in extent and slow in progression. Small bones of the distal extremities are most frequently involved. A granulomatous tissue reaction is also noted here and may be responsible for the peculiar clinical nature of the lesion.

Rhinitis is common and is purulent. Pneumonia is a major manifestation occurring in almost all patients. The disease may be lobar or bronchial in distribution. Ordinarily, the pneumonia is associated with moderate to severe systemic and pulmonary symptoms. Unlike pneumonia occurring in otherwise healthy children, the disease in these patients is persistent despite antimicrobial therapy. Slow resolution over weeks is characteristic. Often the roentgenologic picture is indistinguishable from that observed in other types of pneumonia. On occasion, discrete consolidation, the so-called encapsulated pneumonia associated with nodular densities is observed [51]. Some investigators consider this diagnostic of granulocyte dysfunction.

Onset and Course of Infections in Phagocytic Immunodeficiency
Often the disease becomes evident early in infancy, even in the newborn period. Most often the initial infections are of the skin, although we have observed osteomyelitis as a primary lesion. Unexplained fever is common during this period of time. Or, there may be frank bacteremia, usually with the same organism observed in the skin lesions. Recurrent episodes occur with evident suppurative lymphadenitis. Pneumonia can occur at any time and is most often repetitive. In some individuals, recurrent perianal abscesses are prominent early in the disease.

The disease runs a prolonged course with major infectious episodes, often against a background of chronic skin infection and punctuated by febrile episodes. There is considerable variability in both the frequency and severity of infections. In the classic form of the disease death usually occurs in or before adolescence and is related to an untreatable infection. Antimicrobial therapy may or may not influence individual episodes. Many of the organisms are only partially inhibited by available antibiotics and, in the absence of effective phagocytosis, may resist specific therapy. Many of the skin and pulmonary episodes appear to run their course irrespective of treatment. Occasionally, therapy appears to exert a detectable response, but the variability of the disease and of the individual infectious episodes makes such judgments insecure.

Variations
Variants of chronic granulomatous disease differ in both their infectious patterns and their courses. The major differences are indicated as follows:

1. *Job's syndrome* [13]: Occurs in fair-skinned red-haired females and is characterized by recurrent "cold" staphylococcal abscesses of skin, lymph nodes, lung, liver, and abdominal cavity. Eczema, otitis media, and purulent rhinitis are also seen.

2. *Myeloperoxidase deficiency* [35]: Unusual susceptibility to *C. albicans* infections.

3. *Glucose 6-phosphate dehydrogenase deficiency* [10]: Severe infection with similar spectrum to chronic granulomatous disease.

4. *"Lazy leukocyte" syndrome* [39] (defective chemotaxis): Recurrent, severe infections associated with defective migration of leukocytes in response to chemotactic stimuli.

5. *Splenectomized or decreased splenic function* [17]: Unusual susceptibility to pneumococci and *H. influenzae* with septicemia and metastatic infections noted. Associated with inability to develop opsonizing antibody and therefore inefficient phagocytosis. Also seen in sicklemia, where "autosplenectory" results from recurrent thrombosis or splenic vesicles.

6. *Severe infections* [11]: During certain acute, severe infections phagocyte dysfunction may occur and can result in prolongation of the infection or in new infections.

7. *Chediak-Higashi syndrome* [52]: An autosomal recessive disorder with large cytoplasmic inclusions noted in the phagocytes. Associated with susceptibility to severe pyogenic infections.

8. *Miscellaneous syndromes:* Increasingly, a variety of disorders are being characterized by defective phagocytic function. All are associated with increased susceptibility to certain infectious agents but vary in their form and severity. For example, a partial defect has been described in children with moderately severe, persistent impetigo as their major manifestation.

9. *Congenital Neutropenias* [34]: Both cyclic and noncyclic forms of this condition have been described. The absence, or relative decrease, in numbers of neutrophils results in susceptibility to a wide variety of bacterial agents, including streptococci, pneumococci, and staphylococci. Severe infections of many types are observed, including skin, respiratory, bloodstream, gastrointestinal, and other infections. They tend to be severe, recurrent, and persistent. Many such infants die early in life due to their extreme susceptibility.

Immunologic Factors of Infectious Susceptibility in Phagocytic Disorders
The variability in defects does not permit a single, all-inclusive immunologic explanation for the susceptibility of these children. A discussion of the phagocytic cycle and of defects in it will help to define the variable deficiencies.

Breach of natural barriers by pathogenic bacteria results in tissue destruction that initiates a complex chemical and morphologic sequence, referred to as the inflammatory response. Phagocytes are attracted to the site of entry of microorganisms by these powerful migratory stimuli. Capillary dilatation and leakage of plasma components result in a chemical and cellular response that is inimical to bacteria. Phagocytes ingest and digest bacteria and other microorganisms encountered. This phagocyte function is enhanced by the presence of specific antibody, opsonins, complement, and possibly other factors. Poorly defined stimuli arising from the local bacterial-tissue inter-action result in mobilization of bone marrow, circulatory, and other phago-cytic reserves. Increased numbers of leukocytes become available to partici-pate in the defense against the microbial invader.

Defects in chemotaxis, specific antibody, or complement may interfere with migration or efficiency of phagocytes. These defects permit organisms to multiply locally and to invade and enter the bloodstream. Depending on the extent and nature of the defect, local infection (skin, respiratory tract) can occur or bacteremia and distant infection can supervene.

Absent or very low numbers of neutrophils permit virtually uncontrolled local multiplication and spread. The most severe and lethal infections are found among children lacking neutrophils. The phagocyte ingests bacteria and other microbes on random contact. More efficient, directed contact is afforded by organisms that have interacted with specific antibody or other opsonins. Once ingested, bacteria are destroyed as a result of the metabolic activity of the leukocyte, myeloperoxidase, hydrogen peroxide derived from the respiratory cycle, and a halogen, usually iodine, together result in "kill-ing" of the bacteria. Defects in any of these will render the leukocyte in-capable of bacterial destruction. In chronic granulomatous disease the disability is in the respiratory cycle with absent H_2O_2 production. Bacteria and fungi (viruses ?) fail to be killed, although there are some exceptions; those bacteria that inadvertently produce H_2O_2 allow the neutrophil to de-stroy them. Streptococci are seldom found in infections in patients with chronic granulomatous disease for this reason.

There are other mechanisms involved in bactericidal activity of the leuko-cyte, but these generally play a lesser role in defense. Defects in these mecha-nisms, however, will result in modest susceptibility.

Prevention of Infections in Phagocytic Immunodeficiency
A variety of methods have been applied in an attempt to alter the infectious susceptibility associated with phagocytic dysfunction. Avoidance of micro-organisms is impractical, since most are members of the indigenous flora and are ubiquitous.

Some physicians have sought a regimen of continuous antimicrobial pro-phylaxis to control infections in these children [30]. Most have met with failure. Limited success has been claimed for the administration of chlor-amphenicol [30]. The rationale for this therapy is that chloramphenicol permeates the leukocyte, in contrast to most other antibiotics that are effec-tive for the bacteria involved in this disease. Then the intracellular antimicrobial effects should supplement or replace the bactericidal capacity of the leukocyte. However, unfortunately, this regimen has met with limited success. Many of the organisms are uninfluenced by chloramphenicol; hence infections still occur.

Attempts have been made to correct or improve the basic defect, hence improving the response to bacteria and preventing infections. Agents such as methylene blue, which favorably alter the respiratory cycle in vitro, have failed to change the clinical course in vivo [32].

Recently it was discovered that sulfa drugs, and possibly the combination of trimethaprim and sulfa, enhance the respiratory cycle in phagocytes, probably by increasing the hexose monophosphate shunt activity [33]. In the laboratory this has resulted in enhanced bactericidal activity. In very preliminary results thus far in patients, some beneficial effect has been claimed. However, it is too early to judge the role and efficacy of this form of therapy.

Complement Immunodeficiencies

These are uncommon to rare disorders in which components of the complement system are either absent or functionally inadequate [2, 23]. Many are asymptomatic, and a few have symptoms unassociated with infectious susceptibility. A few disorders have been described with specific infectious susceptibility. They are briefly summarized as follows:

1. Congenital hypercatabolism of C3 [1]: One patient was described who had a lifelong susceptibility to pyogenic organisms (streptococci and meningococci) and to other bacteria (diphtheria bacillus). Restoration to normal C3 function by plasma infusion had a beneficial effect on bactericidal activity and presumably to bacterial defense.
2. Congenital C5 dysfunction [38]: Infants with susceptibility to staphylococci and gram-negative enteric bacilli manifest as severe diarrhea and bacteremia. Administration of fresh plasma and antibiotics improved the children clinically.

Summary

Congenital defects in five categories of immunodeficiencies have been described in relation to the specific infectious susceptibility conferred on the involved children. The spectrum of infectious agents, the types of infection, and current immunologic explanations for the infectious susceptibility have been presented. The means for prevention of these infections, where available, have been detailed and discussed. For more detailed consideration of infections in children with various immunodeficiencies, see Fulginiti and Kempe [21].

References

1. Alper, C. A., et al. Complement defect associated with increased susceptibility to infection. *N. Engl. J. Med.* 282:349, 1970.
2. Alper, C. A., and Rosen, F. S. Genetic aspects of the complement system. *Adv. Immunol.* 14:251, 1971.
3. Anderson, V., et al. Fatal granulomatous disease. *Acta Paediatr. Scand.* 57:110, 1968.
4. Bodey, G. P. Isolation for the compromised host. *J.A.M.A.* 233:543, 1975.
5. Bodey, G. P., and Johnston, D. Microbiological evaluation of protected environments during patient occupancy. *Appl. Microbiol.* 22:828, 1971.
6. Bridges, R. A., Berendes, H., and Good, R. A. A fatal granulomatous disease of childhood. *Am. J. Dis. Child.* 97:387, 1959.
7. Bruton, O. C. Agammaglobulinemia. *Pediatrics* 9:722, 1952.
8. Chandra, R. K., Kaveramma, B., and Soothill, J. F. Generalized, nonprogressive vaccinia associated with IgM deficiency. *Lancet* I:687, 1969.
9. Chilgren, R. A., et al. The cellular immune defect in chronic mucocutaneous candidiasis. *Lancet* I:1286, 1969.
10. Cooper, M. R., et al. Complete deficiency of leucocyte glucose-6-phosphate dehydrogenase with defective bactericidal activity. *J. Clin. Invest.* 51:769, 1972.
11. Copeland, J. L., et al. Bactericidal activity of polymorphonuclear leucocytes from patients with severe bactericidal infections. *Tex. Rep. Biol. Med.* 29:555, 1971.
12. Davis, S. D., et al. The congenital agammaglobulinemia. *Pediatrics* 47:927, 1971.
13. Davis, S. D., Schaller, J., and Wedgwood, R. J. Job's syndrome recurrent, "cold" staphylococcal abscesses. *Lancet* I:1013, 1966.
14. Davis, S. D., Schaller, J., and Wedgwood, R. J. Antibody deficiency syndromes, in B. M. Kagan, and E. R. Stiehm (Eds.), *Immunologic Incompetence.* Chicago: Year Book Medical Publishers, 1971.
15. DiGeorge, A. M. Congenital absence of the thymus and its immunologic consequences: Concurrence with congenital hypoparathyroidism. In D. Bergsma, and R. A. Good (Eds.), *Immunologic Deficiency Diseases in Man.* Baltimore: Williams & Wilkins, 1968.
16. Dubois, R. S., et al. Disaccharidose deficiency in children with immunologic defects. *J. Pediatr.* 76:377, 1970.
17. Ellis, E. F., and Smith, R. T. Role of spleen in immunity. *Pediatrics* 37:111, 1966.
18. Fischoff, J., Whitten, C. F., and Pettit, M. A. A psychiatric study of mothers of infants with growth failure secondary to maternal deprivation, *J. Pediatr.* 79:209, 1971.
19. Fudenberg, H. D., et al. Primary immunodeficiencies. Report of a World Health Organization Committee. *Pediatrics* 47:927, 1971.
20. Fulginiti, V. A., et al. Dissociation of delayed-hypersensitivity and antibody-synthesizing capacities in man. *Lancet* II:5, 1966.
21. Fulginiti, V. A., and Kempe, C. H. The implications of specific infectious susceptibility in immune deficiency syndromes. In *Immunopathology: Sixth International Symposium.* Basel/Stuttgart: Schwabe, 1970.
22. Fulginiti, V. A., et al. Progressive vaccinia in immunologically deficient individuals. In D. Bergsma, and R. A. Good (Eds.), *Immunologic Deficiency Diseases in Man.* Baltimore: Williams & Wilkins, 1968.
23. Gewurz, H., et al. Complement-deficient biological function in complement deficiency in man. *Lancet* II:356, 1966.

24. Glasgow, L. A. Cellular immunity in host resistance to viral infections. *Arch. Intern. Med.* (Chicago) 126:125, 1970.
25. Good, R. A., et al. Immunological deficiency diseases. *Prog. Allergy* 6:187, 1962.
26. Haurowitz, F. The evaluation of selective and instructive theories of antibody formation. *Symp. Quant. Biol.* 32:559, 1967.
27. Haworth, J. C., Hoogstraten, J., and Taylor, H. Thymic alymphoplasia: Report of 13 cases and review of the literature. *Arch. Dis. Child.* 42:40, 1967.
28. Hitzig, W. H., Barundun, S., and Cottier, H. Die schweizerische Form der Agammaglobulinämie. *Ergebn. Inn. Med. Kinderheilk.* 27:79, 1968.
29. Hoyer, J. R., et al. Lymphopenic forms of congenital immunologic deficiency diseases. *Medicine* 47:201, 1968.
30. Huang, N. Personal communication.
31. Jameson, B., et al. Five-year analysis of protective isolation. *Lancet* 1:1034, 1971.
32. Johnson, R. B., Jr., and Baehner, R. L. Improvement of leucocyte bactericidal activity in chronic granulomatous disease. *Blood* 35:350, 1970.
33. Johnston, R. B., Jr., et al. Enhanced bactericidal activity of phagocytes from patients with chronic granulomatous disease in the presence of sulphisoxazole. *Lancet* I:824, 1975.
34. Kauder, E., and Mauer, A. M. Neutropenias of childhood. *J. Pediatr.* 69:147, 1966.
35. Lehrer, R. I., and Cline, M. J. Leucocyte myeloperoxidase deficiency and disseminated candidiasis. *J. Clin. Invest.* 48:1478, 1969.
36. Levine, A. S., et al. Protected environments and prophylactic antibiotics. *N. Engl. J. Med.* 288:477, 1973.
37. Matsaniotis, N., and Economou-Maurou, C. BCG vaccination and profound lymphopenia. *Pediatrics* 34:138, 1964.
38. Miller, M. E., and Nilsson, U. R. A familial deficiency of the phagocytosis-enhancing activity of serum related to a dysfunction of the fifth component of complement (C5). *N. Engl. J. Med.* 282:354, 1970.
39. Miller, M. E., Oski, F. A., and Harris, M. B. Lazy leucocyte syndrome. *Lancet* I:665, 1971.
40. Nezelof, C., et al. L'hypoplasie héréditaire du thymus. La place et sa responsabilité dans une observation d'aplasie lymphocytaire, normoplasmacytaire et normoglobinémique du nourrison. *Arch. Fr. Pediatr.* 21:897, 1964.
41. Ochs, H. D., Ament, M. E., and Davis, S. D. Giardiasis with malabsorption in X-linked agammaglobulinemia. *N. Engl. J. Med.* 287:341, 1972.
42. Penland, W. Z., and Perry, S. Portable laminar air flow isolator. *Lancet* I:174, 1970.
43. Quie, P. G. Chronic granulomatous disease in childhood. *Adv. Pediatr.* 16:287, 1969.
44. Robbins, J. B. *Pneumocystis carinii* pneumonia: A review. *Pediatr. Res.* 1:131, 1967.
45. Saulsbury, F. T., et al. Combined immunodeficiency and vaccine-related poliomyelitis in a child with cartilage-hair hypoplasia. *J. Pediatr.* 86:868, 1975.
46. Stiehm, E. R. Immunodeficiency Disorders. In E. R. Stiehm, and V. A. Fulginiti (eds.), *Immunologic Disorders in Infants and Children.* Baltimore: Williams & Wilkins, 1968.
47. Stoelinga, G. B. A., Van Munster, R. J. J., and Slooff, J. P. Antibody deficiency syndrome and autoimmune hemolytic anemia. *Acta Paediatr. Scand.* 58:352, 1969.
48. Tomasi, T. B., Jr., and Blenenstock, J. Secretory Immunoglobulins. *Adv. Immunol.* 9:1, 1968.

49. Trexler, P. C. An isolator system for the maintenance of aseptic environments. *Lancet* I:91, 1973.
50. White, J. G. The Chediak-Higashi syndrome, a possible lysosomal disease. *Blood* 28:143, 1966.
51. Wolfson, J. J., et al. Bone findings in chronic granulomatous disease of childhood. *J. Bone Joint Surg.* (America) 51:1573, 1969.
52. Wolfson, J. J., et al. Roentgenologic manifestations in children with a genetic defect of polymorphonuclear leucocyte function: Chronic granulomatous disease of childhood. *Radiology* 91:37, 1968.

9. Host Defenses in Protein-Calorie Malnutrition

Robert M. Suskind, Stitaya Sirisinha, Robert Edelman,
Vicharn Vithayasai, Panja Kulapongs,
Claus Leitzmann, and Robert E. Olson

It is well accepted that the malnourished child is more susceptible to infection and that infection is a major factor in the high morbidity and mortality associated with protein-calorie malnutrition (PCM) [24]. It is also well established that infection is often a major factor in precipitating acute nutritional deficiencies [10]. Clinical observations suggest that the malnourished individual's immune system may respond to infection differently from the well-nourished individual's. An organism that may be relatively harmless to the well-nourished child may give rise to a severe or even fatal infection in the malnourished child. When localized infection spreads in a child with PCM, it does so with the development of gangrene and not suppuration [30]. Children with PCM also tend to develop gram-negative septicemia [21].

To better understand the mechanisms by which the malnourished host responds to infection, we initiated several studies at the Anemia and Malnutrition Research Center in Chiang Mai, Thailand, which evaluated the cell-mediated immune system (CMI), phagocytosis, and the killing function of leukocytes (PKF), humoral and secretory immunoglobulins, and the complement and C3 activating system.

Cell-Mediated Immunity (CMI)

Cell-mediated immunity is an important defense against such diseases as tuberculosis, moniliasis, herpes simplex, measles, and chickenpox [24], diseases that may be particularly severe in children with PCM. A possible relationship between the increased incidence of Australian antigenemia in children with PCM and the impaired CMI response has been suggested by Suskind, Olson, and Olson [32]. Harland reported depressed tuberculin skin-test responses in malnourished children who had received BCG [9]. Several other investigators have reported similar defects in the in vivo evaluation of the CMI system in children with PCM [4, 8, 30]. To understand the mechanisms involved more fully, we devised a series of in vivo experiments designed to evaluate the inflammatory, sensitization, and recall limbs of the CMI system.

Initially, there must be intact, circulating, thymus-derived (T) lymphocytes that can be sensitized to the antigen. Later the sensitized lymphocyte must be able to recognize that foreign antigen and respond with the release

Supported by NIH Grant AM 11044.

122.

Table 9-1. Cutaneous Inflammatory Response to 2 mg DNFB

Day Tested	Number of Patients	Skin Response	
		Positive	Negative
1	30	4 (13%) [a]	26
15	5	3 (60%)	2
56	8	6 (75%) [a]	2

[a] Significantly different ($\chi^2 = 9.4$; $P < 0.01$).
Source: Edelman, R., et al. Mechanisms of defective delayed cutaneous hypersensitivity in children with protein-calorie malnutrition. *Lancet* I:506, 1973.

of lymphokines. The released lymphokines will produce a localized inflammatory response. To evaluate the inflammatory response in children with PCM, we applied 2 mg dinitrofluorobenzene (DNFB) to the forearms of 30 children on admission to the hospital. Five additional children were studied on hospital day 15, and eight on day 56 (Table 9-1) [5]. The presence or absence of erythema and induration was determined 2 days after application of DNFB. Of the children studied with DNFB on admission, only 4 out of 30 (13%) had positive inflammatory responses, while on day 56, 6 out of 8 (75%) had positive inflammatory responses. The difference between the two groups was statistically significant ($P < 0.01$). The results of this initial study indicated that the children with PCM were unable to develop a normal inflammatory response, whereas nutritionally recovered children were able to respond.

Next we evaluated the ability to sensitize PCM patients with 2 mg DNFB. Ten children sensitized with DNFB on day 1 and all the children sensitized on days 15 and 56 were rechallenged on day 72 with 100 μg DNFB (Table 9-2). Of those sensitized on admission, only 2 (20%) recalled the initial sensitization, while seven-eighths (87%) of those sensitized on day 56 recalled the

Table 9-2. Attempt to Sensitize PCM Patients with 2 mg DNFB

Day Sensitizing Dose Applied	Number of Patients	Skin Test Response [a]	
		Positive	Negative
1	10	2 [b]	8
15	5	1	4
56	8	7 [b]	1

[a] Skin test dose of 100 μg DNFB applied on day 70 and read on day 72.
[b] Significantly different ($\chi^2 = 4.7$; $P < 0.05$).
Source: Edelman, R., et al. Mechanisms of defective delayed hypersensitivity in children with protein-calorie malnutrition. *Lancet* I:506, 1973.

challenge on day 72. The difference between the two groups was statistically significant at the $P < 0.05$ level. Thus one might conclude that most children with severe PCM do not have circulating lymphocytes that can be sensitized. However, with nutritional repair, the ability to sensitize these children returns.

In another series of tests to determine the recall phenomenon in PCM (Table 9-3), 14 children were given intradermal *Candida albicans* (0.1 ml, 1:100 dilution) on admission to the hospital. Only two of the 14 (14%) showed more than 5 mm induration. On day 29, the remaining 12 children were retested; eight now reacted, bringing the cumulative positive response to 72%. When the last four children were tested again on day 10, all but one responded, bringing the total response to 92%. These figures compare favorably with the 80 to 85% positive skin-test reactions to *Candida* antigen among well-nourished Thai children [35]. The results of this study indicate that most children with severe PCM are not able to recall prior sensitization to a foreign antigen. However, because of the depressed inflammatory response, one cannot say whether the decreased skin-test reactivity is secondary to a depressed recall phenomenon or to the depressed inflammatory response itself.

T lymphocyte function was studied further in a series of experiments in vitro [13]. Initially, the percentage blast cell transformation and incorporation of tritiated thymidine into phytohemagglutinin (PHA) stimulated lymphocytes were determined. The percentage of T and B cell populations in PCM was then evaluated by rosette formation of lymphocytes with sensitized sheep red cells.

Peripheral lymphocytes were separated from whole blood with 6% dextran and cultured in medium 199 with 20% autologous plasma and 0.1 ml PHA solution. After 48 hours of incubation at 37°C, tritiated thymidine (0.1 μCi/1.5 ml of culture) was added to the culture medium. After an additional 18 hours of incubation, material from 10^6 lymphocytes was pre-

Table 9-3. Candida albicans Skin Test Recall Response

Day Tested	Number of Patients	Skin Test Response [a]		Accumulated Percent Positive
		Positive	Negative	
1	14	2	12	14
29	12	8 [b]	4	72
70	4	3 [b]	1	92

[a] Skin tests read 2 days after 0.1 ml of 1:100 antigen injected intradermally; positive means > 5 mm induration.
[b] Significantly different from proportion on day 1; McNemar test corrected for continuity gives 6.12, $P \le 0.02$ for day 29; $\chi^2 = 9.1$, $P < 0.01$ for day 70.
Source: Edelman, R., et al. Mechanisms of defective delayed cutaneous hypersensitivity in children with protein-calorie malnutrition. *Lancet* I:506, 1973.

cipitated with perchloric acid, and the incorporation of tritiated thymidine was measured. The ratio of counts incorporated into the PHA-stimulated versus the unstimulated sample was determined and expressed as the proliferation index. The percentage of blast cell transformation was determined after 72 hours of incubation. The T cell population was determined by quantitation of rosettes formed by incubation of lymphocytes with washed sheep red cells at 0 to 4°C and pH 7.4 to 7.6 [16, 39]. The B cell population was determined by quantitation of the rosette-forming lymphocytes formed during the incubation of sensitized sheep red cells with the patient's lymphocytes [16, 20].

The mean proliferation index of patients on admission was significantly lower than the mean on discharge (P < 0.01) (Figure 9-1). Likewise, the blast cell transformation on admission (46%) was significantly lower than that of the control population and the discharge blast cell transformation (Figure 9-2). By day 8 both the proliferation index and the blast cell transformation had increased significantly. Similarly, the mean percentage of T lymphocytes on admission (28%) was significantly lower than that of recovered patients (Figure 9-3). The increase in the percentage of T cells was significant by day 15 (P < 0.05). The B cell population was not significantly decreased on admission.

The above findings in vitro confirm the studies in vivo, demonstrating

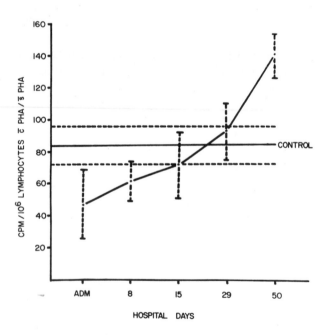

Figure 9-1. Proliferation index (H^3-TDR uptake) by peripheral lymphocytes in children with PCM (mean ± SEM). (From Kulapongs et al. [13].)

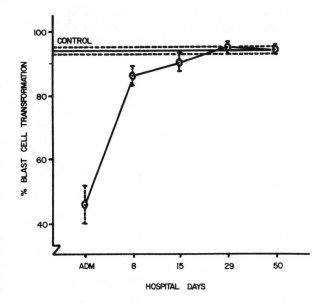

Figure 9-2. Percentage blast cell transformation of PHA-stimulated lymphocytes (mean ± SEM). (From Kulapongs et al. [13].)

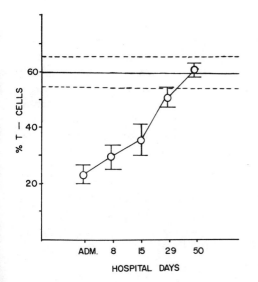

Figure 9-3. Percentage T cells in children with PCM on admission and throughout recovery (mean ± SEM). (From Kulapongs et al. [13].)

depressed CMI function in PCM. The studies confirm those of other investigators [4, 8, 9, 17]. They also indicate that the changes in the CMI system are reversible.

Polymorphonuclear Leukocyte

The leukocyte plays an important role in protecting the host against bacteria. Selvaraj and Bhat [25] and Seth and Chandra [26] found polymorphonuclear leukocyte function to be compromised in children with PCM. Kumate, Hernandez-Yasso, and Vazquez on the other hand, found that the phagocytic and killing function of leukocytes was not impaired in children with PCM [15]; Smith and Lopez made similar observations in malnourished pigs [29].

Because of this controversy regarding leukocyte function, a study was undertaken at the Anemia and Malnutrition Research Center in Chiang Mai, Thailand, to evaluate this parameter in 42 malnourished children (16 with marasmus, 14 with marasmus-kwashiorkor, and 12 with kwashiorkor) [36]. Patients were studied on admission and on days 15, 28, 49, and after day 50. Five milliliters of peripheral heparinized whole blood was added to 2.5 ml dextran 6% in normal saline and kept at room temperature for 45 to 60 min. Then the leukocyte-rich plasma was centrifuged. The cell pellet was washed twice in heparinized sterile saline and then with 0.1% gel Hanks solution, in which it was finally suspended with *Escherichia coli* at a bacteria-to-phagocyte ratio of 1 : 1. The incubation mixture was sampled at 0, 60, and 120 min. Culture plates were counted after 18 hours incubation, and the percentage of killing was calculated by dividing the number of viable bacteria remaining at 60 and 120 min by the initial number of bacteria added to the culture medium. Controls were run with each patient's sample. The mean $\pm$ 2SD PKF value for 199 controls was 97.7 $\pm$ 9.9. Therefore any value of less than 88% was considered abnormal.

Only one out of 16 (6%) children with marasmus had an abnormal PKF on admission, while two out of 14 (14%) with marasmus-kwashiorkor and 3 out of 12 (25%) with kwashiorkor had abnormal PKFs (Figure 9-4). All leukocyte function had normalized by day 15, except in one patient with kwashiorkor, whose PKF remained abnormal until day 28. All the abnormal PKFs were found to be secondary to a defect in leukocyte function that was not corrected by normal control serum. Furthermore, serum from the patients with abnormal PKFs did not inhibit normal control leukocyte function.

The phagocytic index (the number of intracellular bacteria in 200 consecutive neutrophils) was compared in those with abnormal and normal PKFs; *E. coli* was added to the leukocyte suspension in a bacteria-leukocyte ratio of 10 : 1 [36]. A smear of the incubation mixture was made at 10, 20, 30, and 45 min. The average number of intracellular bacteria per neutrophil was reported as the phagocytic index (PI).

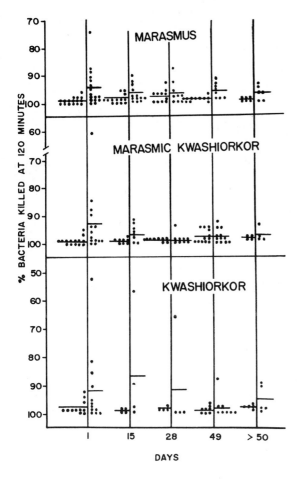

Figure 9-4. Percentage of bacteria killed at 120 min on hospital days 1, 15, 28, 49, and 50 for children with marasmus, marasmus-kwashiorkor, and kwashiorkor. (From Leitzmann et al. [36].)

The mean PI of those with normal and abnormal PKF was not different at 10, 20, or 30 min. At 45 min, however, the mean PI of those with abnormal PKFs was significantly greater than that of the control group (P < 0.01). While the number of bacteria decreased in the control it increased in patients with decreased PKFs, confirming the impression that the defect in the abnormal leukocytes was not in the ability to phagocytize the organisms but in the ability to kill and digest them. One must conclude from these studies in vitro that not all children have as severe a deficit in PKF as those reported by Selvaraj and Bhat [25] and by Seth and Chandra [26]. Indeed, in only 14% of the total was any detectable deficit determined in our test system. Thus our results confirm those of Kumate and Smith and their coworkers [15, 29], who did not find major deficits in their in vitro evaluations of polymorphonuclear leukocyte function.

It has been suggested that the higher ratio of bacteria to leukocyte used by Selvaraj and Bhat [25] may have provided greater stress to the in vitro system, thereby bringing out deficits that would not be apparent in a system using fewer bacteria. Kumate, Hernandez-Yasso, and Vazquez [15] disproved this idea, however, by showing that different ratios produced no difference in results. Aside from differences in patient populations, a possible explanation for the different results may be found in the incubation media. Selvaraj and Bhat [25] used Krebs phosphate buffer, which contains no amino acids; we used Hanks, which contains all the essential amino acids. Although an in vivo system is never completely devoid of amino acids, the complete absence of them might accentuate differences between patients and controls that are in fact artificially established by the system itself.

To evaluate in vivo leukocyte function we placed Rebuck skin windows on the forearms of children with PCM on admission to the hospital and after recovery [14]. Well-nourished infected children, PCM-recovered and

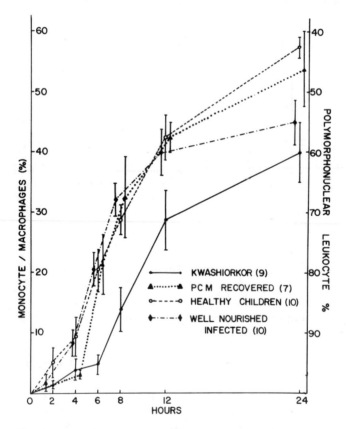

Figure 9-5. Percent macrophage and polymorphonuclear leukocyte response in Rebuck skin windows in children with kwashiorkor, healthy controls, infected well-nourished controls and in children recovered from kwashiorkor (mean ± SEM, 2 to 24 hours after the initial skin abrasion). (From Kulapongs et al. [14].)

normal controls were also studied. A 1-cm superficial abrasion was made on the volar surface of the forearm and a coverslip was placed over the abrasion. The first coverslip was removed after 30 min and additional coverslips were placed over the abrasion at 2, 4, 6, 8, 12, and 24 hours. Each coverslip was stained with Wright's stain and evaluated for cellularity. A differential count was done on each slide. In children with PCM there was no deficit in cellular response nor was there a deficit in the percentage of polymorphonuclear leukocytes (Figure 9-5). However, the children with PCM did not appear to have a normal mononuclear response in that the percentage of monocytes at 18 and 24 hours was significantly lower than in the well-nourished children or those who had recovered from PCM. These results are similar to those of Freyre et al. [7].

In summary, the polymorphonuclear leukocyte in the malnourished child is able to phagocytize bacteria adequately, although its ability to kill adequately appears to be depressed in selected patients. The leukocyte appears to respond appropriately to dermal injury.

Humoral Immune System

Serum Immunoglobulins
There is no unanimous agreement on the effect of PCM on the humoral immune system. Most studies, however, have shown that immunoglobulin levels are not depressed [1, 12, 19]; antibody response appears to vary according to the type and form of antigen used [3, 6, 22]. In the following study, the humoral immune system in children with marasmus and kwashiorkor was evaluated by analysis of the levels of serum immunoglobulins (IgG, IgM, IgA, IgD, and IgE) and by specific antibody response to typhoid immunization [34].

Fourteen children with marasmus, seven with marasmus-kwashiorkor, and seven with kwashiorkor, all 2 to 5 years old, were serially evaluated for immunoglobulin status on admission and on hospital days 8, 29, 50, 71, and 84. Eleven infected but well-nourished children of the same age and from the same socioeconomic background as the children with PCM served as controls. Five of the children had pneumonia and two had fevers of undetermined origin (FUO); the others had herpetic stomatitis, gastroenteritis, diphtheria, and encephalitis. The levels of serum IgG, IgA, IgM, IgD, and IgE were determined by radioimmunodiffusion using commercial immunoplates and reference standards.*

Immunoglobulin values for the marasmus-kwashiorkor and kwashiorkor groups were pooled because no significant difference was found between them. The children with marasmus-kwashiorkor and kwashiorkor (MK-K) tended to have higher IgM, IgA, IgG, and IgD values on admission than

---

* Hyland Laboratories, 3300 Highland Avenue, Costa Mesa, California 92626.

130.

did the children with marasmus (Figure 9-6). IgG levels in both the marasmus and the MK-K groups were significantly higher than those of the controls (P < 0.02 and P < 0.01, respectively). The IgM and IgA levels of those with marasmus and MK-K were not significantly different from the controls'. Eighty percent of the children with marasmus had detectable IgD titers, with a mean titer of 4.0 ± 1.1 mg/100 ml. A similar percentage of children with MK-K had elevated IgD titers, but their mean titer was much higher (13.5 ± 4.3 mg/100 ml). IgD could not be detected in control children. At discharge, IgD was still detectable in the malnourished children.

Sixty-four percent (16 out of 25) of the malnourished children had detectable IgE levels at the time of admission; after recovery only 37% were still positive. Only one of the 10 control children was positive for IgE.

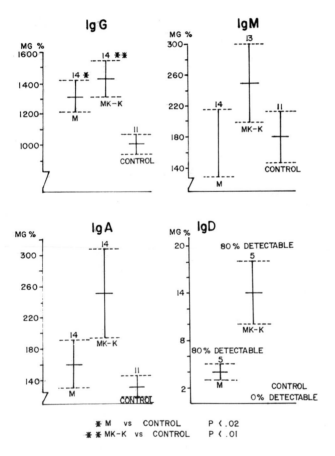

Figure 9-6. Admission IgM, IgA, IgG, and IgD immunoglobulins for 14 children with marasmus and 14 with marasmus-kwashiorkor and kwashiorkor compared with 11 well-nourished infected controls (mean ± SEM).

While the IgE levels tended to decline with dietary treatment, the final level in many children was still higher than in the control population. The elevated serum IgM, IgA, and IgD gradually decreased during hospitalization, while the IgG remained elevated (Figure 9-7).

The results of this study are in agreement with those of several investigators who found either normal or elevated immunoglobulins in children with PCM [1, 12, 19]. However, elevated immunoglobulin levels do not necessarily indicate that the humoral system is intact at the time the malnourished child is admitted to the hospital. One must also look closely at the antibody response to a foreign antigen, such as typhoid antigen. An additional 10 malnourished children (five kwashiorkor, three marasmus-kwashiorkor, and two marasmus) and 10 recovered patients were evaluated for antibody response to intradermal typhoid antigen 8 and 20 to 29 days after immunization. During their first 8 days in the hospital, the malnourished patients were given 1 g protein per kilogram per day. By day 8, calories were gradually increased to 100 cal per kilogram per day. From days 8 to 29 all patients were on 175 cal and 4 g protein per kilogram. The anti-H antibody was measured by radioimmunoassay.

Children with PCM who were immunized on admission showed essentially no increase in antibody titer in the first week, during which they re-

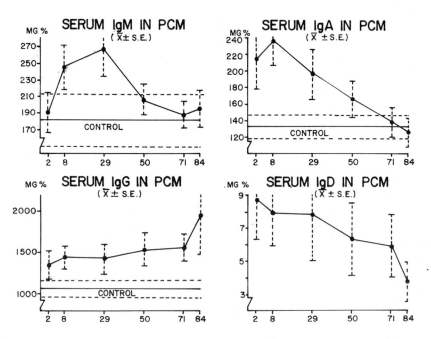

Figure 9-7. IgM, IgA, IgG and IgD (mean ± SEM) malnourished children on admission and during recovery as compared with 11 well-nourished infected children.

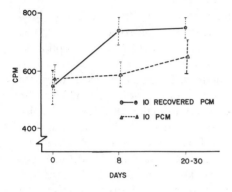

Figure 9-8. Typhoid H antibody response 8 and 20 to 29 days after intradermal typhoid antigen immunization in 10 malnourished and 10 recovered children. CPM = counts per minute. PCM = protein-calorie malnutrition. (From Suskind et al. [34].)

ceived 100 cal and 1 g protein per kilogram (Figure 9-8). The nutritionally recovered children, who were receiving 175 cal and 4 g protein per kilogram, showed a significant increase in antibody activity over the preimmunization level ($P < 0.05$) within a week after immunization. These results confirm those of Wohl, Reinhold, and Rose [37] and Chandra [4], who found decreased antibody responses to typhoid vaccine in malnourished children, and those of Reddy and Srikantia [23] and Mathews et al. [18], who found that children with higher protein intakes had better antibody responses to typhoid immunization than did controls.

Impaired antibody response to a single antigen does not necessarily show that the response to all antigens is depressed in the malnourished child. Normal antibody responses have been reported in children with PCM [4]; Work et al. [38] found normal antibody responses to keyhole-lympet hemocyanin and pneumococcal polysaccharide in children with PCM. Malnourished children have been found to respond adequately to polio and smallpox immunization but poorly to yellow fever vaccine [3]. Elmolla et al. [6], who studied the antibody response to cholera vaccine in children with PCM, suggested that one antibody-producing system may have been affected while the other was intact. Such speculation seems reasonable; the variation in response to different antigens may be due to selective impairment of the various antigenic systems in the malnourished state.

The response to an antigenic stimulus constitutes a much more sensitive and reliable evaluation of the humoral immune system than does the level of circulating immunoglobulins. The fact that malnourished children on admission have depressed antibody responses to typhoid H antigen suggests that the child's nutritional state does affect the antibody response with regard to at least one antigenic stimulus. Of significance is the fact that when the nutritional state of the malnourished child is improved, his antibody response to an antigenic stimulus also improves.

Secretory IgA System
Because of the clinical impression that children with PCM tend to have an increased incidence of respiratory and gastrointestinal tract infections, we

decided to evaluate the status of the secretory immunoglobulin system. The level of secretory IgA (SIgA) was determined in the nasal washings of children with PCM on admission to the hospital and during dietary treatment [28]. Serum IgA was determined simultaneously in the same patients.

To obtain the nasal specimens, the patient was positioned on one side with his neck extended and tilted to one side. Five milliliters of normal saline was slowly instilled into the upper nostril and aspirated from the nasopharynx through a No. 8 French plastic catheter inserted in the lower nostril. The same procedure was repeated with the patient lying on the other side. The concentration of IgG and SIgA in the nasal washing was determined by electroimmunodiffusion. Monospecific antisera to purified salivary IgA (anti-Sc) and to individual serum immunoglobulins were prepared. Absolute values were converted to percent of total protein concentration.

SIgA was the predominant protein in the nasal washings from the malnourished control children (Figure 9-9). Although concentrations of total protein, IgG, and albumin measured in all nasal washings were reduced in children with PCM, only the SIgA concentration was significantly lower in the children with PCM than in the control children. When the data were pooled for given periods of time, the relative concentrations of SIgA on days 1 through 8 and on days 9 through 70 were significantly lower than those of the controls (Figure 9-10). However, the SIgA concentrations in samples taken on days 71 through 84 and on followup were not significantly different from the controls.

The mean serum IgA in the malnourished children on admission was significantly higher than that of the normal children of the same age. During

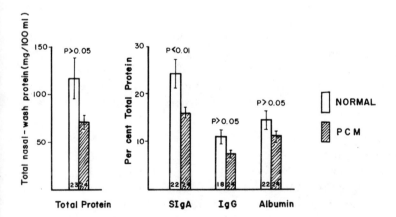

Figure 9-9. Nasal washings in 13 children with PCM. SIgA, IgG, albumin, and total protein expressed as a percent of total protein. (From Sirisinha, S., et al. Secretory and serum IgA in children with protein-calorie malnutrition. In J. Mestecky and A. R. Lawton [Eds.], *The Immunoglobulin A System.* New York: Plenum, 1974.)

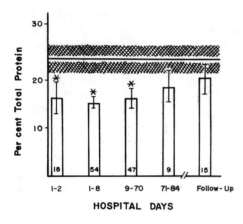

Figure 9-10. Secretory IgA as a percent of total protein on days 1–2, 3–8, 9–70, 71–84, and followup. (* = statistically significant difference from normal; P < 0.05.)

hospitalization these relatively high levels decreased to those of the controls. Electroimmunodiffusion of the serum samples failed to disclose the presence of the secretory component (SC).

This study indicates that children with PCM suffer a slight, but significant, impairment in the production of secretory IgA in the respiratory tract, which requires up to 10 to 12 weeks to repair. This observation suggests that in the malnourished child there is either a failure to synthesize SIgA normally or there is a block in the passage of SIgA from its mucosal surface. The possibility of SIgA returning to the circulation has been excluded by the fact that no reactive anti-SC was detected in the serum.

The production of SIgA is known to involve at least two types of cells: the lymphocytes underlying the mucosa, which produce the IgA, and the epithelial cells, which produce the secretory component. Perhaps one or both cell types is affected in PCM, resulting in decreased SIgA levels and increased susceptibility to mucosal infections. Since IgA is thought to play a role in localizing enteric organisms to the intestinal lumen [31], one might speculate that a reduction in gastrointestinal SIgA, similar to the reduction in the nasal SIgA, could lead to the invasion of gram-negative organisms and development of the septicemia frequently seen in children with PCM.

Complement System

A defect in the complement system is known to be associated with an increased susceptibility to bacterial infection [2], and since children with PCM have an increased incidence of bacterial infections, it might be expected that their complement system is impaired. We therefore evaluated the serum concentrations of the complement proteins in both the classic system and the C3-activating system in children with marasmus and kwashiorkor on admission and during recovery [27]. A second study was developed to evaluate the hemolytic activity of the complement system in malnourished children on admission and after recovery [33].

Complement Components

Ten children with marasmus and 10 with kwashiorkor were studied on days 1, 8, 29, and 71. During the first 8 days of hospitalization, the children received 1 g protein per kilogram of body weight and a gradually increasing caloric intake. On day 8 they were divided into groups and placed on one of four dietary treatments: 100 cal and 1 g protein per kilogram of body weight per day; 100 cal and 4 g protein; 175 cal and 1 g protein; or 175 cal and 4 g protein. All patients received 175 cal and 4 g protein per kilogram of body weight from day 29 through day 70. The concentrations of C1q, C1s, C3, C4, C5, C6, C8, C9, and C3PA were measured by radioimmunodiffusion, using immunoplates containing antiserum specific for the individual complement components.

The mean concentration for eight out of nine components was significantly lower in the 20 children with PCM than in the 19 controls (P < 0.05) (Figure 9-11). Although C4 was lower in the children with PCM, the difference was not significant. The mean concentration of eight of the nine components was lower in the children with kwashiorkor than in those with marasmus, although the difference was statistically significant in only three (C1q, C6, and C8) (Figure 9-12). A marked increase in all the complement proteins except C9 was first noted on day 29 (Figure 9-12). Except for C9, maximum levels were reached by day 71. The late-acting components (C5, C6, C8, and C9) did not appear to increase as readily as did the early-reacting ones. Although C9 continued to be low through day 71, followup blood samples taken several months later indicated an ultimate normalization of this factor.

To evaluate the effect of diet on the various components, the data from the children with marasmus and kwashiorkor were combined. The importance of dietary protein levels was clearly demonstrated. Between days 8 and 29, complement levels increased to normal or above normal in children receiving 175 cal and 4 g protein. In those receiving 175 cal and 1 g protein, complement levels remained unchanged or even decreased (Figure 9-13). Although children on 175 cal and 4 g protein tended to have higher complement levels on day 29 than did those on 100 cal and 4 g protein, the difference was not as dramatic as that produced by different protein intakes.

Although the role of infection in complement utilization could not be ruled out, evidence from this study suggests that serum complement levels were probably reduced because their synthesis was impaired. Furthermore, the present study demonstrated the importance of protein in the resynthesis of the complement components. To determine whether the decrease in the plasma complement concentration affected complement activity, a second study was designed to look at the CH_{50} of serum obtained from children with PCM on admission and during recovery.

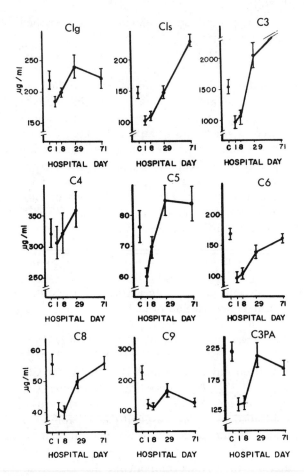

Figure 9-11. Change in complement components with recovery. (From Sirisinha, S., et al. Complement and C3 proactivator levels in children with protein-calorie malnutrition and the effect of dietary treatment. *Lancet* I:1016, 1973.)

CH_{50} Study

Twenty-eight children (4 with marasmus, 10 with marasmus-kwashiorkor, and 14 with kwashiorkor) were evaluated for CH_{50} activity and anticomplementary activity on admission and on days 4, 8, 29, 50, and 71 [33]. The serum CH_{50} activity was determined with a standard assay of total hemolytic complement activity [11]; the results are expressed as the reciprocal of the dilution (in units per milliliter), producing 50% hemolysis of sensitized sheep red blood cells. To determine the anticomplementary activity, the patient's serum was diluted with an equal volume of a standard serum with a known CH_{50} titer. The mixture was incubated at 37°C for 30 min, and the total hemolytic titer was determined as above. For dilution control,

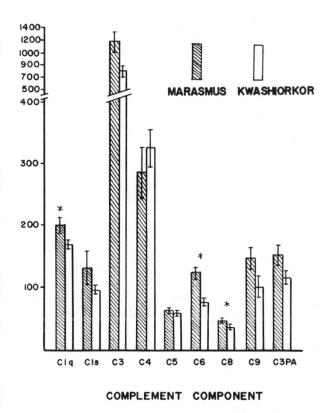

MARASMUS KWASHIORKOR

COMPLEMENT COMPONENT

Figure 9-12. Admission serum complement levels in 10 children with marasmus and 10 with kwashiorkor. (* = difference between marasmus and kwashiorkor groups statistically different; P < 0.05.) (From Sirisinha, S., et al. Complement and C3 proactivator levels in children with protein-calorie malnutrition and the effect of dietary treatment. *Lancet* I:1016, 1973.)

heat-inactivated (56°C, 30 min) standard serum and saline were each mixed with the unheated standard serum and incubated at 37°C for 30 min. The CH_{50} titer of the mixture was then determined.

Since no significant difference was found in the admission CH_{50} titers of patients with marasmus and those with marasmus-kwashiorkor, their data were pooled for statistical analysis (M-MK). On admission there was no significant difference between the CH_{50} titers of the M-MK group and the controls (Figure 9-14). Children with kwashiorkor, however, did have significantly lower CH_{50} titers on admission than did the controls. With improved nutritional status, CH_{50} titers increased significantly in both groups of patients. By day 50, the CH_{50} titers were significantly higher in the previously malnourished children than in the control patients. On day 71 the CH_{50} titers had fallen to levels not significantly different from the control mean. The mean CH_{50} titer of 16 febrile, well-nourished controls was

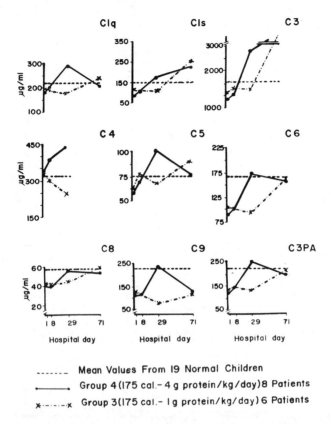

C1q C1s C3

C4 C5 C6

C8 C9 C3PA

Hospital day   Hospital day   Hospital day

------- Mean Values From 19 Normal Children

————— Group 4(175 cal.- 4 g protein/kg/day)8 Patients

x-------x Group 3(175 cal.- I g protein/kg/day)6 Patients

Figure 9-13. The effect of dietary protein on the recovery of complement levels. (From Sirisinha, S., et al. Complement and C3 proactivator levels in children with protein-calorie malnutrition and the effect of dietary treatment. *Lancet* I:1016, 1973.)

significantly higher than that of the well-nourished, nonfebrile controls. The mean CH_{50} titer of the PCM patients was significantly lower than that of the febrile controls on days 1 and 4. On subsequent days there was no significant difference between the groups.

When 33 sera from healthy, febrile controls were each mixed with a standard serum of 960 to 1280 units per milliliter, the CH_{50} activity was always equal to or greater than 480 units per milliliter. Therefore a resultant titer of 320 units per milliliter or less was considered to indicate the presence of anticomplementary (AC) activity (Figure 9-15). Thus 7 out of 27 (25%) had detectable AC activity on day 1; and 7 out of 26 (27%), on day 4. None demonstrated AC activity on days 50 or 71. Decreased CH_{50} activity was significantly correlated with the presence of AC activity on admission (P < 0.01).

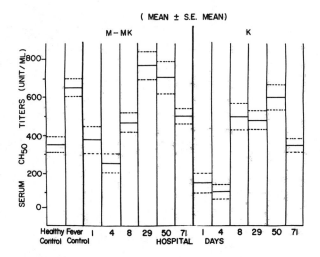

Figure 9-14. Serum CH_{50} activity in units per milliliter in healthy and febrile controls and in children with marasmus, marasmus-kwashiorkor, and kwashiorkor on admission and with recovery (mean ± SEM). (From Suskind et al. [33].)

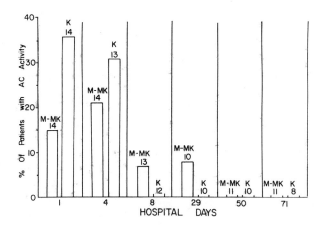

Figure 9-15. Percent of patients with anticomplementary activity on admission and with recovery. (From Suskind et al. [33].)

The CH_{50} study confirms the functional impairment of the complement system that had been suggested by the decrease in the individual complement components. It also demonstrates the presence of a complement activator, which may be partly responsible for the decreased CH_{50} activity. Several substances are known to activate complement; they include circulating immune complexes, endotoxin, macroglobulins, C-esterase inhibitors, and C3 and C6 inhibitors.

Endotoxemia in PCM

In a final study, 28 patients with PCM were prospectively evaluated for the presence of endotoxemia as determined by the limulus assay. Eleven of 28 (40%) had circulating endotoxin on admission. Because of the vigorous treatment there appeared to be no increased mortality or morbidity associated with the circulating endotoxin. However, the very high incidence of endotoxemia in PCM may help to explain the very high mortality in undertreated malnourished children.

Summary

In summary, several host defenses in the malnourished child are compromised: the cell-mediated immune system, the immunoglobulin system, and the complement system. The killing function of the leukocyte appears to be compromised in a relatively small percentage of malnourished children, and a significant percentage of children with PCM show evidence of circulating endotoxemia on admission to the hospital.

References

1. Alvarado, J. Serum immunoglobulins in edematous protein calorie malnourished children. Studies in Guatemalan children at INCAP. *Clin. Pediatr.* 10(3):174, 1971.
2. Alper, C. A., et al. Increased susceptibility to infection associated with abnormalities of complement-mediated functions of the third component of complement (C_3). *N. Engl. J. Med.* 282:349, 1970.
3. Brown, R. E., and Katz, M. Antigenic stimulation in undernourished children. *East Afr. Med. J.* 42:221, 1965.
4. Chandra, R. K. Immunocompetence in undernutrition. *J. Pediatr.* 81:1194, 1972.
5. Edelman, R., et al. Mechanisms of defective delayed cutaneous hypersensitivity in children with protein-calorie malnutrition. *Lancet* I:506, 1973.
6. Elmolla, A., et al. Antibody-production in protein-calorie malnutrition. *J. Trop. Med. Hyg.* 76:248, 1973.
7. Freyre, E. A., et al. Abnormal Rebuck skin window response in kwashiorkor. *J. Pediatr.* 82:523, 1973.
8. Geefhuysen, J., et al. Impaired cellular immunity in kwashiorkor with improvement after therapy. *Br. Med. J.* 4:527, 1971.
9. Harland, P. S. E. G. Tuberculin reactions in malnourished children. *Lancet* II:719, 1965.
10. Hutt, M. S. R. Malnutrition and infection—East African studies. *J. Trop. Pediatr.* 15:153, 1969.
11. Kabat, E. A., and Mayer, M. M. *Experimental Immunochemistry.* Springfield, Ill.: Thomas, 1961.
12. Keet, M. P., and Thom, H. Serum immunoglobulins in kwashiorkor. *Arch. Dis. Child.* 44:600, 1969.
13. Kulapongs, P., et al. In vitro Cell-Mediated Immune Response in Thai Children with Protein-Calorie Malnutrition. In R. Suskind (Ed.), *Malnutrition and the Immune Response.* New York: Raven Press, 1977.

14. Kulapongs, P., et al.   Defective local leukocyte mobilization in children with kwashiorkor. *Am. J. Clin. Nutr.* 30:367, 1977.
15. Kumate, J., Hernandez-Yasso, F., and Vazquez, V.   Neutrophil-mediated immunity in severe malnutrition. *Research Forum: Malnutrition and Infection,* 1971.
16. Lay, W. H., et al.   Binding of sheep red cells to a large population of human lymphocytes. *Nature* 230:531, 1971.
17. Lloyd, A. U. C.   Tuberculin test in children with malnutrition. *Br. Med. J.* 3:529, 1968.
18. Mathews, J. D., et al.   Protein supplementation and enhanced antibody producing capacity in New Guinean school children. *Lancet* II:675, 1972.
19. Najjar, S. S., Stephan, M., and Asfour, R. Y.   Serum levels of immunoglobulins in marasmic infants. *Arch. Dis. Child.* 44:120, 1969.
20. Papamichail, M., et al.   Subpopulations of human peripheral lymphocytes distinguished by combined rosette formation and membrane immunofluorescence. *Lancet* II:64, 1972.
21. Phillips, I., and Wharton, B.   Acute bacterial infection in kwashiorkor and marasmus. *Br. Med. J.* 1:407, 1968.
22. Pretorius, P. J., and De Villiers, L. S.   Antibody response in children with protein malnutrition. *Am. J. Clin. Nutr.* 10:379, 1962.
23. Reddy, V., and Srikantia, S. G.   Antibody response in kwashiorkor. *Indian J. Med. Res.* 52:1154, 1964.
24. Scrimshaw, N. S., Taylor, C. E., and Gordon, J. E.   Interactions of nutrition and infection. *WHO Monogr. Ser.* No. 57, 1968.
25. Selvaraj, R. J., and Bhat, K. S.   Metabolic and bactericidal activities of leukocytes in protein-calorie malnutrition. *Am. J. Clin. Nutr.* 25:166, 1972.
26. Seth, V., and Chandra, R. K.   Opsonic activity, phagocytosis and bactericidal capacity of polymorphs in undernutrition. *Arch. Dis. Child.* 37:282, 1972.
27. Sirisinha, S., et al.   Complement and C3 proactivator levels in children with protein-calorie malnutrition and the effect of dietary treatment. *Lancet* I:1016, 1973.
28. Sirisinha, S., Suskind, R., and Edelman, R.   Secretory immunoglobulins in protein calorie malnutrition. *Pediatrics* 44:166, 1975.
29. Smith, N. J., and Lopez, V.   Immunologic response in severe undernutrition. *International Symposium on Malnutrition and Function of Blood Cells.* Kyoto, Japan, November 1972.
30. Smythe, P. M., et al.   Thymolymphatic deficiency and depression of cell-mediated immunity in protein-calorie malnutrition. *Lancet* II:939, 1971.
31. Stites, D. P., et al.   Selective "dysgammaglobulinemia" with elevated serum IgA levels and chronic salmonellosis. *Am. J. Med.* 54:260, 1973.
32. Suskind, R. M., Olson, L. C., and Olson, R. E.   Protein-calorie malnutrition and infection with hepatitis-associated antigen. *Pediatrics* 51:525, 1973.
33. Suskind, R., et al.   Complement activity in children with protein-calorie malnutrition. *Am. J. Clin. Nutr.* 29:1089, 1976.
34. Suskind, R., et al.   Immunoglobulins and antibody response in children with protein-calorie malnutrition. *Am. J. Clin. Nutr.* 29:836, 1976.
35. Vithayasai, V., Suskind, R., and Edelman, R. Unpublished data, 1973.
36. Leitzmann, C., et al. Phagocytosis and Killing Function of Polymorphonuclear Leukocytes in Thai Children with Protein-Calorie Malnutrition. In R. Suskind (Ed.), Malnutrition and the Immune Response. New York: Raven Press, 1977.
37. Wohl, M. G., Reinhold, J. G., and Rose, S. B.   Antibody responses in patients with hypoproteinemia. *Arch. Intern. Med.* 83:402, 1949.
38. Work, T. H., et al.   Tropical problems in nutrition (discussion). *Ann. Intern. Med.* 79:701, 1973.

39. Wybran, J., Carr, M. C., and Fudenberg, H. H. The human rosette-forming cell as a marker of a population of thymus derived cells. *J. Clin. Invest.* 51: 2537, 1972.
40. Sirisinha, S., et al. Secretory and serum IgA in children with protein-calorie malnutrition. In J. Mestecky and A. R. Lawton (Eds.), *The Immunoglobulin A System.* New York: Plenum, 1974.

10. Prevention of Infection in Patients with Acute Leukemia

Gerald P. Bodey, Victorio Rodriguez,
and Emil J Freireich

The treatment of patients with acute leukemia has improved substantially in recent years due to the introduction of effective chemotherapeutic regimens. However, infectious complications continue to represent a serious threat to these patients. Prolonged and severe neutropenia occurs commonly as a result of their disease or its therapy. In these patients, both the frequency of infectious complications and the mortality rate are related to the degree and duration of neutropenia [1]. Hence methods for protecting patients from infection during periods of neutropenia would be beneficial.

Conventional reverse isolation procedures have not resulted in a substantial reduction in the infectious complications of neutropenic patients, since this approach only protects against transmission of organisms by physical contact. Many potentially pathogenic organisms are capable of surviving routine hospital cleansing procedures and therefore would still represent a hazard to the patient in reverse isolation. Hospital food can be contaminated with pathogenic organisms at the time of delivery to the kitchen or during preparation and serving [12]. Pathogenic organisms also can be transmitted via contaminated air-conditioning ducts [15].

Initial approaches to provide more effective protection for the susceptible patient included the design of special units similar to surgical suites, often with a separate filtered air supply. In one study, patients with malignant diseases or aplastic anemia were treated in an isolation unit equipped with ultraviolet lighting and a low-efficiency air filtration system [18]. Personnel caring for these patients were cultured at regular intervals, and those who were carriers of organisms, such as *Staphylococcus aureus,* were transferred from the unit. This approach is not very practical, since patients who were not "pathogen-free" were excluded from the isolation unit. Nearly all organisms are potentially pathogenic for the neutropenic patient, including common environmental contaminants and organisms comprising the patient's normal endogenous microbial flora.

The most sophisticated approach to the prevention of infection has been the use of single-patient isolation units plus prophylactic antibiotic regimens. The initial isolation unit, introduced for this purpose, was a plastic tent isolator that provided a high-efficiency air filtration system [5, 19]. However, air flow in these units is turbulent and only about 13 air volumes are exchanged per hour. More recently, laminar air flow (LAF) units have been

Supported in part by Grants CA 10042 and CA 05831 and Contract N01-CM-53832 from the National Cancer Institute, National Institutes of Health, U.S. Public Health Service, Bethesda, Maryland 20014.

utilized [2, 20]. Turbulence is at a minimum in these units, and the air volume is exchanged about 150 to 400 times per hour, depending on the air velocity. Most of these isolation units are constructed so that procedures can be performed on the patient through plastic sleeves on the side of the unit, thus reducing or eliminating the possibility of patient contamination via contact with hospital personnel. All items entering the unit, including the patient's food, are presterilized. The units are cleansed at regular intervals with antimicrobial solutions.

Environmental Monitoring

We have evaluated the efficacy of LAF units in reducing environmental microbial contamination during patient occupancy [6]. There was a 600-fold difference in the concentration of organisms in air samples collected from LAF rooms than in those collected from regular hospital rooms (Table 10-1). Only 1% of air samples from LAF rooms contained potentially pathogenic organisms, whereas 59% of samples from hospital rooms contained pathogens such as *S. aureus, Escherichia coli, Klebsiella* species, *Pseudomonas aeruginosa,* and other gram-negative bacilli. Over half the settling plates placed in LAF rooms for 8-hour periods remained sterile. Over 50 times more organisms were deposited on settling plates in regular hospital rooms than in LAF rooms. None of the floor cultures from regular hospital rooms were sterile, whereas 72% of the floor cultures from LAF rooms were sterile. Potential pathogens were cultured from nearly 50% of floor samples collected from regular hospital rooms, but only 3% were cultured from samples collected from LAF rooms.

Table 10-1. Environmental Monitoring of Laminar Air Flow Rooms

	LAF Rooms	Hospital Rooms
Air Sampling		
Volume sampled	140,160	6,360
Organisms per 1000 ft^3	5	3,064
% samples with pathogens	1	59
Settling Plates		
Hours of sampling	23,288	432
Organisms per 8 hours	1.8	100
% sterile samples	57	0
% samples with pathogens	9	26
Floor Cultures		
Number of samples	1,045	120
% sterile samples	72	0
% samples with pathogens	3	47

Although the amount of microbial contamination in **LAF** rooms is significantly lower than in regular hospital rooms, this reduction is not solely a result of the protected environment. Our recent studies indicate that the amount of microbial contamination in protected environment units is dependent on whether or not the patient's endogenous microbial burden is reduced by antibiotic prophylaxis. There is substantially less contamination of floor cultures and settling plates when the units are occupied by patients who are receiving oral nonabsorbable antibiotics than when they are occupied by patients who are not receiving these regimens (Table 10-2). The gastrointestinal flora are greatly reduced or eliminated in patients who are receiving oral antibiotic prophylaxis and, consequently, they deposit fewer organisms into the environment.

Patient Monitoring

The effect of the prophylactic regimens listed in Table 10-3 has been evaluated in 79 patients who received chemotherapy in protected environment units on 91 occasions [7]. Cultures of stool, throat, ears, nose, skin, and urine specimens were obtained before the administration of the antibiotics and at least weekly thereafter. The antibiotic regimens have been effective in eliminating the vast majority of bacteria from each body site (Table 10-4). The oral antibacterial regimen containing gentamicin has been more effective but is considerably more expensive, since a commercial oral preparation is not available. None of the antifungal agents has been very effective in eliminating fungi from the throat or stools.

The overall effects of the prophylactic measures on the various body sites are summarized in Table 10-5. Only one patient had consistently sterile throat and skin cultures. The majority of bacterial organisms that persisted were organisms of low pathogenicity, such as *Lactobacillus* species, diphthe-

Table 10-2. Effect of Oral Antibiotic Prophylaxis on Microbial Contamination of Laminar Air Flow Rooms

	Patients Receiving Oral Antibiotics	Patients Not Receiving Oral Antibiotics
Floor Cultures		
Number of samples	1,910	614
% sterile samples	71	63
% samples with pathogens	5	17
Settling Plates		
Hours of sampling	25,448	11,232
Organisms per 8 hours	4.5	10
% sterile samples	57	43
% samples with pathogens	6	21

Table 10-3. Prophylactic Regimens

Regimen		Administration
Oral Antibiotic		
Antibacterial agents		
Regimen A		Every 4 hours
Paromomycin sulfate	500 mg	
Polymyxin B sulfate	70 mg	
Vancomycin hydrochloride	250 mg	
Regimen B		Every 4 hours
Gentamicin sulfate	200 mg	
Vancomycin hydrochloride	250 mg	
Antifungal agents		Every 4 hours
Amphotericin B	500 mg	
Nystatin	3.6 million units	
Candicidin	100 mg	
Topical Antibiotic		
Spray a		Apply 4 times daily to nose and throat
Neomycin sulfate	100 mg	
Vancomycin hydrochloride	10 mg	
Polymyxin B sulfate	5 mg	
Ointment b		Apply 4 times daily to gums, ears, anterior nares, groin, and perianal areas
Neomycin sulfate	50 mg	
Nystatin	25,000 units	
Vancomycin hydrochloride	5 mg	
Polymyxin B sulfate	2.5 mg	
Antibiotic gel b		Apply into rectum and vagina twice daily
Neomycin sulfate	100 mg	
Nystatin	50,000 units	
Vancomycin hydrochloride	10 mg	
Polymyxin B sulfate	5 mg	
Bacteriostatic Soap Baths		Twice daily
Iodinated soap (G.S.I.) or pHisoHex or P-300		

a Antibiotic concentration per milliliter.
b Antibiotic concentration per gram.

Table 10-4. Effect of Prophylactic Regimens on Bacterial and Fungal Organisms

Body Site	Total Bacterial Strains Isolated	Percent Eliminated	Total Fungal Strains Isolated	Percent Eliminated
Stools	841	97	87	44
Throat	340	80	19	5
Ears	205	82	5	80
Nose	201	81	1	0
Vagina	89	96	6	67
Skin	585	75	23	52

Table 10-5. Effect of Prophylactic Measures on the Microbial Flora of Body Sites

Body Site	Percent of Patients with			
	Persistently Sterile Cultures	Persistent Pathogenic Bacteria	Persistent Fungi	Newly Acquired Organisms
Stool	24	16	66	48
Throat	3	25	60	80
Ears	32	2	7	62
Nose	32	9	7	53
Vagina	60	13	30	43
Skin	2	33	40	87

roids, *Bacillus* species, and *Staphylococcus epidermidis*. However, potentially pathogenic organisms persisted in the stool, throat, and skin cultures of a substantial number of patients. Most of the organisms, newly acquired on one body site by the patients after they entered the protected environment units, had been present on another body site prior to entry. However, 43 patients acquired new potential pathogens such as *Klebsiella* species, *P. aeruginosa,* and *Candida* species. Only two patients acquired new organisms that had been cultured from the protected environment unit before they were cultured from the patients. The newly acquired organisms were cultured from 16 of the 43 patients within the first week after entry into the units. This suggests that these organisms were present on the patients prior to entry but our culture methods failed to detect them. However, 19 patients acquired new organisms after prolonged periods of time in the protected environment units and the source of these organisms could not be identified.

Remission Induction Studies in Acute Leukemia
The most important consideration in the use of a protected environment-prophylactic antibiotic (PEPA) program is whether it protects the patient from infectious complications. Most studies of the PEPA program have been conducted in patients undergoing remission induction chemotherapy for acute leukemia. Our original study compared the results in 33 leukemic patients treated while on the program with matched control patients [4]; 76% of the PEPA patients never developed a major infection, compared to 58% of the control patients. Fatality from infection was 9% among the PEPA patients and 21% among the controls. The amount of time spent with a neutrophil count of less than 100 per cubic millimeter was 33% for the PEPA patients, but only 14% for the control patients. Since the frequency of major infectious complications is related to the severity and duration of neutropenia, the patients on the PEPA program were at greater risk. Hence the proportion of days spent with infection was calculated in rela-

tion to the neutrophil count (Table 10-6). At every level of circulating neutrophils, the proportion of days spent with both local and major infection was lower for the PEPA patients.

The complete remission rates for the two groups of patients were not significantly different, but they also favored the PEPA patients (61% versus 49%). However, the differences in duration of remission and survival were significantly different. The median duration of complete remission was 55 weeks for the PEPA patients and 26 weeks for the control patients (P < 0.05). This difference was presumably due to the fact that the patients on the PEPA program received more intensive chemotherapy, since they had less frequent infectious complications. The median duration of survival was 34 weeks and 23 weeks, respectively (P < 0.05).

Subsequently we initiated a prospective randomized trial of the PEPA program during remission induction therapy of acute leukemia to extend our earlier experience [16]. When a protected environment unit was available, patients were randomized to receive induction chemotherapy in a protected environment unit with oral prophylactic antibiotics (PEPA), with parenteral antibiotics (PESA), or outside a protected environment unit with parenteral antibiotics (SA). When no protected environment unit was available, patients were randomized to receive oral antibiotics (PA) or parenteral antibiotics (SA). Seventy-two patients were entered on this study at the time of the analysis.

Since the numbers are too small in each group for meaningful comparisons, the patients are combined as follows: PEPA + PESA versus SA + PA, and PEPA + PA versus PESA + SA. The proportion of patients treated in and out of the protected environment units who developed major infectious complications was similar (Table 10-7). However, only 14% of the former group developed fatal infections compared to 32% of the latter group. Also, patients treated in the protected environment units had fewer episodes of

Table 10-6. Frequency of Infection Related to Neutrophil Count

	PEPA Patients			Control Patients		
Neutrophil Count/mm³	Total Days	Percent Days with Local Infection	Percent Days with Major Infection	Total Days	Percent Days with Local Infection	Percent Days with Major Infection
Less than 100	555	20 a	18	328	27 a	21
101 to 1000	842	10 a	7 a	1036	14 a	14 a
More than 1000	460	9	8 a	1074	10	14 a

PEPA = protected environment, prophylactic antibiotic.
a Statistically significant differences between PEPA and control patients.

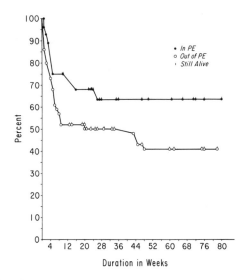

Figure 10-1. Survival of patients following onset of remission induction chemotherapy for acute leukemia. The small lines indicate the period of observation for patients who are still alive.

major infection per patient and a lower proportion of days spent with infection, but these differences were not statistically significant. The complete remission rates for patients treated in and out of the protected environment units were 71% and 45%, respectively (P = 0.06). There were no differences in the duration of remission between these two groups, but only 9 of the 40 patients relapsed. The differences in the duration of survival were statistically significant, favoring the patients treated in protected environments, as shown in Figure 10-1 (P = 0.04). Although there were no statistically significant differences between the PA and SA groups, the results consistently favored the SA group (Table 10-7). Hence this study also indicates that the PEPA program is beneficial and suggests that parenteral antibiotic prophylaxis is superior to oral antibiotic prophylaxis.

Several other comparative studies of remission induction therapy in patients with acute leukemia have been completed recently. All these studies have demonstrated that patients treated with the PEPA program develop fewer major infections than controls [13, 17, 21]. The proportion of days spent with major infection also is lower in the PEPA patients (Table 10-8). In one of these studies, the complete remission rate was higher for the PEPA patients, which is in agreement with the results of our current study. Also, the duration of survival has been better for the PEPA patients than for control patients in these studies.

A variety of studies has been reported in which oral prophylactic antibiotics have been administered to patients receiving antileukemic therapy

Table 10-7. Preliminary Results of Prospective Randomized Remission Induction Study

	In PE		Out of PE		PA		SA	
	No.	%	No.	%	No.	%	No.	%
Patients entered	28		44		29		43	
Patients developing major infection	15	54	27	61	18	62	24	56
Episodes per patient	0.6		0.8		0.8		0.7	
Fatal infections	4	14	14	32	7	24	11	26
Days on study	1611		1938		1390		2159	
Days with < 100 neutrophils/mm^3	627	39	872	45	633	46	866	40
Days with major infection	204	13	369	19	273	20	300	14
Patients achieving complete remission	20	71	20	45	14	48	26	60

PE = protected environment; PA = prophylactic antibiotic; SA = parenteral antibiotics.

in conventional hospital rooms. The majority of these studies compare the infectious complications in this group of patients with nonrandomized, unmatched, control patients whose histories were all that was seen [8, 11, 14]. Even in prospective randomized studies, the results have been conflicting. For example, Levine et al. found no differences in infectious complications between patients receiving prophylactic antibiotics and control patients [17], whereas Schimpff et al. found substantial differences favoring the former group [13]. However, these latter favorable results are tempered by the fact that these investigators have observed an increase in the number of antibiotic resistant organisms on their wards [9]. Presumably, this is a consequence of the use of oral prophylactic antibiotics and represents a threat, not only to the patients receiving prophylaxis but also to all other patients exposed to these resistant organisms. Because of the conflicting results and the potential hazard, oral antibiotic prophylaxis for patients outside protected environment units should not be recommended.

Remission Consolidation Therapy
The favorable results obtained during remission induction therapy led us to investigate the PEPA program during early consolidation therapy. The objective of this study was to attempt to administer several courses of intensive chemotherapy early in remission, when the number of leukemic cells was greatly reduced and before the remaining cells developed resistance. It was anticipated that this approach might result in prolonged, complete remissions. Twenty-six patients who had achieved complete remission with vincristine, prednisone, and arabinosyl cytosine (OAP) were eligible for this study. Following one course of maintenance therapy, the patients were randomized to receive their early consolidation therapy in one of the following groups: PEPA, protected environment without oral

Table 10-8. Summary of Studies of the PEPA Program during Remission Induction Therapy of Acute Leukemia

Study	Percent Days Spent with Infection at Neutrophil Count/mm³			Percent Patients with Major Infection	Percent Patients with Fatal Infection	Percent Patients Achieving Complete Remission
	< 100	101–1000	> 1000			
PEPA Patients						
Levine et al. [13]	12	8	3	14	0	45
Yates and Holland [21]	9	—	—	25	5	33
Schimpff et al. [17]				17	17	54
Control Patients						
Levine et al. [13]	40	10	12	50	24	43
Yates and Holland [21]	12	—	—	80	19	31
Schimpff et al. [17]				62	52	24

prophylactic antibiotics (PE), oral prophylactic antibiotics without protected environment (PA), and controls. Six patients were not entered on the study because they had physical or psychological characteristics that prevented them from being placed into a protected environment unit. An additional seven patients were excluded because the study was abandoned after one patient died. Hence these 13 patients received conventional maintenance therapy with OAP plus BCG immunotherapy, and their remission duration and survival can be compared with that of the 13 patients who received early consolidation therapy followed by the same maintenance therapy.

Remission consolidation therapy consisted of three courses of OAP therapy. Dosage of arabinosyl cytosine was gradually escalated by increasing the duration of therapy from 6 to 8 to 10 days if the patient did not develop a major infectious complication. If major infection followed a course of therapy, the duration of arabinosyl cytosine administration was reduced to the previous dosage schedule, which had not been associated with infection. The interval between courses was determined by recovery from myelosuppressive toxicity.

The results of this study are summarized in Table 10-9. Five of the eight patients treated in the protected environment units received full escalation of arabinosyl cytosine up to 10 days during the third course, compared to only one of five patients treated outside the protected environment units. Four patients developed six episodes of major infection. One patient in the PEPA group and one in the control group experienced two episodes of major infection. Five of the six infections were caused by gram-negative bacilli and one control patient developed toxoplasmosis. The proportion of days spent with major infection was substantially higher for the control group. The proportion of days spent with severe neutropenia was similar

Table 10-9. Results of Early Consolidation Therapy

	PEPA	PE	PA	Control
Patients entered	6	2	3	2
Patients escalated fully	3	2	0	1
Patients developing major infection	1	1	1	1
Episodes per patient	0.3	0.5	0.3	1.0
Fatal infections	0	1	0	0
Days on study	540	148	209	167
Days with < 100 neutrophils/mm^3	104	36	62	36
Percent days with major infection	6	7	7	14
Percent days with major infection and < 100 neutrophils/mm^3	4	28	23	28

PEPA = protected environment, prophylactic antibiotic; PE = protected environment; PA = prophylactic antibiotic.

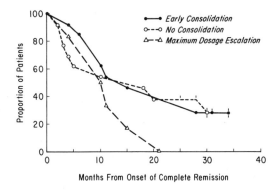

Figure 10-2. Duration of complete remission from onset of remission for patients with acute leukemia. Comparison between 13 patients who received early consolidation therapy and 13 patients who received only conventional maintenance therapy.

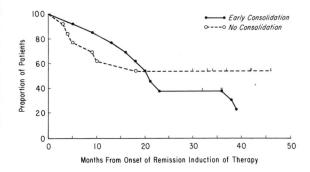

Figure 10-3. Duration of survival for patients on the early consolidation study compared to patients who received only conventional maintenance therapy.

in all groups, but the PEPA patients spent substantially less of this time with major infection. One patient in the PE group developed fatal *E. coli* septicemia, which resulted in the abandonment of this study. Although only a few patients were entered, the results consistently favored the patients in the PEPA group over the control group.

Unfortunately, early consolidation therapy did not improve duration of complete remission or survival (Figures 10-2 and 10-3). The median duration of remission was 15 months for the patients who received early consolidation therapy and 18 months for the patients who received only conventional maintenance therapy. Even for those patients who received maximum dosage escalation during early consolidation, the median duration of remission was only 11 months. The median duration of survival was 21 months for the former group and more than 30 months for the latter group. It is possible that early consolidation therapy interfered with recovery of im-

munologic competence following induction therapy. Host immune mechanisms appear to assist in preventing recurrence of leukemia, and BCG
immunotherapy during remission has been demonstrated to prolong the
duration of chemotherapy-maintained remissions [10].

Late Intensification Therapy

Late intensification therapy has been a most encouraging approach to pro-
longing remissions in patients with acute leukemia. The objective of this
study is to administer several courses of intensive chemotherapy with new
agents when the number of leukemic cells is at a minimum. Hopefully, this
therapy might eliminate the "last" leukemic cell and cure the patient. Nine-
teen patients who had been in continuous complete remission on maintenance therapy for 1 to 2 years were given three courses of therapy at gradually escalating doses [3]. Most of the patients received the combination of
vincristine, prednisone, 6-mercaptopurine, and methotrexate (POMP). The
interval between courses depended on recovery from the toxicity of the
previous course. On completion of the late intensification therapy, these
patients received no further chemotherapy, although 12 received BCG immunotherapy. All 19 patients received their late intensification therapy
while on the PEPA program to minimize the risk of infectious complications.

Sixteen of the 19 patients completed three courses of late intensification
therapy and the majority were able to tolerate dosage escalation during
subsequent courses. The duration of remission and survival for these 19
patients is shown in Figure 10-4. The median duration of complete remission following cessation of late intensification therapy has not been reached
but will exceed 30 months. Likewise, the median total duration of remission
has not been reached but will exceed 45 months. Only eight of these patients have relapsed, at 19 to 68 months from the onset of complete remission. All the remaining 11 patients have been in remission for at least 46
months with a median observation period of 67 months. Thirteen patients

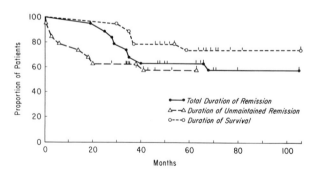

Figure 10-4. Results of late intensification therapy in 19 patients with acute leukemia.

are still alive and the median observation period for these patients is 68 months.

Toxicity from late intensification therapy consisted primarily of myelo-suppression and liver impairment. Myelosuppression occurred in 17 of the 19 patients. The patients spent a median of 46% of the late intensification period with a neutrophil count less than 1000 per cubic millimeter and 15%, with a neutrophil count less than 100 per cubic millimeter. Six patients developed fever during periods of neutropenia, but none had documented infections. Eleven patients developed transient liver function abnormalities and seven developed stomatitis.

Since myelosuppressive toxicity was generally not severe and no patients developed documented infections, the PEPA program is no longer used during late intensification therapy. Subsequent experience has indicated that the PEPA program is not necessary. However, it is unlikely that we would have initiated a study of intensive chemotherapy for patients in re-mission without being able to minimize the potential risk of infectious com-plications until the magnitude of that risk was known.

Future Prospects for Prophylaxis of Infection in Patients with Acute Leukemia

All the studies conducted in patients undergoing remission induction therapy for acute leukemia have demonstrated beneficial effects from the PEPA program. However, since infections still occur in patients on this program, further research is necessary to develop more effective regimens for patient sterilization. Neutropenia and other impairments in host defense mecha-nisms are associated with other disease processes, and these patients may also benefit from a similar program. Studies are currently in progress to ascertain the value of the PEPA program in patients undergoing chemo-therapy for other types of malignant diseases. The ultimate role of this tool for prevention and localization of infection awaits future investigations.

References

1. Bodey, G. P., et al. Quantitative relationships between circulating leukocytes and infection in patients with acute leukemia. *Ann. Intern. Med.* 64:328, 1966.
2. Bodey, G. P., Freireich, E. J., and Frei, E., III. Studies of patients in a laminar air flow unit. *Cancer* 24:972, 1969.
3. Bodey, G. P., et al. Late intensification Therapy for patients with acute leukemia in remission. *J.A.M.A.* 235:1021, 1976.
4. Bodey, G. P., et al. Protected environment—prophylactic antibiotic program in the chemotherapy of acute leukemia. *Am. J. Med. Sci.* 262:138, 1971.
5. Bodey, G. P., et al. Studies of a patient isolator unit and prophylactic anti-biotics in cancer chemotherapy. *Cancer* 22:1018, 1968.
6. Bodey, G. P., and Johnston, D. Microbiological evaluation of protected en-vironments during patient occupancy. *Appl. Microbiol.* 22:828, 1971.
7. Bodey, G. P., and Rosenbaum, B. Effect of prophylactic measures on the

microbial flora of patients in protected environment units. *Medicine* 53:209, 1974.

8. Dietrich, M., et al. Antimicrobial therapy as part of the decontamination procedures for patients with acute leukemia. *Eur. J. Cancer* 9:443, 1973.

9. Greene, W. H., et al. *Pseudomonas aeruginosa* resistant to carbenicillin and gentamicin. *Ann. Intern. Med.* 79:684, 1973.

10. Gutterman, J. U., et al. Chemoimmunotherapy of adult acute leukemia: Prolongation of remission in myeloblastic leukemia with bacillus Calmette-Guerin. *Lancet* II:1405, 1974.

11. Keating, J. J., and Pennington, D. G. Prophylaxis against septicaemia in acute leukemia: The use of oral framycetin. *Med. J. Aust.* 2:213, 1973.

12. Kominos, S. D., et al. Introduction of *Pseudomonas aeruginosa* into a hospital via vegetables. *Appl. Microbiol.* 24:567, 1972.

13. Levine, A. S., et al. Protected environments and prophylactic antibiotics. A prospective controlled study of their utility in the therapy of acute leukemia. *N. Engl. J. Med.* 288:477, 1973.

14. Reiter, B., et al. Use of oral antimicrobials during remission induction in adult patients with acute nonlymphocytic leukemia (abstract). *Clin. Res.* 21:652, 1973.

15. Rengrose, R. E., et al. A hospital outbreak of *Serratia marcescens* associated with ultrasonic nebulizers. *Ann. Intern. Med.* 69:719, 1968.

16. Rodriguez, V̂., et al. Protected environments (PE) and prophylactic antibiotics in remission induction therapy of adults with acute leukemia (abstract). *Proc. Am. Assoc. Cancer Res.* 15:340, 1974.

17. Schimpff, S. C., et al. Infection prevention in acute nonlymphocytic leukemia. *Ann. Intern. Med.* 82:351, 1975.

18. Schneider, M., et al. Pathogen-free isolation unit—three years' experience. *Br. Med. J.* 1:836, 1969.

19. Schwartz, S. A., and Perry, S. Patient protection in cancer chemotherapy. *J.A.M.A.* 197:623, 1966.

20. Whitfield, W. J. Microbiological studies of laminar air flow rooms. Sandia Corp. reprint SC-DC-66-2277. Albuquerque. N.M., September 1966.

21. Yates, J. W., and Holland J. F. A controlled study of isolation and endogenous microbial suppression in acute myelocytic leukemia patients. *Cancer* 32:1490, 1973.

11. Changes in Host Defenses in the Immunosuppressed Patient After Kidney Transplantation

Peter J. Morris

Nonspecific and specific immunity against infection may be suppressed in many conditions, such as congenital immune deficiency diseases, Hodgkin's disease, major burns, chemotherapy for cancer, or suppression of graft rejection. This may be due to suppression of any one of a number of mechanisms involved in the host's defenses against infections. Many of these problems are discussed elsewhere in this symposium, and this paper will confine remarks to the effects of azathioprine and steroids on these defense mechanisms, for these drugs form the backbone of immunosuppressive drug therapy in renal transplantation.

There is no doubt that patients receiving azathioprine and prednisolone after renal transplantation have defective defenses against infection, for infection is the commonest cause of death in these patients. We are all aware that viral and fungal infections, which we tend to attribute to a depression of cell-mediated immunity, are seen frequently in such patients [3, 10, 27, 32, 44, 46, 55, 56, 57, 61, 63, 64] but it should not be forgotten that bacterial infections are also a major problem in transplant patients. This is well illustrated by the Australasian renal transplant registry figures, where infection is the major single cause of death. However, death has been attributed to bacterial infection more often than viral and fungal infections (Figure 11-1). These figures probably attribute a falsely low cause of death to viruses and fungi, particularly in the early years of transplantation, where viral and fungal identification was often inadequate; but they do show that there is an increased susceptibility to all infections in patients on immunosuppressive drug therapy after transplantation.

I intend to discuss changes that occur in specific immunologic host defenses, namely cellular and humoral immunity, in immunosuppressed transplant patients, and then briefly describe the available information about nonspecific immune mechanisms, such as polymorph and macrophage function, interferon, and complement.

Cellular Immunity

There is a considerable amount of information available concerning changes in various immunologic responses in patients who are suppressed with azathioprine and steroids after renal transplantation. There is also supple-

Part of the work described in this paper was supported by the National Health and Medical Research Council of Australia and the Medical Research Council of England.

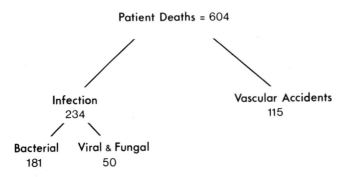

Renal Allografts = 1889

Patient Deaths = 604

Infection
234

Vascular Accidents
115

Bacterial
181

Viral & Fungal
50

Figure 11-1. Australasian Transplant Registry figures, showing that infection is the major single cause of death following renal transplantation. (By permission of Professor A. G. R. Sheil.)

mentary information concerning the effect of azathioprine alone in different immunopathic diseases.

We have studied a number of aspects of cellular immunity in 77 patients who were surviving with a functioning renal transplant from 6 months to 6 years after transplantation [59]. These patients were being treated with daily maintenance doses of immunosuppressive drugs, namely 2.5 mg/kg of azathioprine and 10 mg per day of prednisolone. Antilymphocyte globulin was not used in these patients.

The following immunologic assessments of cellular immunity were performed: absolute lymphocyte counts, T and B cell estimations, PHA responsiveness of peripheral blood lymphocytes, skin tests with *Candida,* PPD, mumps *Trichophyton,* and DNCB.

Thymus Derived (T) and Bone Marrow Derived (B) Lymphocytes
Lymphocytes were isolated from heparinized blood using an Isopaque-Ficoll gradient [8]. The number of T cells in peripheral blood was estimated by counting the lymphocytes forming rosettes with sheep red cells as described by Jondal, Holm, and Wigzell [31]. B cells were estimated by the presence of immunoglobulin receptors using immunofluorescent labeling, again as described by Jondal et al. [31]. These results in the transplant patients were compared with those obtained from 19 healthy volunteers.

First, there was a significant lymphopenia in the transplant patients, since the mean lymphocyte count in these patients was approximately half of that in the controls (Table 11-1). This lymphopenia appeared to be due to a decrease in T cells, while the absolute number of B cells remained un-

Table 11-1. The Distribution of T and B Cells in Normal Subjects and in Renal Transplant Patients at Times Ranging from 6 to 72 Months after Transplantation

Cells	Normals	Transplants
Lymphocytes/mm³	2100 ± 300	788 ± 608
T cells (%)	48.1 ± 10.1	47.4 ± 14.9
B Cells (%)	23 ± 4.5	38.2 ± 14.2

changed. Thus the normal ratio of T to B cells of 2 : 1 was reduced in the transplant patients, which was less marked in patients who were transplanted at least 2 years before these studies (Table 11-2). These results are in contrast to those of Campbell et al. [11], who found a modest but significant lymphopenia in patients with inflammatory bowel disease, who had been treated with azathioprine (2.5 mg/kg) alone for 1 year, whose ratio of T and B cells was not altered. This difference might be due to the prednisolone given to the transplant patients. There are no data concerning T and B cell distribution in patients on long-term steroid therapy, but both Fauci and Dale [19] and Yu et al. [74] have shown that a single dose of prednisolone or hydrocortisone will produce a lymphopenia, in which a depression is predominantly found in the T lymphocytes.

PHA Response

The response to PHA (Burroughs Wellcome) in doses of 5, 20, and 100 μg was measured by the uptake of tritiated thymidine at 72 hours [20]. Any response falling below the level of 1 standard deviation of an established control group was considered to be depressed. Only 17 (26%) of the 65 patients tested showed suppressed PHA responses. Thus if PHA responsiveness is considered an index of T cell function [13, 52, 53] then the majority of these patients did not show a depression of T cell function despite their apparent decrease in T cell numbers.

There is a great variation in the reports of PHA responsiveness in pa-

Table 11-2. The Ratio of T to B Cells in Normal Subjects and in Kidney Transplant Patients at Different Times After Transplantation. Only the Altered Ratio for the Most Recently Transplanted Group is Significantly Altered Because of the Wide Variance in the Other Groups

Group	Number	Mean T : B Ratio
Normals	19	2.08 : 1
Transplants	75	1.54 : 1
6–18 months	25	1.40 : 1 *
18–30 months	26	1.62 : 1
30–72 months	24	1.69 : 1

* $P < 0.05$.

tients receiving azathioprine, either with or without steroids. Moderate suppression of PHA responses after transplantation was found by Ming, Ming, and Dammin [45], while they were found to be unchanged by Abdou, Zweiman, and Casella [1] and Daniels et al. [15]. Denman et al. [18] also found that patients with rheumatoid arthritis or Still's disease had depressed PHA responses, but they returned to normal after treatment with azathioprine. In our studies PHA responsiveness was reduced in 75% of our dialysis patients before transplantation, compared to 26% after transplantation, suggesting that uremia has a much greater depressive effect on PHA responsiveness than the maintenance doses of azathioprine and steroids used in these patients. This marked depression of PHA responsiveness in uremic patients has been noted by many workers [29, 47], and this depression has been attributed to a dialyzable factor in uremic serum by Newberry and Sanford [48]. However, Kasakura and Lowenstein [33] found no reduction in PHA response in uremia, nor any effect of uremic plasma on PHA response, but did show a reduction in the response of uremic lymphocytes to allogeneic cells. Thus, in general, it is reasonable to conclude that PHA responsiveness, an in vitro measure of T cell function, is depressed in only a relatively small proportion of patients receiving azathioprine and small maintenance doses of prednisolone.

Skin Testing

Further testing of cellular immunity was carried out by delayed hypersensitivity skin tests with *Candida* (Bencard), mumps (Eli Lilly), *Trichophyton* (Bencard), tuberculin 1 : 1,000 (Commonwealth Serum Laboratories), and to primary skin sensitization with 0.1 ml solutions of 50 μg and 2,000 μg of dinitrochlorobenzene (DNCB) in acetone. The DNCB reactions were graded 0 to 4 as described elsewhere [59].

The hypersensitivity skin reactions were depressed to a striking extent in the transplant patients, compared to the normals, and gave a mean of 0.6 positive reactions per patient, compared to 2.5 positive reactions in the normal volunteers (Table 11-3). Thirty six patients gave no reaction to any of the antigens. On the other hand, the mean DNCB reaction score was 2.9, which does not represent a marked depression of this primary sensitization reaction. Only three normals were tested as controls and their mean reaction score was 3.7. This discrepancy between the skin reactions to the four antigens that represent secondary responses and the primary sensitization to DNCB is difficult to explain on immunologic grounds, since it would be expected that the primary response would be easier to suppress than the sensitized response. The low reaction rate to the skin-test antigens might be explained on technical grounds, for the skin of these patients is particularly fragile because of their steroid therapy. It is difficult therefore to give a true intradermal injection, and injection of the test antigen subcutaneously would tend to give falsely negative results. However, Toh et al. [70] did show suppression of delayed hypersensitivity responses to five skin-test

Table 11-3. The Results of Skin Hypersensitivity Reactions in 33 Normal Subjects and 60 Kidney Transplant Patients, and DNCB Responses in 3 Normal Subjects and 51 Transplant Patients

	Percent Normals [a]	Percent Transplants [a]
Candida	63	18
Mumps	66	15
Trichophyton	36	8
Tuberculin	82	22
Positive reactions per subject	2.5	0.6
Mean DNCB score [b]	3.7	2.9

[a] The number of patients giving a positive reaction is expressed as a percentage of those tested.
[b] Out of a possible 4.0.

antigens in patients with autoimmune disorders on azathioprine and prednisolone but not in patients on prednisolone alone, where, presumably, fragile skin would have been a problem again. Thus the skin-test reactions in our patients may have been genuinely negative, while the minimal depression to DNCB may be due to the very strong nature of this form of primary sensitization. Maibach and Epstein [42] also failed to show a depression of contact sensitivity to DNCB in volunteers receiving 100 mg azathioprine per day.

In general, then, these studies of cellular immunity showed a reduction of the numbers of T cells and a spectrum of responses to various T cell functions. Bacterial infections occurred in 42% of these patients, while viral and fungal infections occurred in 22%. Correlations were sought between the occurrence of such infections and the various immune responses tested. Significant associations at the 5% level were seen between susceptibility to viral infections and depression of the T cell count and PHA response in the same patient, while negative *Candida* responses were significantly associated with an increased incidence of mucocutaneous candidiasis. However, these associations were not striking, bearing in mind that the comparison of a large number of variables, as here, can lead to the occurrence of some significant associations by chance. Of some interest was the failure to observe any association between the development of cancers (mostly skin cancers), which occurred in seven patients (9%), and a depression of the various immune responses.

Cellular immune responses have been studied in other situations in patients receiving azathioprine with or without steroids. However, these patients generally had autoimmune diseases, which makes it more difficult to evaluate the role of azathioprine and steroids in an uncomplicated situation. For example, Swanson and Schwartz [66] showed that the delayed hypersensitivity reaction to keyhole-limpet hemocyanin, following a primary injection at the commencement of azathioprine therapy, was suppressed. Toh et al. [70], in their study of inpatients with a variety of autoimmune disorders, found that azathioprine and prednisolone therapy significantly suppressed skin-test reactions, while prenisolone in doses of 3 to 20 mg per day did not. Similarly, Dawkins and Mastaglia [16] found that patients with polymyositis, treated with either prednisolone in doses greater than 20 mg per day or azathioprine 150 mg per day, showed a suppression of direct lymphocyte cytotoxicity directed against target muscle cells, while lesser doses of prednisolone had no effect. Again, skin hypersensitivity reactions were suppressed by the larger immunosuppressive doses only. However, Folb and Trounce [21] have studied the response of *Candida* in transplant patients on azathioprine and prednisolone. They found that the response of lymphocytes in culture was significantly depressed but that the humoral response, as measured by agglutinating and fluorescent antibodies, was normal. Debray-Sachs et al. [17] measured the response of transplant recipient lymphocytes to allogeneic lymphocytes, both from the living related donor and unrelated third parties. All patients were receiving azathioprine only. Seven of the eight patients tested gave normal expected responses.

I can draw only tentative conclusions from data of this type, but in general they suggest that the combined therapy of azathioprine and prednisolone suppresses cellular immunity to a variable extent in different patients and that the most marked features of this suppression that can be demonstrated are the absolute reduction in T cells and the depression of hypersensitivity skin reactions.

Certainly the common occurrence of viral and fungal infections in transplant patients is strong indirect evidence that cellular immunity is depressed. That specific cellular immunity is a major defense mechanism against viral infection has been convincingly demonstrated in a number of experimental models. For example, Blanden [6] has shown that mice treated with antithymocyte serum before subcutaneous injection of ectromelia virus (a member of the pox virus group, which gives rise to mousepox, a generalized disease) showed a greatly increased mortality, although the neutralizing antibody and interferon responses were not impaired, nor was the ability of macrophages to clear blood-borne viruses in these mice (Figure 11-2). The main activity of such an antithymocyte serum would be to suppress the cellular arm of the immune response. This definitive role of cellular immunity was elegantly confirmed by Blanden [7] by showing that spleen cells, but not serum, from immune donors, could suppress ectromelia virus growth in the infected nonimmune recipient and that this protective effect of the immune spleen cells was abolished by treatment of the cells with anti-θ ascitic fluid. Hirsch and Murphy [28] have studied the effect of antilymphocyte serum on a number of viral infections in mice and, in general, found that the extent of the disease, mortality, and oncogenesis were increased, suggesting that cellular immunity was an important factor

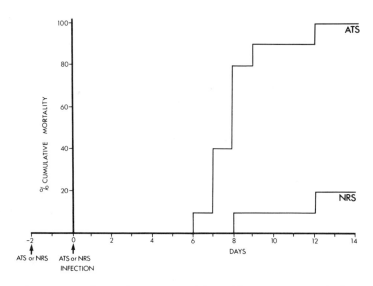

Figure 11-2. Effects of treatment with antithymocyte serum before subcutaneous injection of ectromelia virus (mousepox) showing greatly increased mortality in presence of antithymocyte serum. (From Blanden, R. V. Mechanisms of recovery from a generalized viral infection: Mousepox. I. The effects of anti-thymocyte serum. *J. Exp. Med.* 132:1035, 1970).

in the host's defense mechanisms in these viral infections. Volkert and Lundstedt [72] have also shown that ALS treatment of mice that have recovered from a lymphocytic choriomeningitis (LCM) viral infection leads to a marked reactivation of the infection with viremia in the presence of normal complement-fixing antibody titers. Bach et al. [4] have shown in man an alarming incidence of viral and fungal infections in renal transplant patients treated with antilymphocyte globulin in addition to azathioprine and prednisolone, and they attribute this reaction mainly to the use of antilymphocyte globulin.

Cellular immunity also plays an important role in the host defense mechanisms against obligatory intracellular bacteria [37, 38, 43]. This has been demonstrated in experimental mouse models using *Mycobacterium ulcerans, Mycobacterium leprae, Mycobacterium tuberculosis,* and *Listeria monocytogenes.* In these infections the cellular immune response leads to activation of macrophages, which in turn are responsible for bacterial destruction. If cellular immunity is depressed, then the macrophages fail to take part in the response. It is of interest that an immune response to one intracellular bacterium will increase the resistance to infection with another such bacterium at the height of the immune response, showing that once macrophages have been activated, their action is not specific for the bacteria triggering the initial immune responses [5]. North [49] has shown that a single injection of cortisone given to mice at the time of infection with *L. mono-*

cytogenes leads to unrestricted bacterial multiplication, but he attributes this to suppression of macrophage division and the delay in accumulation at the foci of infection rather than to the suppression of cellular immunity.

The intracellular bacterial infections have not proved to be a frequent problem in renal transplant patients, but tubercular and listerial infections are a serious and often lethal complication when they do occur.

Humoral Immunity

Specific antibody plays a major role in the host's defenses against most bacterial infections but a less important role in intracellular bacterial, viral, and fungal infections. The major action of antibody against bacteria is one of opsonization, thus facilitating adherence of the coated bacterium to the polymorph or macrophage allowing phagocytosis. This action is mediated by IgG, for IgM-coated bacteria adhere weakly to macrophage surfaces. Complement also augments this effect, since there are complement receptor sites on the macrophage surface as well as IgG receptor sites. Certain types of gram-negative bacteria that have a lipoprotein outer wall are susceptible to lysis by antibody and complement, and in this situation IgM is quite efficient. Antibody can also neutralize viruses by spatially inhibiting their attachment to cell surface receptors, preventing infection of a cell. Antibody provides its greatest protective effect in those viral infections where the virus has to travel through the bloodstream before it reaches the tissue that it finally infects. Poliomyelitis provides such an example.

The effect of azathioprine and steroids on antibody production is unpredictable, and this may be explained by the large number of studies of antibody responses that have been carried out in patients with immunopathologic disorders treated with these drugs. Swanson and Schwartz [66] tested patients with autoimmune disorders and found that the primary response to keyhole-limpet hemocyanin comprised a prolonged IgM response with no IgG response, while a secondary response to diphtheria toxoid was completely suppressed. The immunosuppressive effect was unrelated to the leukopenia that occurred in some patients. Similarly, Stocker, McKenzie, and Morris [65] found that the lymphocytotoxic response to histocompatibility antigens was converted from IgG before transplantation to IgM after transplantation in patients on azathioprine and prednisolone, while Tiong and Morris [68] found that the rise in heterophil antibody titer that occurred after renal transplantation was an IgM response only. Rowley, Mackay, and McKenzie [60] showed that although the primary response to monomeric flagellin from *Salmonella adelaide* was mainly IgM, both in transplant patients on azathioprine and steroids and in healthy volunteers, the secondary response was predominantly IgM in the transplant patients compared to IgG in controls. However, the same group failed to show any difference in the response to flagellin in patients with autoimmune disease who were treated with azathioprine and steroids [35]. Maibach and Epstein [42], using normal volunteers, showed that azathioprine produced some depression of the primary response to plague vaccine but completely suppressed the secondary and, presumably, IgG response. Denman et al. [18] also found a normal antibody response to influenza virus, tetanus toxoid, and *Brucella* in rheumatoid patients treated with azathioprine at dosage levels sufficient to maintain a persistent lymphocytopenia. Taylor and Morris [67] found that renal transplant patients on azathioprine and steroids gave a greater spectrum of responses to vaccination with influenza virus during an epidemic than normal controls, since more patients than controls failed to mount a response at all to one vaccination.

In an interesting recent study Mackay, Dwyer, and Rowley [39] showed that the humoral response to flagellin in patients with immunopathic disorders treated with azathioprine was depressed only moderately, although there was relatively more IgM present. The numbers of lymphocytes binding iodinated flagellin, presumably B cells, were unchanged. Levy et al. [36] demonstrated that azathioprine does not alter immunoglobulin levels but that immunoglobulin synthesis is moderately reduced, from which he concludes that the constant level of immunoglobulins is maintained by decreased catabolism.

These changes in antibody responses have been demonstrated in many instances in patients treated with steroids in addition to azathioprine, but it seems reasonable to attribute the changes to azathioprine rather than to steroids. Although steroids inhibit antibody responses in steroid-sensitive species, such as the mouse and the rat, the responses in steroid-resistant species, such as man, guinea pig, and monkey, are inhibited only by very large doses of steroids [12]. However, Butler and Rossen [10] showed that a short course of predisolone causes a decrease in IgG due to increased catabolism, but this was not related to specific antibody production.

From this large amount of often contradictory data about humoral responses in patients treated with azathioprine either with or without steroids, it seems reasonable to conclude that such patients can mount a humoral response against antigenic challenge, but this response tends to comprise IgM rather than IgG, and that secondary responses, i.e., immunologic memory, may be abolished. That there will be a varying response to different antigens is not surprising, since azathioprine does appear to affect T cell functions rather than B cell functions in the human, as shown earlier in this chapter, and T cells in the mouse have been shown to be very sensitive to azathioprine [3]. Since many antibody responses are thymic dependent, it is these responses that will be depressed by azathioprine rather than the thymic independent antibody responses.

It is possible now to relate the above data to the susceptibility of renal transplant patients to bacterial infections. First, suppression of a secondary humoral response to bacterial infection will increase the susceptibility of such patients by delaying their response to infection. Second, the development of a humoral response that is predominantly IgM suppresses the ability of the host to opsonize invading bacteria, for IgM is a poor opsonizing antibody, as mentioned already. There are other nonspecific immune factors in the host's defense mechanisms against infection that may be altered, but depression of specific immunity against bacterial infections may be an important effect of azathioprine therapy.

Patients can mount a humoral response to viral infections, which is well illustrated in figures 11-3 and 11-4. A transplant patient in the early weeks of transplantation, at which time large doses of prednisolone and azathioprine are being administered, can mount both a primary response to cytomegalovirus (CMV) and a secondary response, due to reactivation of the virus. In this case the response is certainly due in part to IgG because the antibody titer is measured by complement fixation, and IgM is a poor complement fixer in this particular situation [69]. However, immunofluorescent assay shows that the IgM titer also rises. Reference has already been made to the role of cellular immunity in the host's defenses against viral infections, and the direct role of antibody is probably to limit systemic spread of the virus; thus the importance of this role will depend on the type of viral infection. For example, antibody provides the major line of defense against the spread of the poliomyelitis virus. However, in both CMV and herpes virus hominis infections, an elevation of antibody titer in the presence of continuing infections and continuing virus isolation or excretion may be seen in the immunosuppressed transplant patient (Figure 11-3, 11-4, and 11-5). This suggests that humoral antibody may not be of great importance in the host's defense mechanisms. Despite the above evidence, Simmons et al. [63] have suggested that the only patients to die of CMV infection after transplantation were those patients who failed to develop any antibody response to CMV, which might reflect a severe generalized immunodepression in such patients. However, there is a possible exception to this conclusion concerning the importance of humoral antibody, which is discussed separately in the next section.

Antibody-Mediated Cellular Immunity (AMCI)

This is an in vitro phenomenon [40] in which antibody is specifically attached to a target cell and then target cell killing is mediated by a population of lymphocytes that have receptors for determinants on the FC part of the antibody. The effector cells are known sometimes as K cells. They have some characteristics of B cells, but probably represent a separate mononuclear cell population. All the subclasses of IgG can take part in this phenomenon but IgM cannot. If this phenomenon is relevant to in vivo defense mechanisms, it could well be important in cells infected with virus, where viral expression on the cell surface would enable antibody to attach, thus allowing destruction of the infected target cell by K cell activity. Recent in vitro evidence suggests that such a mechanism might be important in viral infections. For example, Shore et al. [62] and Rager-Zisman and Bloom [54] have both shown that cells infected with herpes simplex virus

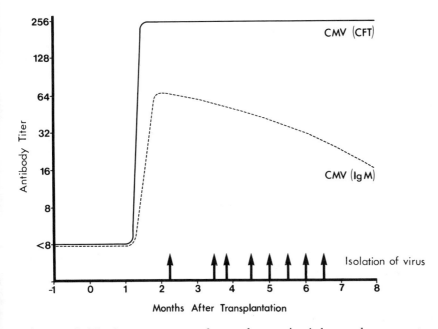

Figure 11-3. The immunosuppressed transplant patient's humoral response to cyto-megalovirus (CMV) infection.

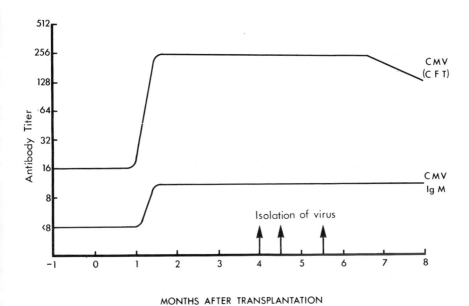

Figure 11-4. The immunosuppressed transplant patient's humoral response during reactivation of cytomegalovirus (CMV) infection.

168.

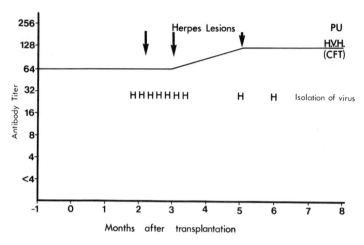

Figure 11-5. The occurrence of herpes virus hominis lesions in an immunosuppressed transplant patient in the presence of antibody.

may be destroyed by nonspecific effector cells in the presence of antibody directed against the virus.

If then AMCI does play a role in host defenses as discussed above, it is not difficult to envisage how immunosuppression might depress this activity. For example, the specific part of the reaction is dependent on IgG antibody. Thus if IgM is the predominant antibody response to many antigens in the presence of azathioprine treatment, then AMCI would be suppressed. That this might occur is suggested by studies of AMCI before and after transplantation [14, 71], for antibody against the major histocompatibility complex (HLA) could be demonstrated in all patients before transplantation but in virtually none after transplantation. This finding is most readily explained on the basis of the absence of IgG antibody, for the effector cells were from a normal unrelated donor with known K cell activity.

In addition, azathioprine appears to have a direct, suppressive effect on K cell activity. This was shown by Campbell et al. [11] in a series of patients with inflammatory bowel disease treated with azathioprine alone (Figure 11-6). Thus if AMCI is an important defense mechanism against viral infections, then azathioprine therapy can depress this type of response by two possible actions.

Nonspecific Defense Mechanisms
The polymorphonuclear leukocyte plays a major role in the host's bacterial defense mechanisms, because it can phagocytose bacteria and destroy them by lysozymal activity. Phagocytosis is enhanced by opsonization of the bacteria by antibody, as discussed previously. Defects in this mechanism can therefore be seen at the level of phagocytosis or at the level of bacterial

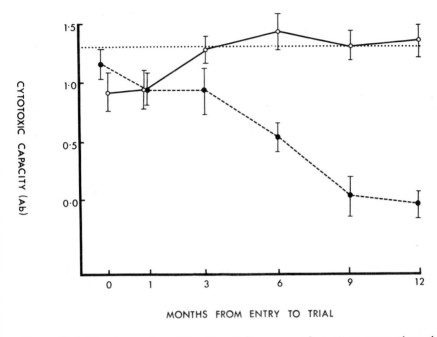

CYTOTOXIC CAPACITY (Ab)

MONTHS FROM ENTRY TO TRIAL

Figure 11-6. The depression of K cell activity expressed as mean cytotoxic activity in a series of patients with inflammatory bowel disease treated with azathioprine alone or a placebo. (From Campbell, A. C., et al. Immunosuppression in the treatment of inflammatory bowel disease. II. The effects of azathioprine on lymphoid cell populations in a double blind trial in ulcerative colitis. *Clin. Exp. Immunol.* 24:249, 1976.)

destruction in the phagolysosome. Defects in the latter mechanism are seen in the Chediak-Higashi anomaly, which results in increased susceptibility to bacterial infections. There is not a great deal of information about the effect of azathioprine on polymorph function, but it appears that polymorph function is not altered. For example, Baardsen, Midtvedt, and Trippestad [2] showed that the phagocytosis of *Escherichia coli* in germ-free rats was not altered by azathioprine. Similarly, MacLennan and Morris [41] have shown that polymorph function both in patients with inflammatory bowel disease treated with azathioprine and in patients in the early months after kidney transplantation is quite normal.

Although steroids do appear to reduce the polymorph infiltration of an acute inflammatory reaction [23, 73], their effect on polymorph function is variable. Fuenfer, Olson, and Polk [22] demonstrated differing effects on phagocytic-bactericidal activity of polymorphs, depending on the type of steroid tested. For example, hydrocortisone sodium succinate produced inhibition of this polymorph activity, while methylprednisolone did not produce any of these inhibitory effects. Thus the increased susceptibility of the immunosuppressed renal transplant patient cannot be attributed in general to defective polymorph function.

Reticuloendothelial function has been studied in more detail in immuno-suppressed animals and patients. 6-mercaptopurine, an active breakdown product of azathioprine, has been shown by several workers to reduce the monocyte infiltration of skin windows [30, 50]. However, in vivo clearance of colloidal gold in rabbits [34] and carbon particles in mice [25] is not altered by azathioprine. Palmer, Rifkind, and Brown [51] demonstrated that clearance of heat-aggregated serum albumin was relatively normal in renal transplant patients receiving azathioprine and steroids.

A number of studies of the effect of cortisone on the reticuloendothelial system have been reviewed by Germuth [23]; he concludes that cortisone inhibits the accumulation of macrophages in an inflammatory area, but he did not feel there was any convincing evidence that cortisone influences the functional activity of the reticuloendothelial system. However, more recently Rinehart et al. [58] have demonstrated an in vitro depression of monocyte bactericidal activity as well as decreased phagocytosis of crypto-cocci in the presence of hydrocortisone succinate or methylprednisolone succinate.

Two other important factors in the host's defense mechanisms are com-plement and interferon. Complement is needed for antibody-mediated lysis of bacteria or for the attachment of opsonized bacteria and antibody com-plement complexes to complement receptors on macrophages. However, there is no evidence that azathioprine or steroids affect complement activity. Interferon inhibits intracellular viral replication and is produced by cells themselves in response to viral infection. Thus interferon probably plays a role in recovery from viral infection. Interferon levels may be depressed by steroids [24, 26], depending on the nature of the viral infection, but were not altered in mice infected with ectromelia and treated with antilympho-cyte serum [6]. It seems unlikely that alteration in interferon production is a major factor in the increased susceptibility of transplant patients to viral infections.

Conclusion

A renal transplant patient treated with azathioprine and prednisolone to suppress renal allograft rejection represents a unique example of a patient in whom defense mechanisms against infection are altered by drugs in the absence of underlying disease (since this is corrected by the transplant). These patients are more susceptible to infection, which is the cause of one-third of deaths in renal transplant patients. Bacterial, viral, and fungal in-fections are all seen more frequently. The major changes produced by the immunosuppressive drugs are directed at specific immune responses, rather than nonspecific immunity mediated by such mechanisms as phagocytosis, interferon, complement, and lysozyme activity. Changes in both specific humoral and cellular immunity can be demonstrated. The more profound changes occur in cellular immunity as shown by a decrease in T cell numbers and depression of some T cell functions. This depression of cellular immunity explains the increased susceptibility of such patients to viral, fungal, and obligatory intracellular bacterial infections. The changes in humoral immunity are more subtle and vary from little change in antibody response to a shift toward IgM rather than IgG responses. This shift toward IgM antibody production has important implications, which need to be explored further, for these changes could result in inefficient opsonization of bacteria as well as a depression of antibody-mediated cellular immunity, a phenomenon that could be an important defense mechanism in viral infections.

Acknowledgments

I am grateful to my colleagues Ian MacLennan M.D., and John Tobin M.D., for allowing me to cite some of their unpublished work.

References

1. Abdou, N. I., Zweiman, B., and Casella, S. R. Effects of azathioprine therapy on bone marrow-dependent and thymus-dependent cells in man. *Clin. Exp. Immunol.* 13:55, 1973.
2. Baardsen, A., Midtvedt, T., and Trippestad, A. Influence of azathioprine on humoral defence factors against *Escherichia coli* in germ free and monocontaminated rats. *Acta Pathol. Microbiol. Scand.* Section B. 81:799, 1973.
3. Bach, J. F., and Dardenne, M. Antigen recognition by T lymphocytes: II. Similar effects of azathioprine, anti-lymphocyte serum, and anti-thetac serum on rosette-forming lymphocytes in normal and neonatally thymectomised mice. *Cell. Immunol.* 3:11, 1972.
4. Bach, M. C., et al. Influence of rejection therapy on fungal and nocardial infections on renal transplant recipients. *Lancet* I:180, 1973.
5. Blanden, R. V., Mackaness, G. B., and Collins, F. M. Mechanisms of acquired resistance in mouse typhoid. *J. Exp. Med.* 124:585, 1966.
6. Blanden, R. V. Mechanisms of recovery from a generalized viral infection: Mousepox. I. The effects of anti-thymocyte serum. *J. Exp. Med.* 132:1035, 1970.
7. Blanden, R. V. Mechanisms of recovery from a generalized viral infection: Mousepox. II. Passive transfer of recovery mechanism with immune lymphoid cells. *J. Exp. Med.* 133:1074, 1971.
8. Boyum, A. Isolation of mononuclear cells and granulocytes from human blood. *Scand. J. Clin. Lab. Invest.* 97(Suppl.):77, 1968.
9. Burton, J. R., et al. Aspergillosis in four renal transplant recipients. Diagnosis and effective treatment with amphotericin B. *Ann. Intern. Med.* 77:383, 1972.
10. Butler, W. T., and Rossen, R. D. Effects of corticosteroids on immunity in man. *J. Clin. Invest.* 52:2629, 1973.
11. Campbell, A. C., et al. Immunosuppression in the treatment of inflammatory bowel disease. II. The effects of azathioprine on lymphoid cell populations in a double blind trial in ulcerative colitis. *Clin. Exp. Immunol.* In press.
12. Claman, H. N. Corticosteroids and lymphoid cells. *N. Engl. J. Med.* 287:388, 1972.

13. Clot, J., Massip, H., and Mathieu, O. In vitro studies on human B and T cell purified populations. Stimulation by mitogens and allogeneic cells and quantitative binding of phytomitogens. *Immunology* 29:445, 1975.
14. d'Apice, A., and Morris, P. J. The role of antibody dependent cell mediated cytotoxicity in renal allograft rejection. *Transplantation* 18:20, 1974.
15. Daniels, J. C., et al. In vitro reactivity of human lymphocytes in chronic uraemia: Analysis and interpretation. *Clin. Exp. Immunol.* 8:213, 1971.
16. Dawkins, R. L., and Mastaglia, F. L. Cell-mediated cytotoxicity to muscle in polymyositis. Effect of immunosuppression. *N. Engl. J. Med.* 288:434, 1973.
17. Debray-Sachs, M., et al. Mixed lymphocyte culture in human renal allograft recipients. *Cell. Immunol.* 7:181, 1973.
18. Denman, E. J., et al. Failure of cytotoxic drugs to suppress immune responses of patients with rheumatoid arthritis. *Ann. Rheum. Dis.* 29:220, 1970.
19. Fauci, A. S., and Dale, D. C. The effect of in vivo hydrocortisone on subpopulations of human lymphocytes. *J. Clin. Invest.* 53:240, 1974.
20. Fitzgerald, M. G. The establishment of a normal human population dose response curve for lymphocytes cultured with PHA. *Clin. Exp. Immunol.* 8:421, 1971.
21. Folb, P. I., and Trounce, J. R. Immunological aspects of *Candida* infection complicating steroid and immunosuppressive drug therapy. *Lancet* II:112, 1970.
22. Fuenfer, M. M., Olson, G. E., and Polk, H. Effect of various corticosteroids upon the phagocytic bactericidal activity of neutrophils. *Surgery* 78:27, 1975.
23. Germuth, F. G. The role of adrenocortical steroids in infection, immunity and hypersensitivity. *Pharmacol. Rev.* 8:1, 1956.
24. Giron, D. J., et al. Further studies on the influence of steroids on viral infection in mice. *Am. Soc. Microbiol.* 8:151, 1973.
25. Gotjamanos, T. The effect of azathioprine on phagocytic activity and morphology of reticuloendothelial organs in mice. *Pathology* 3:171, 1971.
26. Haahr, S. The occurrence of virus and interferon in spleen, serum and brain in steroid-treated mice under experimental infection with West Nile virus. *Acta Pathol. Microbiol. Scand.* 75:303, 1969.
27. Hill, R. B., Rowlands, D. T., Jr., and Rifkind, D. Infectious pulmonary disease in patients receiving immunosuppressive therapy for organ transplantation. *N. Engl. J. Med.* 271:1021, 1964.
28. Hirsch, M. S., and Murphy, F. A. Effects of anti-lymphoid sera on viral infections. *Lancet* II:37, 1968.
29. Huber, H., et al. In vitro reactivity of human lymphocytes in uraemia—A comparison with the impairment of delayed hypersensitivity. *Clin. Exp. Immunol.* 5:75, 1969.
30. Hurd, E. R., and Ziff, M. Studies on the anti-inflammatory action of 6-mercaptopurine. *J. Exp. Med.* 128:785, 1968.
31. Jondal, H., Holm, G., and Wigzell, H. Surface markers on human T and B lymphocytes. I. A large population of lymphocytes forming nonimmune rosettes with sheep red blood cells. *J. Exp. Med.* 136:207, 1972.
32. Kanich, R. E., and Craighead, J. E. Cytomegalovirus infection and cytomegalic inclusion disease in renal homotransplant recipients. *Am. J. Med.* 40:874, 1966.
33. Kasakura, S., and Lowenstein, L. The effect of uremic blood on mixed leukocyte reactions and on cultures of leukocytes with phytohemagglutinin. *Transplantation* 5:283, 1967.
34. Kaufman, D. B., and McIntosh, R. M. The effects of azathioprine on reticuloendothelial clearance. *Clin. Res.* 19:221, 1971.
35. Lee, A. K. Y., et al. Measurement of antibody-producing capacity to flagellin

in man. IV. Studies in autoimmune disease, allergy and after azathioprine treatment. *Clin. Exp. Immunol.* 9:507, 1971.

36. Levy, J., et al. The effect of azathioprine on gamma globulin synthesis in man. *J. Clin. Invest.* 51:2233, 1972.

37. Mackaness, G. B. The immunological basis of acquired cellular resistance. *J. Exp. Med.* 120:105, 1964.

38. Mackaness, G. B. The influence of immunologically committed lymphoid cells on macrophage activity in vivo. *J. Exp. Med.* 129:973, 1969.

39. Mackay, I. R., Dwyer, J. M., and Rowley, M. J. Differing effects of azathioprine and cyclophosphamide on immune responses to flagellin in man. *Arthritis Rheum.* 16:455, 1973.

40. MacLennan, I. C. M. Antibody in the induction and inhibition of lymphocyte cytotoxicity. *Trans. Rev.* 13:67, 1972.

41. MacLennan, I. C. M., and Morris, P. J. Unpublished observations, 1976.

42. Maibach, H. I., and Epstein, W. L. Immunologic responses of healthy volunteers receiving azathioprine. *Int. Arch. Allergy* 27:102, 1965.

43. McGregor, D. D., Koster, F. T., and Mackaness, G. B. The mediator of cellular immunity. 1. The life-span and circulation dynamics of the immunologically committed lymphocyte. *J. Exp. Med.* 133:389, 1971.

44. Merigan, T. C., and Stevens, D. A. Viral infections in man associated with acquired immunological deficiency states. *Fed. Proc.* 30:1858, 1971.

45. Ming, P. L., Ming, S. C., and Dammin, G. J. Effect of uremia and azathioprine on lymphocyte response to phytohemagglutinin. *Fed. Proc.* 27:432, 1968.

46. Montgomerie, J. Z., et al. Herpes-simplex-virus infection after renal transplantation. *Lancet* II:867, 1969.

47. Nakhla, L. S., and Goggin, M. J. Lymphocyte transformation in chronic renal failure. *Immunology* 24:229, 1973.

48. Newberry, W. M., and Sanford, J. P. Defective cellular immunity in renal failure: Depression of reactivity of lymphocytes to phytohemagglutinin by renal failure serum. *J. Clin. Invest.* 50:1262, 1971.

49. North, R. J. The action of cortisone acetate on cell-mediated immunity to infection. Suppression of host cell proliferation and alteration of cellular composition of infective foci. *J. Exp. Med.* 134:1485, 1971.

50. Page, A. R. Anti-inflammatory activity of 6-mercaptopurine. *Fed. Proc.* 21:276, 1962.

51. Palmer, D. L., Rifkind, D., and Brown, D. W. ^{131}I-labeled colloidal human serum albumin in the study of reticuloendothelial system function. III. Phagocytosis and catabolism compared in human leukemic and immunosuppressed human subjects. *J. Infect. Dis.* 123:465, 1971.

52. Phillips, B., and Weisrose, E. The mitogenic response of human B lymphocytes to phytohaemagglutinin. *Clin. Exp. Immunol.* 16:383, 1974.

53. Potter, M. R., and Moore, M. PHA stimulation of separated human lymphocyte populations. *Clin. Exp. Immunol.* 21:456, 1975.

54. Rager-Zisman, B., and Bloom, B. R. Immunological destruction of herpes simplex virus I infected cells. *Nature* 251:542, 1974.

55. Reynolds, E. S., Walls, K. W., and Pfeiffer, R. I. Generalized toxoplasmosis following renal transplantation. *Arch. Intern. Med.* 118:401, 1966.

56. Rifkind, D. The activation of varicella-zoster virus infections by immunosuppressive therapy. *J. Lab. Clin. Med.* 68:463, 1966.

57. Rifkind, D., Faris, T. D., and Hill, R. B. *Pneumocystis carinii* pneumonia. Studies on the diagnosis and treatment. *Ann. Intern. Med.* 65:493, 1966.

58. Rinehart, J. J., et al. Effects of corticosteroids on human monocyte function. *J. Clin. Invest.* 54:1337, 1974.

59. Rogers, L., et al. Immune responsiveness in dialysis and transplant patients. In preparation.

60. Rowley, M. J., Mackay, I. R., and McKenzie, I. F. C. Antibody production in immunosuppressed recipients of renal allografts. *Lancet* II:708, 1969.

61. Schober, R., and Herman, M. M. Neuropathology of cardiac transplantation. *Lancet* I:962, 1973.

62. Shore, S. L., et al. Detection of cell-dependent cytotoxic antibody to cells infected with herpes simplex virus. *Nature* 251:350, 1974.

63. Simmons, R. L., et al. Cytomegalovirus: Clinical virological correlations in renal transplant recipients. *Ann. Surg.* 180:623, 1974.

64. Spencer, E. S., and Andersen, H. K. Clinically evident, nonterminal infections with herpesviruses and the wart virus in immunosuppressed renal allograft recipients. *Br. Med. J.* 3:251, 1970.

65. Stocker, J. W., McKenzie, I. F. C., and Morris, P. J. IgM activity in human lymphocytotoxic antisera after renal transplantation. *Nature* 222:483, 1969.

66. Swanson, M. A., and Schwartz, R. S. Immunosuppressive therapy. The relation between clinical response and immunologic competence. *N. Engl. J. Med.* 277:163, 1967.

67. Taylor, H., and Morris, P. J. Unpublished observations, 1971.

68. Tiong, T. S., and Morris, P. J. Human heterophil antibodies against erythrocytes. II. Gross reactivity with human A and B substances. *Clin. Exp. Immunol.* 10:179, 1972.

69. Tobin, J. Personal communication, 1975.

70. Toh, B. H., et al. Depression of cell-mediated immunity in old age and the immunopathic diseases, lupus erythematosus, chronic hepatitis and rheumatoid arthritis. *Clin. Exp. Immunol.* 14:193, 1973.

71. Williams, K., and Morris, P. J. Retrospective screening for lymphocyte-dependent antibody in recipients of renal transplants. *Clin. Exp. Immunol.* 27:191, 1977.

72. Volkert, M., and Lundstedt, C. The provocation of latent lymphocyte choriomeningitis virus infections in mice by treatment with antilymphocytic serum. *J. Exp. Med.* 127:327, 1968.

73. Wiener, S. L., et al. The mechanism of action of a single dose of methylprednisolone on acute inflammation in vivo. *J. Clin. Invest.* 56:679, 1975.

74. Yu, D. T. Y., et al. Human lymphocyte subpopulations. Effect of corticosteroids. *J. Clin. Invest.* 53:565, 1974.

12. Host Defects Caused by Surgical Operation

John F. Burke

The two factors of primary importance in infection are the bacteria and the host. Since the mere presence of bacteria in the tissue of a patient does not always mean that an infection will result, it is clear that the body resists the attempts of bacteria to grow in living tissue. This capacity of resistance to bacterial infection suggests that infection can be reduced in at least three ways: by reducing the number of bacteria to levels the host can cope with, by raising the capacity of the host's defensive mechanisms to a level whereby the number of bacteria presented may be successfully resisted, or a combination of the two.

This latter area offers the most promising field for work. Combined with attempts to eliminate bacteria from the surgical environment, analysis of the nature of host resistance will provide the greatest likelihood of understanding the means of preventing wound infection and, in particular, the means of preventing infection following surgery.

Changes in surgical practice over the years clearly indicate that the problems of preventing postoperative bacterial infection are far different from those encountered in the early Listerian era. Following the discovery of aseptic and antiseptic techniques that substantially reduced postoperative bacterial infection, the application of surgical therapy was greatly widened. As surgical and anesthetic techniques improved and as the understanding of normal physiology and pathophysiology expanded, an increasingly broader group of diseases have become repairable by surgical means. Concomitantly, this change in the population of patients to include increasingly more patients with serious risk of infection has resulted in an increase in the overall problems of prevention of sepsis. Despite this fact, improvements in the techniques of preventing postoperative infections have kept pace with the increasing challenge of a more susceptible patient population, and the occurrence of infection has remained, generally, about the same [3].

Expansion of knowledge concerning sterilization and aseptic techniques as well as the use of antibiotic substances have served to provide better control of infection. Expanded physiologic and biochemical knowledge has made it possible to increase the indications for surgical therapy to include patients who are at a much higher risk of developing infection. The patients who, in the past, were too poor a risk to undergo surgery because of physiologic or chemical imbalance no longer are, due largely to our increased ability to deal effectively with their problems. However, although much can be done to restore physiologic and chemical balance, we are not yet able to restore the balance of natural resistance to bacterial invasion. Hence many patients, although well prepared for surgery in the cardiovascular pulmonary sense, remain at high risk for developing postoperative sepsis

175

because of unrepaired host defense defects. A patient may have all systems, except his normal resistance against bacteria, restored to near-normal function before undergoing an extensive surgical procedure but, because his resistance to bacterial invasion cannot be brought to the same near-normal state, the small number of bacteria that enter the wound may multiply, invade, and produce postoperative wound sepsis.

The number of patients undergoing surgical procedures with reduced resistance against bacterial invasion is increased as the indication for surgery widens, and this gives great urgency to the efforts being made to understand and modulate the basic principles of host defense. It is becoming increasingly clear that the further development of surgical therapy is directly related to the surgeon's ability to restore the patient preoperatively to a normal state that includes a normal resistance to bacteria. The answer to the problem of postoperative bacterial complications appears to be in a fuller understanding of the process involved in host resistance, leading to the ability to maintain or restore physiologic and immunologic parameters, coupled with the principles of aseptic and surgical technique so carefully learned.

The present state of knowledge concerning host resistance against bacterial invasion, although incomplete, provides a starting point for an examination of key concepts. Traditionally, the factors that can be mustered by the organism to defend itself against infection have been divided into specific and nonspecific factors, depending on their activity in relation to a single organism. Specific host resistance is active against a particular microorganism that is related, essentially, to a previous experience of the host with that microorganism. Nonspecific host resistance, on the other hand, is that category of defense activity that does not depend on a previous experience of the host. It is this category that is of primary importance in preventing postoperative surgical problems [7, 8].

The role of natural, nonspecific resistance against bacterial invasion has always been underrated in an overall evaluation of the treatment of prevention of infection. In reality, the ability to treat or prevent bacterial infection depends almost entirely on the host's natural defensive mechanisms. They can only be supplemented; as yet they cannot be replaced. Furthermore, these mechanisms do not exist alone but are completely dependent on a near-normal level of cardiorespiratory and metabolic activity to maintain normal function. When intact, tissue resistance against bacterial invasion provides adequate protection in almost all situations met in daily life. However, this natural resistance to bacterial invasion varies from one tissue to another and according to its physiologic state. Therefore decreased host resistance frequently accompanies disease and is further diminished by anesthesia or the surgical procedure itself. In the patient undergoing operation, resistance to bacterial invasion is reduced by two key factors not seen in other patients. These must be kept in mind in examining means of supplementing resistance. First, the integument is open during surgical procedures and, hence, the normal defense mechanism that prevents bacterial contamination of tissue has been breached (this basic point reminds us that host resistance varies from one place on the patient to another). Second, the effect of surgical operation and anesthesia in themselves tend to reduce host defense.

The location of the surgical operation or the nature of the trauma will influence the number of organisms that gain entrance. At operation the technical skill and care with which the surgeon deals with the wound is a crucial element, minimizing tissue trauma, maintaining local tissue resistance, and thus preventing postoperative septic complications.

To the extent that contributing factors to decreased host resistance can be identified, it is possible to consider means to repair or supplement to restore a near-normal level of host resistance. In a series of studies, Miles [6] identifies some of these factors that "interfere" with normal resistance. Essentially, the studies demonstrated that while host defensive forces are effective when functioning, they can also be easily blocked. More importantly, the discovery of the importance of timing in response to bacterial lodgment was seen as crucial. A further consideration of these studies will demonstrate these points.

In the experiments to observe the effects of interference with normal host resistance, the expected decrease in bacterial killing and resultant increase in lesion size were observed. An important observation in the first experiments was that the ability to interrupt the host's usual suppression of a developing lesion was limited to the first few hours following bacterial contamination. In three distinct cases — i.e., when the bacteria were injected into the dermis during the time the animal was in shock; in the period of local adrenalin ischemia; or closely following injection of the complement blocking agent, sodium polyanethol sulphonate (Liquoid) — the resulting mature lesions were substantially larger and more severe than the control lesions. The increase in size and severity of the lesions corresponded to an increase in the number of bacteria that survived in the tissue. The ability of bacteria to create an inflammatory lesion appeared to be enhanced by the blocking of the host defenses. In addition, it was observed that the lesions initiated at the same time as, or shortly after, the blocking of a component of the antibacterial defenses were considerably enhanced. However, lesions that were several hours old before shock, before adrenalin ischemia was initiated, or before sodium polyanethol sulphonate was injected were not enhanced, even though they would not reach a maximum size for an additional 20 (or more) hours. At 24 hours these lesions, subjected to blocking agents 4 or more hours following bacterial contamination, were the same size as the controls [5].

From these experiments three concepts emerged. First, certain tissue antibacterial mechanisms that are inhibited by a reduced or absent local blood flow, or by anticomplementary substances, allow bacterial survival in the tissue in unusual proportions, resulting in a considerably enlarged area of tissue damage. Second, these particular antibacterial mechanisms exert the major portion of their ability to control the lesion within the first 3 hours following tissue contamination. Third, it is during this short early period that the ultimate size of the lesion is determined. Thus, in the normal state, tissue defenses appear to act immediately, and if a lesion is to be prevented, the anti-bacterial activity must be effective in a short period of time. If, as was done in laboratory experiments, defenses are made inoperative before the contaminating bacteria are killed, the bacteria are allowed to multiply, resulting in an increased area of tissue damage and a larger mature lesion.

This short period, "the decisive period," is that time during which inhibition of certain defense mechanisms results in lesion enhancement [6]. The importance of understanding the existence of this decisive period is greatest in respect to determining the means for increasing host resistance through the use of such exogenous substances as antibiotics, which could add to the host's natural defensive abilities. As a corollary to an understanding of the decisive period, the time of maximum enhancement was found when the tissue defenses were inhibited maximally; that is, the block was carried out immediately before or at the same time the tissue was contaminated with bacteria. The susceptibility of enhancement steadily declined to the end of the decisive period, when the lesion could not be enhanced at all. An example of this development is shown in Figure 12-1, which demonstrates the effect of local adrenalin ischemia on the ability of the dermis to control a standard inoculum of viable staphylococci.

The premise that there is a period of intense, highly effective host antibacterial activity beginning immediately on the arrival of bacteria in tissue, which contains bacterial invasion in less than 4 hours, suggests that there is

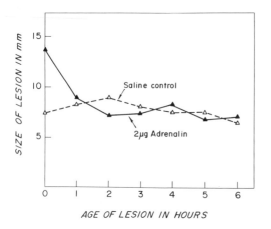

Figure 12-1. The decreasing susceptibility of a staphylococcal lesion to enhancement to a larger lesion size by adrenalin delivered to the tissue at various times following tissue contamination with staphylococci.

value in examining the possibility of enhancing this host defensive activity during this 4-hour decisive period. The implications are great for clinical medicine, particularly in surgery, where infection following operations may severely complicate the patient's recovery. Theoretically, antibiotic substances could augment the natural mechanisms of bacterial resistance in tissue. Their bactericidal or bacteriostatic activity does not interfere with natural host mechanisms but affects bacteria directly. The two antibacterial activities, natural host resistance and antibiotics, should actually be additive or, ideally, synergistic in preventing or reducing the size of the final bacterial lesion. In experimental and clinical studies this has, in fact, proved to be the case. There is a definite period of time during which it is possible to augment the host's antibacterial mechanisms by the use of an antibiotic. The "effective period of preventive antibiotics" [2] occurs when the antibacterial activity of the drug is coordinated with that of the host to produce more effective overall bacterial killing and a smaller final lesion size. Again, a 4-hour period is observed, beginning at the time of bacterial contamination of tissue. However, the effect on lesion size is opposite from that observed when an agent is used to block host resistance during the decisive period. The decisive period, as demonstrated by adrenalin ischemia, compared with the effective period, as demonstrated by the effect of penicillin on an experimental staphylococci lesion, is shown in Figure 12-2. The same biological characteristics are involved in both cases. If penicillin is given at the same time the wound is contaminated, the resultant lesion is similar to the lesion produced by an autoclaved, killed bacterial suspension. On the other hand, if the tissue is contaminated by bacteria but the penicillin is not administered until 4 hours after the bacterial contamination, the lesion

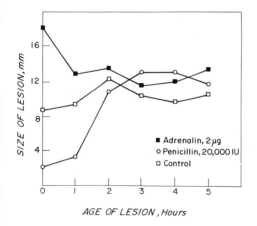

Figure 12-2. Comparison of the decreasing susceptibility to increase in lesion size of staphylococcal dermal lesions to adrenalin ischemia, the "decisive period," and the decreasing susceptibility of staphylococcal lesions to lesion size suppression by systemic penicillin, the "effective period."

is similar to the infection seen in an animal given no penicillin but contaminated with a staphylococcal suspension.

Experiments designed to gather data on blocking or enhancement of the host mechanism and to determine the decisive or effective period of antibacterial activity in tissues reveal three major points. First, nonspecific host resistance against bacterial invasion is a composite of a number of distinct factors, at least some of which operate locally at the site of the bacterial contamination. Second, the interaction between host forces and bacteria begins the moment bacteria arrive in the tissue. There is no "grace period." Third, all the host's defensive forces studied have shown a definite period of intense effective activity, beginning at the moment of contamination and ending within the first few hours following the arrival of bacteria. This means that a number of important components of the host's ability to defend itself against bacterial invasion, which tend to limit the ultimate lesion size, are able to prevent bacterial growth in contaminated tissue for only a short and specific period of time following contamination. Growth of bacteria and the development of the bacterial lesion in itself appear to provide some protection for the bacteria within the lesion.

The overwhelming weight of experimental evidence points to the moment of contamination as the time when the host's defensive mechanisms, if functioning, are most effective. Their effectiveness decreases during the next few hours, and the matter of success or failure in the tissue's struggle to prevent a bacterial lesion is essentially decided within the first hours following the arrival of bacteria in the tissue. The knowledge obtained from these studies of the manner in which the host defends himself against bacteria clearly indicates that if antibacterial potential is to be effectively supplemented, use must be made of that period of time during which contamination of the tissue takes place. These concepts have been successfully incorporated into the surgical clinic as the concept of preventive antibiotics with demonstrated reduction in postoperative infection rate [1, 2, 9].

In summary, three concepts stand out that may serve to channel further research and still serve as functional guidelines for preventing infection caused by surgical procedures: all efforts aimed at dealing with the problem of bacterial infection must concentrate on increasing the patient's natural resistance; such efforts must take place in the period before the onset of surgical or anesthetic trauma; and delivery of any treatment designed to supplement host resistance must be accomplished in the first few hours following bacterial contamination.

References

1. Bernard, H. R., and Cole, W. R.   The prophylaxis of surgical infection: The effect of prophylactic antimicrobial drugs on the incidence of infection following potentially contaminated operations. *Surgery* 56:151, 1964.
2. Boyd, R. J., Burke, J. F., and Colton, T.   A double blind clinical trial of prophylactic antibiotics in hip fracture patients. *J. Bone Joint Surg.* [A] 55:1251, 1973.

3. Burke, J. F.   The effective period of preventive antibiotic action in experimental incisions and dermal lesions. *Surgery* 50:1, 161, 184, 1961.
4. Burke, J. F.   Wound infection and early inflammation. *Monogr. Surg. Sci.* 1(4):301, 1964.
5. Burke, J. F., and Miles, A. A.   The sequence of vascular events in early infectious inflammation. *J. Pathol.* 76:1, 1958.
6. Miles, A. A.   Nonspecific defense reactions in bacterial infection, *Ann. N.Y. Acad. Sci.* 66:356, 1956.
7. Miles, A. A., Miles, E. M., and Burke, J. F.   The value and duration of defense reactions of the skin to the primary lodgement of bacteria. *Br. J. Exp. Pathol.* 38:79, 1957.
8. Miles, A. A., and Niven, J. S. F.   Enhancement of infection during shock produced by bacterial toxins and other agents. *Br. J. Exp. Pathol.* 31:1, 1950.
9. Polk, H. C., Jr., and Lopez-Mayor, J. F.   Postoperative wound infection. *Surgery* 66:97, 1969.

13. *The Etiology and Prevention of Deep Wound Infection Following Total Hip Replacement*

William H. Harris

Total Hip Replacement: A High-Risk Operation

For the purposes of this symposium I will discuss only total hip replacement, rather than total joint replacement in general, because the other major joint implants, such as total knee replacement, have not as yet been done in sufficiently large numbers over a long enough period of time to provide good data for the problems addressed.

Patients receiving total joint replacement are an excellent group to study among the population of infection-prone hospital patients for three major reasons. The first, of course, is the high incidence of infection. The second is that they differ importantly from many of the other populations of patients that are discussed elsewhere in this textbook. They are usually healthy adults undergoing an elective operation for a benign condition. This means that the variables involved in their response to surgery are often fewer and less complicated than certain of the other patient populations. In most instances infection is not complicated by the disease being treated. Malnutrition, immunosuppression, immunodepletion, severe metabolic disturbances, marrow suppression, and the like are not involved.

Third, the total number of patients in this category and the duration of followup are extensive enough to provide a broad population base for the evaluation of individual factors. In addition, of course, they require intense study because of the magnitude and chronicity of the disaster that results from deep wound infection following a total joint replacement.

The risks of infection following total hip replacement then, are more directly related to (1) the general risks of infection associated with clean surgery, and (2) the special risk related to the massive foreign implant. What is the risk of infection following total hip replacement? First, there is the risk reflected by the early experience of a number of surgeons in this type of surgery. Second, there is the risk under current surgical conditions. Table 13-1 shows the prevalence of deep wound infection following total hip replacement in early experiences with this type surgery in four major centers.

Is this an unusually high infection rate? Unfortunately, no comparable control data from these same centers have been published for other types of hip surgery done by these same surgeons under the same conditions and at the same time. Comparison with other reports from other centers is the only recourse, but that, obviously, is hazardous. The study by Boyd, Burke, and Colton [3] at the Massachusetts General Hospital showed a sepsis rate of 4.8% in surgery for hip fractures in cases not receiving antibiotics. On the other hand, Niemann and Mankin reported a 41% prevalence of deep

Table 13-1. Comparison of Incidence of Deep Wound Sepsis Reported in Various Studies

Author	Percent Deep Wound Sepsis
Charnley and Eftekhar [7]	8.9
Wilson et al. [36]	13 [a]
Patterson and Brown [30]	8.2
Moczynski et al. [26]	9

[a] Wilson et al. initially reported 12 septic cases in the first 100 total hip replacements. Subsequently an additional patient also developed deep wound sepsis.

wound sepsis in emergency hip surgery (endoprosthesis insertion) in an elderly population of institutionalized patients [28]. Fogelberg, Zitzmann, and Stinchfield [15] reported a 10% prevalence of deep wound sepsis in a series of patients undergoing elective hip surgery (Vitallium cup arthroplasty) in otherwise healthy patients in a university teaching center population of private patients. In contrast with this, Aufranc did 989 consecutive Vitallium cup arthroplasties with only two cases of deep wound sepsis in a comparable population [1]. Hinchey and Day reported only a 1.4% incidence of deep wound sepsis in his series of patients undergoing endoprosthetic replacement for femoral neck fracture [22].

Despite these wide variations in the sepsis rate from other centers, the lack of valid control data for the series of total hip replacements noted, and the high incidence of infection, it is generally accepted that the sepsis rate for experienced surgeons doing other surgery of the hip is substantially lower than the 8 to 13% figures noted for total hip replacement (Table 13-1).

The fact that the same surgeons listed in Table 13-1 have been able to reduce their sepsis rate to approximately 1% by taking certain preventive steps, which we will discuss later, tends to confirm that these initial rates were unusually high and points out that this type of surgery carries with it a particularly high risk of infection.

The second special feature of infection following total hip replacement is the unusually high prevalence of "late sepsis." Different authors have used different time periods to define "early" and "late" manifestations of sepsis postoperatively. Charnley and Eftekhar considered any infection appearing for the first time 3 months after the operation as a "late" infection [7]. Muller reported his data using 1 year as a cut-off between early and late infections [27]. In any event, substantial numbers of patients, who developed deep wound sepsis following total hip replacement, have a prolonged interval that is free of the manifestations of infection following their surgery, varying from 3 months to as long as 5 years. In Charnley and Eftekhar's experience 60% of the patients with deep wound sepsis experienced their first manifestations of the infection "late" [7]. In Muller's series [27] this feature is even more striking. In a group of 643 total hip replacements done in 1964, the prevalence of deep wound sepsis after 1 year was less than 1%. After 2 years it was 3%, and after 4 years it was 4%. In other words, 80% of the patients with deep wound sepsis experienced infection initially at least 1 year after the surgery.

While in some instances it is probable that late appearance of infection was due to sepsis that was metastatic from a remote source of internal infection [25], the vast majority of these infections have not been so documented. Three bits of indirect evidence support the concept that most of these cases represent late manifestations of infection that gained entrance to the hip area at the time of the surgery. First, Charnley and Eftekhar were able to reduce the prevalence of late infection almost in parallel with the reduction of early infection by a series of changes they made in the operating room environment from 1959 to 1969 [7]. If the majority of cases of late sepsis were secondary to intercurrent bacteremia, such would not be the case. Second, the type and frequency of the bacteria responsible for late infections are very similar to the type and frequency of the bacteria associated with early infections, suggesting a common source for both [7].

Third, these bacteria, identified with late wound sepsis, are substantially different in type and frequency from the bacteria found in the intercurrent bacteremias that occur in a general medical population. All these points are indirect reasons, but they do support the concept of a delayed manifestation of sepsis from organisms that were introduced at the time of the surgery.

Experience with infection after total hip replacement calls attention to three other special features. First, among the bacteria that are commonly found as the infecting agents in deep wound sepsis following total hip replacement is *Staphylococcus epidermidis,* formerly thought to be a nonpathogen. This finding is common in other forms of infection in immunosuppressed or immune-depleted patients; that is, so called nonpathogens are common causative organisms of deep wound sepsis following total hip replacement. Second, "What makes this surgery different?" We freely discuss a "decrease in host resistance" brought about by the massive implant, but what is the real meaning of this phrase? What can and should be done about it? Does this decrease in resistance underlie both the overall high risk of infection and the development of late sepsis from within the wound? Third, why is this implant a site for metastatic infections? The bacteria from the bacteremia obviously are distributed in myriad sites throughout the body without establishing an infection. Even with the transient increase in vascularity that occurs in the repair process after total hip replacement, the absolute number of bacteria lodging at the total hip replacement site are not excessive compared to other more vascular sites in the body where infections do not develop. Again the response is the soothing but incomplete explanation of a decrease in resistance brought about by the massive implant.

Of course, neither of these phenomena, the late manifestations of infection in the hip and the localization of metastatic infection around a total hip replacement following total hip surgery, is unique to total hip replacement. They both have been well documented in association with Vitallium cup arthroplasty, hip nailing, hip fractures, osteotomy of the hip, and the like. What is surprising is the high frequency of these occurrences following total hip replacement, even though they are still uncommon on an absolute scale.

Factors Involved in the High Frequency of Infection

Four factors are widely held to contribute to the high risk of infection following total hip replacement. The first three are self-explanatory and the fourth appears to be so but, in actuality, is poorly understood. These factors are (1) unrecognized preexisting infection, (2) the massive nature of the surgery, (3) poor risk factors in the population undergoing total hip replacement, and (4) decreased resistance secondary to the massive implant.

Infection in the hip of the adult patient following any hip surgery can be extremely subtle indeed [17, 20], and it frequently leads to failure of a previous hip reconstruction. Thus many patients come to total hip replacement as a result of failure of a previous hip operation, from which deep wound sepsis has already been established in the joint *but has not been diagnosed clinically*. Deep wound sepsis may be present in the hip for months or years without any of the customary clinical manifestations, even including elevation of the sedimentation rate. It should be noted, however, that the elevated sedimentation rate is the most reliable of the various laboratory tests available. Obviously such patients increase the postoperative sepsis rate following total hip replacement if this low-grade sepsis remains undetected preoperatively.

Obviously, also, as a more aggressive attack is being made on the treatment of patients with *recognized* sepsis [35], using total hip replacement as the method of salvage, the risks of postoperative infection rise rapidly. However, this is not the group under discussion.

Second, total hip replacement can be a very extensive operative procedure, quite independent of the insertion of the implant itself. This is particularly so if a reoperation is being done because of failure of another total hip replacement. This procedure can require extensive exposure with massive tissue damage, protracted operating time, prolonged retraction of tissues, and creation of substantial dead space. All these factors increase the risk of infection as a general phenomenon, independent of the type of reconstruction that is done [12, 14, 23].

Third, certain correlations have been made with the population at risk, which appear to be valid. As noted previously, patients who are having a reoperation appear to have a higher incidence of wound infection. Some authors have felt that those patients with obesity, diabetes, rheumatoid arthritis, ankylosing spondylitis, and those receiving steroids are at higher risk of deep wound infection. Crawford, Hillman, and Charnley at one time felt that anticoagulation increased the risk of wound sepsis [11] but they subsequently reversed their opinion on that subject [9]. In our experience it is not the anticoagulation per se but the accuracy of the regulation that is important. Well-regulated anticoagulation does not significantly increase the incidence of wound sepsis [18, 19, 32].

Prevention

The prevention of deep wound sepsis after total hip replacement can be considered under four major headings: (1) detection of existing infection, (2) ordinary measures of surgical technique and environmental control, (3) extraordinary measures of surgical technique and environmental control, and (4) steps to increase the resistance to infection.

Detection of existing infection is really only a problem in those cases of the subtle forms of sepsis mentioned previously. We have just completed a prospective study of preoperative aspiration of the hip before total hip replacement in 138 hips in which prior operations had been performed [29]. All aspirations were carried out in the operating room under general anesthesia. All seven cases of unrecognized infection were detected and the organism was identified accurately. Moreover, we found that in each septic case at least one other factor was present. These associated factors were (1) a history suggesting wound infection, (2) an increase in bone resorption, (3) an increase in periosteal new bone formation, (4) settling or migration of an implant, and (5) elevation of the sedimentation rate.

Our study demonstrated that in the absence of all these five factors, no aspiration is needed. In the presence of one or more of these factors, aspiration is required. However, many false-positive cultures were also found. Primarily, these were gram-positive organisms that grew only in the thioglycolate broth. We concluded that a positive culture of an aerobic organism that grows in the thioglycolate broth only and is not confirmed by growth on any of the solid media can safely be ignored as a contaminant as long as none of the five associated features are present.

The high rate of sepsis after total hip replacement, coupled with the magnitude of the disability and suffering associated with it, has made surgeons pay stricter attention to the usually recommended measures of good surgical technique and environmental control. This means that a variety of steps are receiving renewed attention, ranging from the use of two layers of rubber gloves to the restriction of the number of people present in the operating room. None of these measures are new, but unfortunately the application of many of these general disciplines had often become lax. The institution of tighter discipline alone has been of considerable value.

A series of extraordinary measures have also been initiated by certain surgeons. Charnley and Eftekhar [7] have promoted three major extraordinary measures: (1) the use of sequential sterile packs during the case, which reduced the re-use of instruments during the operation, (2) the use of body exhaust systems and more comprehensive, more occlusive operating gowns [8], and (3) the use of an enclosure within the operating room in conjunction with the unidirectional flow of sterile air passing over the operating field [7]. Another approach is the renewed interest [37] in the use of ultraviolet light in the operating room to improve the bacteriologic environment [21].

The short summary of all the long and sometimes acrimonious debates on the advantages of these extraordinary measures is this: Without any doubt, these measures substantially reduce the number of viable pathogenic bacteria in the air over the wound. As Burke has shown [6], this is the final common pathway for the entrance of most of the bacteria causing deep wound infections. However, no vigorous scientific proof that wound infections have been reduced because of these extraordinary measures has yet been generated. This proof would require prospective, simultaneous, controlled studies of very large populations, followed for at least 3 years, and such data do not exist. Charnley and Eftekhar have shown in a retrospective, uncontrolled study [7] a progressive decrease in the infection rate, which paralleled closely the institution of sequential steps that progressively improved the bacteriologic environment in their operating room. This is suggestive of a cause-and-effect relation between the improved operating room environment and the decrease in the frequency of deep wound sepsis. However, without a prospective, randomized, simultaneous control group, rigid proof is still lacking. In addition, Charnley's study contained many questionable variables. A substantial number of his "septic" cases had no bacterial growth. Moreover, the reduction in infections caused by *Staphylococcus* organisms in his study was probably not significant. Many other variables were changed in an unregulated way. And, finally, he subsequently changed the interpretation of some of the findings of that study himself [9].

In addition, surgeons at other institutions have been able to match the low frequency of infection that Charnley achieved using his extraordinary measures without using these extraordinary techniques. For example, the early infection rate at the Mayo Clinic of 0.6% [10] compares favorably with the "less than 1%" deep sepsis rate that Charnley currently achieves [9]. Obviously, such a comparison involves all the variables inherent in work done at two different institutions. In addition, the surgeons at the Mayo Clinic use prophylactic antibiotics, while Charnley does not, and the surgeons at the Mayo Clinic operate in the customary operating rooms, while Charnley works in a specialized greenhouse.

Unresolved, then, by such comparisons is the question of whether the Mayo Clinic experience would be even better using a greenhouse and whether or not Charnley's experience could be further improved if he used prophylactic antibiotics. In the face of these questions, the arguments on the advantages of vertical versus horizontal flow and the advantages of enclosed unidirectional flow versus nonenclosed unidirectional flow seem to be secondary.

Nevertheless, Charnley's suggestive data on the efficacy of these extraordinary measures and the proof that the bacteriologic environment over the wound is significantly improved are strong support for the use of these measures. If ordinary measures, however, lead to an infection rate at the 1% level, the demonstration of the statistical significance of the advantages of the extraordinary measures will require very large samples indeed. To obtain these data, however, is important for three reasons. First, the average medical expense associated with a septic total hip replacement is estimated to be at least $25,000, setting aside the associated suffering. Second, the installation of these expensive extraordinary measures in operating rooms throughout the nation is a fact of life, whether scientifically valid or not. Third, even greater protection against infection is needed because we are now doing increased numbers of more complex and more protracted cases that would not even have been contemplated for total hip replacement 5 years ago.

Finally, a number of steps have been taken to increase the resistance of the normal patient to the development of deep wound sepsis. The first of these is the routine use of prophylactic systemic antibiotics. While this highly debated issue was formerly confused by the misuse of the word prophylactic, it is now clear that the term, *prophylactic,* in association with the systemic use of antibiotics must mean the administration of the antibiotics just before and during the operation. It is also quite clear that they are effective in reducing the deep sepsis rate in major musculoskeletal surgery. The studies of Burke [5] showed the importance of the early administration of the systemic antibiotics in reducing the incidence of established infection. The studies of Bowers, Wilson, and Greene [2] showed that the contaminated hematoma in an experimental osteotomy could be sterilized by systemic antibiotics. The studies of Boyd, Burke, and Colton [3] and Fogelberg, Zitzmann, and Stinchfield [15] have demonstrated the efficacy and safety of prophylactic, systemic antibiotics in major orthopedic surgery. Further support is given by the studies of Pavel et al. [31] and Ericson, Lidgren, and Lindberg [13].

Charnley and his associates do not use systemic prophylactic antibiotics and, as noted above, have a frequency of deep wound sepsis which is comparable to that of the Mayo Clinic, where prophylactic antibiotics are used but the extraordinary environmental control methods are not employed.

The case for the efficacy of topical antibiotics in the wound is less secure. Glotzer and Goodman [16] have experimental data on the guinea pig that indicate the efficacy of topical antibiotics and Scherr, Dodd, and Buckingham [33] have shown that short exposure to topical antibiotics is effective in killing bacteria. However, no controlled prospective studies on the efficacy of the topical use of antibiotics in musculoskeletal wounds in man exist.

Finally, considerable interest is focused on the implanting of antibiotics in the methylmethacrylate that is used as the cement in total joint replacement. Strangely enough the antibiotic is very slowly released from the cement over a long period of time, leading to a prolonged local level of the antibiotic that substantially exceeds the minimal inhibitory concentration [4, 34] for many pathogens. This prolonged release is not associated with deterioration of the physical properties of the cement, at least to date [24]. This slow release does not result in significant systemic blood levels or urine levels of the antibiotics after the first 48 hours. Gentamycin is the drug that has been studied most extensively, but oxacillin and other antibiotics have been shown to behave in a similar manner. Again, a substantial gap remains between the demonstration of the release of the antibiotics in amounts capable of producing local inhibition of bacterial growth and the factual demonstration that this phenomenon leads to a decrease in deep wound sepsis. In most cases intracement antibiotics have been used in patients who already have deep wound sepsis. However, substantial numbers of patients have received gentamycin-containing cement on a prophylactic basis as well. But there has never been a controlled prospective study done in either situation.

Therefore, because of the problem of metastatic localization of infection at the site of total hip replacement, we have adopted the identical prophylactic antibiotic regimen that is routinely used in the protection of patients with a rheumatic valvular heart disease when they are exposed to situations associated with bacteremia.

References
1. Aufranc, O. E. Personal communication, 1968.
2. Bowers, W. H., Wilson, F. C., and Greene, W. B. Antibiotic prophylaxis in experimental bone infections. *J. Bone Joint Surg.* [A] 55:795, 1973.
3. Boyd, R. J., Burke, J. F., and Colton, T. A double-blind clinical trial of prophylactic antibiotics in hip fractures. *J. Bone Joint Surg.* [A] 55:1251, 1973.
4. Buchholz, H. W., et al. Infections prophylaxe and operative behandling der schlerchenden tiefen infection bie der totalen endoprosthese. *Chirug.* 43:446, 1972.
5. Burke, J. F. The effective period of preventive antibiotic action in experimental incisions and dermal lesions. *Surgery* 50:161, 1961.
6. Burke, J. F. Identification of the sources of staphylococci contaminating the surgical wound during operation. *Ann. Surg.* 158:898, 1963.
7. Charnley, J., and Eftekhar, N. Postoperative infection in total prosthetic replacement arthroplasty of the hip-joint, with special reference to the bacterial content of the air of the operating room. *Br. J. Surg.* 56:641, 1969.

8. Charnley, J., and Eftekhar, N. Penetration of gown material by organisms from the surgeon's body. *Lancet* I:172, 1969.

9. Charnley, J. Postoperative infection after total hip replacement with special reference to air contamination in the operating room. *Clin. Orthop.* 87:187, 1972.

10. Coventry, M. B., et al. 2,012 total hip arthroplasties: A study of postoperative course and early complications. *J. Bone Joint Surg.* [A] 56:273, 1974.

11. Crawford, W. J., Hillman, F., and Charnley, J. A clinical trial of prophylactic anticoagulant therapy in elective hip surgery. Internal publication No. 14, Center for Hip Surgery, Wrightington Hospital, Wiggan, England, 1968.

12. Dupont, J. A., and Charnley, J. Low-friction arthroplasty of the hip for the failures of previous operations. *J. Bone Joint Surg.* [B] 54:77, 1972.

13. Ericson, C., Lidgren, L., and Lindberg, L. Cloxacillin in the prophylaxis of postoperative infections of the hip. *J. Bone Joint Surg.* [A] 55:808, 1973.

14. Fitzgerald, R. H., Jr., et al. Bacterial colonization of wounds and sepsis in total hip arthroplasty. *J. Bone Joint Surg.* [A] 55:1242, 1973.

15. Fogelberg, E. V., Zitzmann, E. K., and Stinchfield, F. E. Prophylactic penicillin in orthopaedic surgery. *J. Bone Joint Surg.* [A] 52:95, 1970.

16. Glotzer, D. J., and Goodman, W. S. Topical antibiotic prophylaxis in contaminated wounds. *Arch. Surg.* 100:589, 1970.

17. Harris, W. H., and Aufranc, O. E. Mold arthroplasty in the treatment of hip fractures complicated by sepsis. *J. Bone Joint Surg.* [A] 47:31, 1965.

18. Harris, W. H., Salzman, E. W., and DeSanctis, R. W. The prevention of thromboembolic disease by prophylactic anticoagulation. *J. Bone Joint Surg.* [A] 49:81, 1967.

19. Harris, W. H., et al. Prevention of venous thromboembolism following total hip replacement. *J.A.M.A.* 220:1319, 1972.

20. Harris, W. H. Total hip replacement for failed endoprosthesis and cup arthroplasty: Technical considerations. In A.A.O.S. Instructional Course Lectures, Vol. 23. St. Louis: Mosby, 1974. Pp. 154–163.

21. Hart, D., et al. Post-operative wound infections: A further report on ultraviolet irradiation with comments on the recent [1964] National Research Council Cooperative Study Report. *Ann. Surg.* 67:728, 1968.

22. Hinchey, J. J., and Day, P. L. Primary prosthetic replacement in fresh femoral-neck fractures. *J. Bone Joint Surg.* [A] 46:223, 1964.

23. Lazansky, M. G. Complications revisited. The debit side of total hip replacement. *Clin. Orthop.* 95:96, 1973.

24. Levin, P. D. The effectiveness of various antibiotics in methylmethacrylate. *J. Bone Joint Surg.* [B] 57:234, 1975.

25. Mallory, T. H. Sepsis in total hip replacement following pneumococcal pneumonia. A case report. *J. Bone Joint Surg.* [A] 55:1753, 1973.

26. Moczynski, G., et al. Evaluation of total hip replacement arthroplasties. *Clin. Orthop.* 95:213, 1973.

27. Muller, M. D. Late complications of total hip replacement. In W. H. Harris (Ed.), *The Hip: Proceedings of the Second Open Scientific Meeting of the Hip Society*. St. Louis: Mosby, 1974. Pp. 319–327.

28. Niemann, M. W., and Mankin, H. J. Fractures about the hip in an institutionalized patient population. *J. Bone Joint Surg.* [A] 50:1327, 1968.

29. Patel, D., Karshmer, A., and Harris, W. H. The role of preoperative aspiration of the hip prior to total hip replacement. In C. M. Evarts (Ed.), *The Hip*. Proceedings of the Fourth Open Scientific Meeting of the Hip Society. St. Louis: Mosby, 1976. Pp. 219–223.

30. Patterson, F. P., and Brown, S. C. The McKee-Farrar total hip replacement. Preliminary results and complications of 368 operations performed in five general hospitals. *J. Bone Joint Surg.* [A] 54:257, 1972.

31. Pavel, A., et al. Prophylactic antibiotics in clean orthopaedic surgery. *J. Bone Joint Surg.* [A] 56:777, 1974.
32. Salzman, E. W., Harris, W. H., and DeSanctis, R. W. Reduction in venous thromboembolism by agents affecting platelet function. *N. Engl. J. Med.* 284:1287, 1971.
33. Scherr, D. D., Dodd, T. A., and Buckingham, W. W. Prophylactic use of topical antibiotic irrigation in uninfected surgical wounds. *J. Bone Joint Surg.* [A] 54:634, 1972.
34. Wahlig, H., and Buchholz, H. W. Knochenzement and Gentamycin. *Acta Traumatol.* 3:247, 1973.
35. Wilson, P. D., Jr., Aglietti, P., and Salvati, E. A. Subacute sepsis of the hip treated by antibiotics and cemented prosthesis. *J. Bone Joint Surg.* [A] 56:879, 1974.
36. Wilson, P. D., et al. Total hip replacement with fixation by acrylic cement. A preliminary study of 100 consecutive McKee-Farrar prosthesis replacements. *J. Bone Joint Surg.* [A] 54:207, 1972.
37. Wright, R. L., and Burke, J. F. Effect of ultraviolet radiation on postoperative neurosurgical sepsis. *J. Neurosurg.* 31:533, 1969.

14. Infections and Their Prevention in Surgical Cancer Patients

Demetrius H. Bagley and Alfred S. Ketcham

There is no bibliographic scarcity of reports dealing with the controversial subject of antibiotic use in surgery, particularly as it relates to prophylaxis. The literature is similarly abundant in reports from medical oncologists who stress the overwhelming lethality of infection in cancer patients being treated with chemotherapy [36, 39, 46]. The potential infectious complications that can be associated with the surgical manipulation of cancer have been given little attention in terms of antibiotic usage, either prophylactic or therapeutic, and have been associated with the experiences of general surgical services, often in the treatment of a predominance of nonmalignant entities. At the initiation of these studies, which are reviewed and reported in this chapter, there was a supposition that cancer patients might experience different infectious problems than the usual surgical patient. The surgical candidate for cancer cure ordinarily has a different nutritional and physiologic status than the usual surgical patient, but he seldom is burdened with the severe hematologic depressions invariably associated with chemotherapy. Whether his propensity to develop infectious complications is related to immunosuppression, apparently associated with the basic flaw that allowed cancer to develop, or his frequent status of being a radiation failure, or a previous surgical failure is conjecture. This report may fail to answer these questions but will stress the overall significance of infectious problems in cancer patients treated by surgical modalities.

Infection is frequently the immediate cause of death in the cancer patient, exemplified by a report by Inagaki, Rodriguez, and Bodey [22]. Infection was the predominant and immediate explanation for death in 47% of 816 patients, while 25% died of organ failure and 4% died of carcinomatosis.

In a smaller series, the authors have examined the causes of death in patients treated surgically at the Surgery Branch of the National Cancer Institute. In a personal experience of patients treated by pelvic exenteration for carcinoma of the uterine cervix, 17 of 28 patients or 60%, dying in the postoperative period died from infectious complications [28]. In a subsequent review of the experience of the same surgical oncology service, which included patients with pelvic neoplasms, melanomas, sarcomas, and head and neck tumors, there were 3 of 7 deaths (40%) attributed primarily to infection [27].

An impression that cancer patients undergoing surgical operations appear to have an increased susceptibility to infection has been supported by a statistically marginal but interesting study by Cohen, Fekety, and Cluff, who reviewed wound infections in surgical patients and found that although cancer patients comprised only 24% of the patients studied, they

Table 14-1. Correlation of Postoperative Wound Infection with Preoperative Staphylococcal Carrier State

Preoperative Host-Staphylococcal Relationship	Patients	Patients without Infection	Patients with Infection	Staphylococcal Infections	Autogenous Infections	Heterogenous Infections	Nonstaphylococcal Infections
Asymptomatic nasal carriers	49	32	17	13	13	0	4
Carriers with minor skin infections	19	17	2	2	2	0	0
Carriers with staphylococci in necrotic tumor	11	2	9	9	9	0	0
Total carriers	79	51	28	24	24	0	4
Noncarriers	93	86	7	2	0	2	5
Patients without preoperative cultures	75	69	6	4	0	4	2
Total	247	206	41	30	24	6	11

accounted for 31% of the infections recorded [12]. If there is an association between malignant disease and postoperative infectious complications, many factors may play a role. It has been shown that age, length of surgery, and nutritional deprivation may predispose to infection, and these certainly are factors characteristic of the cancer patient [42].

The authors have reported an early experience that fully demonstrated the significance of infection in surgical cancer patients and the role of antibiotic prophylaxis. A retrospective infection rate ranged from 22 to 30%, and 73% of the infections were with *Staphylococcus aureus*. Of 247 patients who underwent major surgery, 172 had nasal cultures taken preoperatively to determine their infectious carrier states [29]. Table 14-1 shows the relation between the carrier states and the subsequent wound infections, in which 24 of the 30 staphylococcal infections that occurred did so in patients carrying the organism preoperatively (presumably into the operating room). Review of the antibiotic therapy of these patients revealed that wound infections developed in 23% of the patients receiving antibiotics and in 8% of the patients not receiving antibiotic therapy. Although previous studies had suggested that antibiotic usage increased the risk of postoperative infection, it was clear that in such patient reviews, only those more highly at risk of infection had received antibiotics.

Because of these impressions, a prospective double-blind controlled study was undertaken to define further the role of staphylococcal carriage and preventive antibiotics in the development of wound infection in the surgical cancer patient. Patients were cultured on admission to evaluate carrier status. Then they were divided into five groups by anatomic location of the operative site, and on the day of operation they were randomized in double-blind fashion into an antibiotic or placebo group. The antibiotic used was chloramphenicol at a dosage of 2 g every 6 hours, given for 10 days postoperatively.

The study was terminated after 79 patients had been included in the protocol, for it became clear that there was an alarmingly higher infection rate than had been observed previously. There was a 14% infection rate in the group treated with antibiotics and a 54.3% rate in the placebo group (Table 14-2). Postoperative antibiotic prophylaxis was effective in both the

Table 14-2. Postoperative Staphylococcal Wound Infections by Treatment and Carrier Status

	Treatment					
	Antibiotic		Placebo		Totals	
Carrier Status	No.	%	No.	%	No.	%
Carrier	3 of 15	20.0	10 of 14	71.4	13 of 29	44.8
Noncarrier	3 of 28	10.7	9 of 21	42.9	12 of 49	24.5
Treatment Totals	6 of 43	14.0	10 of 35	54.3	25 of 78	32.1

Table 14-3. Incidence of Staphylococcal Wound Infection by Anatomic Area and Treatment

Anatomic Area	Antibiotic			Placebo		
	Total	Number Infected	Percent Infected	Total	Number Infected	Percent Infected
Head and neck	9	2	22.2	11	6	54.5
Thorax	5	1	20.0	4	1	25.0
Abdominal	8	0	0.0	5	2	40.0
Pelvic	17	2	11.8	14	10	71.4
Groin and extremities	4	1	25.0	1	0	0.0
All areas	43	6	14.0	35	19	54.3

carrier and noncarrier groups. Table 14-3 lists the infection rate by anatomic location and treatment. Subsequent studies have shown little value in postoperative antibiotic therapy alone, but they have demonstrated the effectiveness of preoperative and intraoperative treatment [25, 40, 41]. One possible factor for this result is that the large dose of antibiotic used may have been sufficient to render an antibacterial effect, even when given only in the postoperative period. Another possible factor is the antibiotic that was used. Chloramphenicol has been shown to be particularly effective against anaerobic organisms that may have been prevalent in infections of the high risk regions: the head, neck, and pelvic regions [8].

In a subsequent blind study by the authors [30], two antibiotic regimens were compared. One group of patients received chloramphenicol for 3 days preoperatively and 7 days postoperatively. A second group received a placebo for 3 days preoperatively and chloramphenicol for 7 days postoperatively. The results of this study are summarized in Table 14-4. The addition of the preoperative antibiotic decreased the incidence of infection from 17.4 to 8.9%. The differences between the groups achieved statistical significance in comparison to the carrier patients.

Patients colonized by culturable amounts of *S. aureus* have a 28% increased risk of infection over noncarriers. Ninety-three percent of these

Table 14-4. Number and Percent of Postoperative Infections by Treatment and Carrier Status

Carrier Status	Preoperative and Postoperative Antibiotic		Postoperative Antibiotic Only		Totals	
	No.	%	No.	%	No.	%
Carrier	1 of 14	7.1	6 of 18	33.3	7 of 32	21.9
Noncarrier	3 of 31	9.7	2 of 28	7.1	5 of 59	8.5
Treatment Totals	4 of 45	8.9	8 of 46	17.4	12 of 91	13.2

patients became infected with the same phage-type organism that colonized the patient preoperatively [26]. The highest correlation occurred in patients who had staphylococci cultured from their necrotic tumors and subsequently developed infections.

Dor and Klastersky [14] have more recently examined the effect of prophylactic antibiotics in preventing infections in patients undergoing head and neck surgery for cancer. In a double-blind study, the value of ampicillin and cloxacillin given in the perioperative period was compared to a placebo. Bacterial infection developed in 17.3% of the antibiotic treated patients and in 36% of those receiving placebos.

At present, the authors have continued the use of prophylactic antibiotics in patients undergoing major surgical operations for malignancies. A wide-spectrum antibiotic is begun preoperatively, continued in dosages that are sufficient to maintain high levels during the operation, and then administered for a variable period postoperatively. The choice of antibiotic is governed by the site of operation and the potential pathogens to be encountered, by the presence of preexisting infection, or by particularly heavy colonization. Of interest is the fact that in spite of the continued use of chloramphenicol in nearly all patients undergoing cancer surgery over a period of 8 years, no hematologic disturbances were ever identified by the careful monitoring of the hematology service. Equally interesting is the fact that in spite of the intensive use of this antibiotic, it always remained the drug of choice for the usual hospital organisms. It was the drug to which the predominant hospital organisms and organisms causing infectious complications within the surgical service were most sensitive. This fact is attributed to the high-dose, short-course regimen that was used and seldom ever extended beyond the 10-day period of administration.

The surgical wound both in cancer patients and in general surgical patients remains the most common site of infection in the postoperative period [1]. Wound infections range in severity from a minor inflammatory response that may resolve spontaneously to a deep active infection that may be life-threatening and contribute significantly to postoperative morbidity. Several prospective double-blind controlled studies have now shown that wide-spectrum antibiotics used on a preventive basis in the preoperative and intraoperative period can decrease the rate of wound infection [25, 40, 41]. However, to be effective, the antibiotic must reach the site of infection at the interior of the wound to provide sufficient antibacterial levels.

Previous studies in animal models have shown that several antibiotics given in a single dose can achieve significant concentrations in the wound fluid [2, 6]. However, there are problems associated with such studies that prevent their immediate extrapolation to the clinical situation. First, the antibiotic was usually given as a single intravenous bolus injection. Second, the models employed a subcutaneously implanted capsule that possesses inherent difficulties of interpretation because of dilutional factors during repeated sampling. Third, there are the potential species differences.

In an attempt to extend these observations to the human model, the authors have examined the concentration of antibiotic achieved in wound fluid during the early postoperative period [4]. Patients undergoing lymph node dissection for malignant disease received one of six antibiotics. Three cephalosporins (cephalothin, cefazolin, and cephapirin) were studied as well as ampicillin, oxacillin, and clindamycin. The drug was given in a standard dose as an intravenous bolus at 6-hour intervals. The antibiotic was begun 8 hours preoperatively and continued intraoperatively and postoperatively. The patients had closed suction drainage wound catheters (Hemovacs) placed at the time of surgery. Routine care of these catheters included constant suction and intermittent manual aspiration of the wound fluid. The fluid was collected, stored in liquid nitrogen, and subsequently bioassayed for antibiotic concentration.

Figure 14-1 shows the concentration of cephalothin in wound fluid and serum on the first postoperative day during administration of 1 g of the drug intravenously every 6 hours. The first fluid sample, taken 1 hour after antibiotic administration, contained cephalothin 8.3 μg/ml. By 90 min, the concentration reached a maximum of 9.4 and subsequently decreased so that less than 2.5 μg/ml was present by 5 hours after administration. A similar pattern was seen with cephapirin. Cefazolin, which has prolonged serum levels, produced higher concentrations and a flatter curve with significant antibacterial activity even at 6 hours following administration. The patterns obtained with ampicillin, oxacillin, and clindomycin were similar to those of the rapidly cleared cephalosporins. Each drug achieved antibacterial levels at the standard dosages employed. Only cefazolin maintained sufficient levels to inhibit the majority of susceptible gram-negative organisms throughout the 6-hour period between injections. This was related

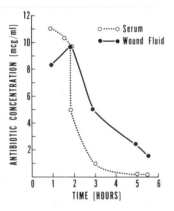

Figure 14-1. The concentration of cephalosporin in wound fluid and serum on the first postoperative day during administration of 1 g of the drug intravenously every 6 hours.

to the sustained blood levels. Protein binding of these antibiotics in the wound fluid was similar to that reported for serum samples.

These studies confirm the applicability in the clinical setting of results from previous animal models describing antibiotic levels in wound fluid. They also demonstrate the differences achieved with these drugs after repeated rather than single administration. Significant wound fluid levels were achieved with all drugs studied. The fluid concentration was related to the serum concentration, but at times, the wound fluid level surpassed the serum levels.

Recently, the spectrum of infective organisms in hospitalized patients has shifted to the gram-negative bacteria [18]. Other authors have described these changes in general surgical patients [3, 47]. Levine, Graw, and Young [36] and others [19] have found that in patients with hematopoietic and lymphoreticular malignancies, there has been a marked increase in infections from gram-negative bacilli, such as *Klebsiella, Serratia,* and *Escherichia coli,* as well as several fungi. Infection with *Pseudomonas aeruginosa* was the single most frequent cause of death from infection. It has been suggested that this change in the pattern of the infective organisms is the result of exposure to the hospital environment and prior antibiotic therapy [24, 33, 43]. There are several studies of bacterial colonization in patients that describe the bacterial alterations that develop during hospitalization and antibiotic treatment [50, 51]. However, these studies have examined the patterns of colonization in hospitalized patients receiving antibiotics for a preexisting infection. Such patients already have immunologic and bacterial alterations accompanying the infection. Thus it is difficult to relate these findings to potential changes in bacterial colonization during the prophylactic use of antibiotics in surgical cancer patients.

In an attempt to define more specifically the changing bacterial environment of patients undergoing surgical treatment of cancer, the sources of bacterial contamination in the physical environment have been examined as well as the spectrum of organisms colonizing the patient before and after treatment. As an integral part of this prospective study, bacterial colonization of the surgical wound was examined and a bacteriologic survey was performed prior to the actual patient study [21]. Surfaces of tables and floors in patient rooms were sampled as well as sinks, tubs, humidifiers, and water fountains. Surfaces were cultured with Rodac surface plates, utilizing blood agar and egg yolk media. Moist swabs from the plumbing fixtures were cultured in broth media and plated on blood agar. The organisms were identified by standard bacteriologic methods.

Fifty-three dry surfaces were sampled, and essentially all these samples grew *Staphylococcus albus,* various spore formers, or a mixture of these organisms. Forty-one wet surfaces were sampled: 16 samples (39%) contained large numbers of *Pseudomonas* species and 11 (27%) contained *Flavobacterium* species (Table 14-5). Whitby and Rampling [52] have reported a slightly higher culture rate of *P. aeruginosa* (53%) from similar hospital lo-

Table 14-5. Bacteria in the Environment of the Cancer Patient

Surface	Culture Number	Organisms	Number
Dry	53	*Staphylococcus albus*	28
		Spore formers	4
		Mixture	21
Wet	41	*Staphylococcus albus*	7
		Pseudomonas species	16
		Flavobacterium species	11
		Mixture	5
		No growth	2

cations. They noted that, in comparison, these bacteria were rarely cultured from the patient's home environment.

As a part of this study, the bacterial colonization of patients was studied when they were admitted to the hospital and during their surgical treatment, which included the perioperative use of prophylactic antibiotics [5]. All patients admitted for surgical treatment of localized malignancy were eligible for the study. Patients allergic to penicillin, those who had a pre-existing infection requiring antibiotic treatment, and those who had received antibiotics during the 2 weeks prior to admission were excluded. Cultures were obtained at six intervals: (1) at admission, (2) 1 day preoperatively, (3) 2 days postoperatively, (4) 7 days postoperatively, (5) 14 days postoperatively, and (6) 21 days postoperatively. Eight sites were sampled: (1) anterior nares, (2) oropharynx, (3) incision, (4) tumor, (5) standard skin site at xyphoid, (6) vagina, (7) rectum, and (8) urine. All cultures were obtained by a single physician and were examined by standard bacteriologic techniques. All patients received cephalothin at a dosage of 1 g intravenously every 6 hours, begun 8 hours prior to surgery, and continued for 24 hours after completion of the operation. At that time, patients were randomized into one of two groups based on their hospital number. The first group received no further antibiotic; the second group continued to receive a cephalosporin antibiotic, either cephalothin at the same dosage or cephalexin at 500 mg orally every 6 hours for 7 days postoperatively. No other antibiotics were given unless clinically indicated, in which case the patient was discontinued from the study. Eighty-eight patients entered the study and were cultured in the preoperative period. Twenty-five were then excluded because of a change in tumor therapy, drug allergy, or failure to be treated according to the protocol of the study. Twenty-eight patients were in the 1 day antibiotic group and 35 were in the 7-day group. Table 14-6 compares the groups according to sex, histology, and site of tumor. Table 14-7 lists the organisms found on pharyngeal culture at admission, when there was a localized malignancy, prior to extended hospitalization. Essentially all patients had alpha streptococci and *Neisseria* species in the

Table 14-6. Distribution of Patients

	Study Groups		
	1 Day	7 Days	Discontinued
Sex			
Males	15	21	14
Females	13	14	11
Histologic diagnosis			
Melanoma	12	14	7
Sarcoma	5	4	5
Squamous or basal			
cell carcinoma	6	10	9
Adenocarcinoma	5	5	1
Other	0	2	3
Site of tumor			
Head and neck	10	7	10
Chest	2	5	2
Abdomen	4	9	4
Extremity	12	14	9
Total	28	35	25

oropharynx at admission. Only 4.7% of the patients had *S. aureus*. Gram-negative bacilli were less commonly found in the pharynx; 3% had *E. coli* on the pharyngeal culture and only single patients had *Proteus, Klebsiella,* or *Enterobacter* species. No patients had pharyngeal cultures that grew *Citrobacter* or *Pseudomonas* species at admission. Yeast was cultured in 7.8% of patients.

Rosenthal and Toger [44] reported results from normal controls, using culture techniques that included broth culture selective for gram-negative

Table 14-7. Organisms on Pharyngeal Culture at Admission

Organism	Percent of Patients with Positive Cultures
Alpha *Streptococcus*	98.4
Neisseria species	96.7
Gamma *Streptococcus*	56.2
Diphtheroids	31.2
Micrococcus	31.2
Hemophilus, hemolytic	32.8
Hemophilus, nonhemolytic	23.4
Beta *Streptococcus*	12.5
Staphylococcus epidermidis	10.9
Staphylococcus aureus	4.7

organisms, showing that 18% of patients cultured had *Enterobacteriaceae* or
P. aeruginosa cultured from the pharynx. Using the agar plate method, 6%
had these organisms in culturable amounts. Others [24, 43] have reported
rates of 2 to 11.5% for these organisms, using agar plates. These rates are
comparable to the reported 7.9%.

The sequential cultures demonstrate the floral changes that occur during
14 days of hospitalization without antibiotic treatment and after a surgical
procedure with antibiotic treatment. Most organisms showed no change in
frequency during the early hospitalization. Alpha and gamma streptococci,
Neisseria species, diphtheroids, micrococci, and nonhemalytic *Hemophilus*
occurred at the same frequency on admission and 14 days later. There were
small increases in the colonization rate of other organisms, including the
gram-negative bacilli and *S. aureus*.

With surgical operation and antibiotic treatment, some organisms decreased in frequency (Table 14-8). The frequency of these three organisms
continued to remain low or decrease in the patients receiving a full 7-day
course of antibiotic treatment. The rate of colonization tended to increase
toward the preoperative level in the patients who received a single day of
antibiotic treatment. These observations suggest that the postoperative
changes in colonization rate resulted at least partially from the antibiotic
treatment and not just as postoperative alterations.

The frequency of colonization with some organisms increased during
postoperative antibiotic treatment with an initial increase on the second
postoperative day, which remained the same or increased further after a
full week of postoperative antibiotic therapy (Table 14-9). The frequency
of colonization generally decreased by the seventh postoperative day in
patients receiving only 1 day of antibiotic therapy. The increased colonization by *Pseudomonas* species continued in both treatment groups.

Table 14-10 presents the relative incidence of *Enterobacteriaceae* in
sequential pharyngeal cultures. There is an increased proportion of these
organisms relative to the total organisms present after preoperative hospitalization and postoperatively. There was a similar increase in incidence
of all *Enterobacteriaceae* or those that were generally resistant to cephalosporins.

Table 14-8. Pharyngeal Organisms Decreasing in Frequency during Postoperative
Antibiotic Therapy

	Percent of Patients Colonized				
				7 Days Postoperative	
Organism	Admission	Preopera-tive	2 Days Post-operative	1 Day	1 Week
Gamma *Streptococcus*	56.2	57.1	31.1	57.1	24.2
Diphtheroids	31.2	30.2	19.7	42.8	6.1
Hemophilus, hemolytic	32.8	42.9	13.1	28.6	15.2

Table 14-9. Pharyngeal Organisms Increasing in Frequency during Postoperative Antibiotic Therapy

	Percent of Patients Colonized				
				7 Days Postoperative	
Organism	Admission	Preopera-tive	2 Days Post-operative	1 Day	1 Week
Escherichia coli	3.1	4.8	8.2	3.6	6.1
Enterobacter species	1.6	1.9	4.9	3.6	12.1
Klebsiella species	1.6	4.8	11.5	3.6	9.1
Citrobacter species	0	0	3.3	0	3.1
Pseudomonas species	0	1.9	4.9	10.7	3.0

The presence of resistant *Enterobacteriaceae* on rectal cultures is shown in Table 14-11. The incidence remained stable during preoperative hospitalization but increased in the postoperative period. By the seventh postoperative day, the incidence of positive cultures decreased in the group receiving 1 day of antibiotic therapy. Colonization in the patients given antibiotics for 1 week postoperatively remained elevated through the first and second postoperative weeks.

In summary, there were organisms that were sensitive to the antibiotic administered which decreased in frequency during postoperative antibiotic therapy. Others, particularly gram-negative bacilli, increased postoperatively. The changes were minimized in patients receiving 1 day of antibiotic therapy. Gram-negative organisms that were both sensitive and resistant to the cephalosporin employed colonized patients increasingly during the postoperative period. These results suggest that diminution of the more sensitive normal bacterial flora may permit the overgrowth of other organisms that are generally more resistant, although still clinically sensitive to the antibiotic used. These changes may be minimized with a shorter course of antibiotics.

The relation between infections and the host immune system has been discussed previously. Alterations in the status of immune reactivity have

Table 14-10. Pharyngeal Cultures with Enterobacteriaceae

	Percent of Organisms Present				
				7 Days postopera-tive	
Organism	Admission	Preopera-tive	2 Days Post-operative	1 Day	1 Week
All *Enterobacteriaceae*	2.0	4.0	10.2	7.1	8.9
Resistant *Enterobacteriaceae*	0.4	1.8	4.9	5.5	4.1

Table 14-11. Rectal Cultures with Resistant Enterobacteriaceae

Time	Percent Bacteria Present
Admission	12.6
Preoperative	12.1
2 days postoperative	19.4
7 days postoperative	
1 day group	15.6
1 week group	18.9
14 days postoperative	
1 day group	15.8
1 week group	21.3

been related to varying susceptibility to infection. The immunologic altera-tions that occur in the cancer patient have been the subject of many recent studies. Each portion of the immune mechanism has been studied, particu-larly in relation to the response to the patient's tumor. The status of the cellular immune response has been correlated with prognosis. An intact cellular response is associated with a favorable prognosis, while a depressed response is more often associated with a poor prognosis. The ability of patients to become sensitized to denitrochlorobenzene (DNCB), a contact allergen, reflects the status of the cellular immune response. The response to DNCB is gradable and has been correlated both with the clinical course and clinical stage of cancer patients [11, 15, 16, 31]. Patients with poor or no sensitization to DNCB more frequently have advanced tumors or subse-quent progression of disease.

The nature of the inflammatory response elicited in these tests has been the subject of some controversy [10, 23]. By comparison with the inflamma-tory response aroused by croton oil, a nonspecific irritant, Roth et al. [45] have shown no correlation between skin reactivity to DNCB and croton oil in previously untreated cancer patients. Although the lack of sensitization to DNCB was clearly correlated with the stage of disease, no such relation existed with the lack of inflammatory response to croton oil. In contrast, Dizon and Southam [13] have reported that patients with advanced cancer have a decreased cellular response following abrasions of the skin.

Studies of nonspecific inflammatory response in tumor-bearing animal models have also failed to present consistent results. Mahoney and Leigh-ton [38] demonstrated that a foreign body implanted within transplanted tumors in rodents failed to provoke a normal inflammatory response. Yet inflammation in normal tissue elsewhere in the tumor-bearing animal re-mained active. Bernstein, Zbar, and Rapp [9] have reported that guinea pigs with large intramuscular tumors have decreased skin inflammatory reactivity to nonspecific agents as well as impaired delayed cutaneous hypersensitivity. The authors suggested that since lymphocytes from the tumor-bearing ani-mals functioned normally in response to antigen in vitro, the defect in skin reactivity could be the result of impairment of a nonspecific component of cellular immunity.

Fauve et al. [17] have reported that mice bearing a teratocarcinoma can be effectively immunized against *Listeria monocytogenes* (a process dependent on activation of macrophages by sensitized T lymphocytes). However, the tumor cells produce a substance that prevented a local inflammatory response and repulsed macrophages in vitro. These authors concluded that in their model, there was no general impairment of immunity but, rather, a local antiinflammatory effect.

In a series of reports, North et al. [39a, b; 50a] have shown that subcutaneous injection of tumor cells in mice produced a circulating factor that impaired the host response to *L. monocytogenes*. Although the return and even enhancement of the antibacterial response paralleled the development of concomitant antitumor immunity, the tumor itself remained a privileged site for bacterial growth.

The antibacterial activity of macrophages from cancer patients remains a subject of controversy. Baum et al. [7] reported a decrease in the phagocytic activity of macrophages from patients with breast cancer. More recently King, Bain, and Lo Buglio [32] reported normal staphylocidal activity in monocytes from patients with solid tumors.

There is similar variability in studies of humoral immune responses in human cancer patients. Lytton, Hughs, and Fulthorpe [37] examined the secondary response to tetanus toxoid and showed that patients with malignant solid tumors gave a lower response than those with nonneoplastic diseases. Other reports have shown a decreased antibody response to flagellin from *Salmonella* species [34]. Still others have failed to demonstrate any alteration in the response to yellow fever, tularemia, or *E. coli* antigens [35, 49]. Therefore it remains difficult to predict the status of the humoral immune response in cancer patients or to assess the role of any alterations in altering the hosts' response to infection.

Descriptions of blocking factors in the serum of cancer patients [20, 48] have produced significant theoretical concern in the field of tumor immunotherapy. However, the specificity of the blocking phenomenon has not been fully studied, and the possibility that it may affect the antibacterial immune response has not been evaluated. Blocking factors may prove to be of major or insignificant importance in the response of the cancer patient to infection.

Table 14-12 summarizes the reported alterations in the immune status of

Table 14-12. Changes in Immune Function in Solid Tumor Patients

Nonspecific inflammation	±
Cellular immunity	↓
Macrophage function	±
Blocking factors	?

patients with solid tumors. It is clear that the role of each factor in the response to infection and its alterations in the solid tumor patient must be defined further before specific therapies can be devised to counteract these deficiencies.

References

1. Alexander, J. W. Nosocomial infections. *Curr. Probl. Surg.* August, 1973.
2. Alexander, J. W., et al. Concentration of intravenously administered antibiotics in experimental surgical wounds. *J. Trauma* 13:423, 1973.
3. Altemeier, W. A., et al. Changing patterns in surgical infections. *Ann. Surg.* 178:436, 1973.
4. Bagley, D. H., et al. Antibiotic levels in human wound fluid. In press.
5. Bagley, D. H., et al. Bacterial flora of the surgical cancer patient. In press.
6. Baker, G., and Hunt, T. K. Penicillin concentration in experimental wounds. *Am. J. Surg.* 115:531, 1968.
7. Baum, M., et al. Macrophage phagocytic activity in patients with breast cancer. *Br. J. Surg.* 60:899, 1973.
8. Beazley, R. M., Polakavetz, S. H., and Miller, R. M. *Bacteroides* infection in a university surgical service. *Surg. Gynecol. Obstet.* 135:742, 1972.
9. Bernstein, I. D., Zbar, B., and Rapp, H. J. Impaired inflammatory response in tumor bearing guinea pigs. *Natl. Cancer Inst.* 49:1641, 1972.
10. Bleumink, E., Nater, J. P., and The, H. DNCB₁-reactivity and skin irritation. *N. Engl. J. Med.* 288:322, 1973.
11. Catalona, W. J., Sample, W. F., and Chretien, P. B. Lymphocyte reactivity in cancer patients: Correlation with tumor histology and clinical stage. *Cancer* 31:65, 1973.
12. Cohen, L. S., Fekety, F. R., and Cluff, L. E. Studies of the epidemiology of staphylococcal infections. VI. Infections in the surgical patient. *Ann. Surg.* 159:321, 1964.
13. Dizon, Q. S., and Southam, C. M. Abnormal cellular response to skin abrasion in cancer patients. *Cancer* 16:1288, 1963.
14. Dor, P., and Klastersky, J. Prophylactic antibiotics in oral, pharyngeal and laryngeal surgery for cancer: A double-blind study. *Laryngoscope* 83:1992, 1973.
15. Eilber, F. R., and Morton, D. L. Impaired immunologic reactivity and recurrence following cancer surgery. *Cancer* 24:362, 1970.
16. Eilber, F. R., Nizzl, A., and Morton, D. L. Sequential evaluation of general immune competence in cancer patients, correlation with clinical course. *Cancer* 35:660, 1975.
17. Fauve, R. M., et al. Inflammatory effects of murine malignant cells. *Proc. Natl. Acad. Sci.* 71:4052, 1974.
18. Finland, M. Changing ecology of bacterial infections as related to antibacterial therapy. *J. Infect. Dis.* 122:419, 1970.
19. Gaya, H., et al. Changing patterns of infections in cancer patients. *Cancer* 9:401, 1973.
20. Hellstrom, I., et al. Blocking of all mediated tumor immunity by sera from patients with growing neoplasms. *Int. J. Cancer* 7:226, 1971.
21. Herrmann, L. G., Bagley, D. H., and Ketcham, A. S. Unpublished observations, 1974.
22. Inagaki, J., Rodriguez, V., and Bodey, G. P. Causes of death in cancer patients. *Cancer* 33:568, 1974.

23. Johnson, M. W., Maibach, H. I., and Salmon, S. E.   Skin reactivity in patients with cancer: Impaired delayed hypersensitivity or faulty inflammatory response. *N. Engl. J. Med.* 284:1255, 1971.
24. Johnson, W. G., Pierce, A. K., and Sanford, J. P.   Changing pharyngeal flora of hospitalized patients. *N. Engl. J. Med.* 281:1137, 1969.
25. Johnstone, F. R. C.   An assessment of prophylactic antibiotics in general surgery. *Surg. Gynecol. Obstet.* 116:1, 1963.
26. Ketcham, A. S.   Antibiotics in cancer surgery. *Chic. Med.* 67:1075, 1964.
27. Ketcham, A. S., et al.   Unpublished data.
28. Ketcham, A. S., et al.   Pelvic exenteration for carcinoma of the uterine cervix. *Cancer* 26:513, 1970.
29. Ketcham, A. S., et al.   The role of antibiotic therapy in control of staphylococcal infections following cancer surgery. *Surg. Gynecol. Obstet.* 114:345, 1962.
30. Ketcham, A. S., Lieberman, J. E., and West, J. T.   Antibiotic prophylaxis in cancer surgery and its value in staphylococcal carrier patients. *Surg. Gynecol. Obstet.* 117:1, 1963.
31. Khoo, S. K., and MacKay, E. V.   Immunologic reactivity of female patients with genital cancer: Status in preinvasive, locally invasive and disseminated disease. *Am. J. Obstet. Gynecol.* 119:1018, 1975.
32. King, G. W., Bain, G., and LoBuglio, A. F.   The effect of tuberculosis and neoplasia on human monocyte staphylocidal activity. *Cell. Immunol.* 16:389, 1975.
33. Kunin, G. M., Tuposi, T., and Craig, S. A.   Use of antibiotics. A brief exposition of the problem and some tentative solutions. *Ann. Intern. Med.* 79:555, 1973.
34. Lee, A. K. V., Rowley, M., and MacKay, I. R.   Antibody-producing capacity in human cancer. *Br. J. Cancer* 24:454, 1970.
35. Levin, R. H., Landy, M., and Frei, E.   The effect of 6-mercaptopurine on immune response in man. *N. Engl. J. Med.* 271:16, 1964.
36. Levine, A. S., Graw, R. S., and Young, R. C.   Management of infections in patients with leukemia and lymphoma: Current concepts and experimental approaches. *Semin. Hematol.* 9:141, 1972.
37. Lytton, B., Hughes, L. E., and Fulthorpe, A. J.   Circulating antibody response in malignant disease. *Lancet* 1:69, 1964.
38. Mahoney, M. J., and Leighton, J.   The inflammatory response to a foreign body within transplantable tumors. *Cancer Res.* 22:334, 1962.
39. Mirsky, H. S., and Cuttner, J.   Fungal infection in acute leukemia. *Cancer* 30:348, 1972.
39a. North, R. J., Kirstein, D. P., and Tuttle, R. L.   Subversion of host defense mechanisms by murine tumors. I. A circulating factor that suppresses macrophage-mediated resistance to infection. *J. Exp. Med.* 143:559, 1976.
39b. North, R. J., Kirstein, D. P., and Tuttle, R. L.   Subversion of host defense mechanisms by murine tumors. II. Counter-influence of concomitant antitumor immunity. *J. Exp. Med.* 143:574, 1976.
40. Pavel, A., et al.   Prophylactic antibiotics in clean orthopedic surgery. *J. Bone Joint Surg.* [A] 56:777, 1974.
41. Polk, H. C., Lopez-Mayor, J. F.   Postoperative wound infection: A preoperative study of determinant factors and prevention. *Surgery* 66:97, 1969.
42. Post-operative wound infections: The influence of ultraviolet irradiation of the operating room and of various other factors. National Academy of Sciences, National Research Council, Division of Medical Sciences, Ad Hoc Committee of the Committee on Trauma. *Ann. Surg.* 160 (Suppl. 2), 1964.

43. Rahal, J. S., et al. Upper respiratory tract carriage of gram-negative enteric bacilli by hospital personnel. *J.A.M.A.* 214:754, 1970.
44. Rosenthal, S., and Toger, I. B. Prevalence of gram-negative rods in the normal pharyngeal flora. *Ann. Intern. Med.* 83:355, 1975.
45. Roth, J. A., et al. Lack of correlation between skin reactivity to dinitrochlorobenzene and croton oil in patients with cancer. *N. Engl. J. Med.* 293:388, 1975.
46. Schimpff, S. C., et al. Origin of infection in acute nonlymphocytic leukemia. Significance of hospital acquisition of potential pathogens. *Ann. Intern. Med.* 77:707, 1972.
47. Schlenker, J. D., and Barrios, R. Gram-negative pneumonias in surgical patients. *Arch. Surg.* 106:267, 1973.
48. Sjögren, H. O., et al. Elution of blocking factors from human tissues capable of abrogating tumor-cell distribution by specifically immune lymphocytes. *Int. J. Cancer* 9:274, 1972.
49. Southam, C. M. The immunologic status of patients with nonlymphomatous cancer. *Cancer Res.* 28:1433, 1968.
50. Spencer, R. C., and Philip, J. R. Effect of previous antimicrobial therapy on bacteriological findings in patients with primary pneumonia. *Lancet* II:349, 1973.
50a. Spitalny, G. L., and North, R. J. Subversion of host defense mechanisms by malignant tumors: An established tumor as a privileged site for bacterial growth. *J. Exp. Med.* 145:1264, 1977.
51. Tillotson, J. R., and Finland, M. Bacterial colonization and clinical superinfection of the respiratory tract complicating antibiotic treatment of pneumonia. *J. Infect. Dis.* 119:597, 1969.
52. Whitby, J. L., and Rampling, A. *Pseudomonas aeruginosa* contamination in domestic and hospital environments. *Lancet* I:15, 1972.

15. *Acute Susceptibility to Infection in Trauma and Shock and Its Prevention*

John R. Border, J. LaDuca, and R. Seibel

Because of the confusion and uncontrolled nature of most literature reports on sepsis, this chapter describes exactly how our trauma service is operated with respect to the problem of infection and attempts to relate these activities to basic principles. This discussion will certainly lead to some disagreements with other authorities and publications.

Trauma patients are widely reputed to have an increased incidence of infections. Also, trauma is associated with multiple local conditions that are conducive to sepsis and to multiple systemic alterations that both contribute to the local development of sepsis and alter the systemic response to it. The predominant means of preventing sepsis is management of the local conditions that contribute to its development, which can be supplemented by systemic management that enhances local resistance to sepsis. The onset of infection requires the proper local combination of bacterial contamination plus bacterial nutrient. This combination allows the bacterial colony to grow until it can invade the tissues and produce infection.

An infection may be defined as a self-perpetuating colony of bacteria that induces local pathologic tissue changes. Since bacterial growth requires nutrients not provided by living tissue, this definition implies that, in a stable infection, the bacteria colony can produce sufficient tissue necrosis to provide the nutrient required for bacterial growth. Thus enlarging infections imply an excess of bacterial nutrient (i.e., dead tissue), which can be caused by necrosis produced at the time of trauma or by virulent bacteria. Clearly this process is accentuated by the conditions observed in closed-space infections, such as abscesses, and is diminished by drainage of closed-space infections. Therefore it may be presumed that the physical pressure in a closed-space infection together with its associated high concentration of bacteria also contributes to inducing tissue necrosis.

The systemic response to a closed-space infection is also alleviated by drainage. Thus the systemic response is also related to the conditions of a closed-space infection, and probably occurs secondary to pain, toxins, and bacteremia. Clearly, all the characteristics of the systemic septic response can be induced by stimuli, such as electric stimulation of the hypothalamus or hematomas, that have nothing to do with infection, and clearly the systemic septic response can occur in multiple trauma patients who recover without any area of sepsis ever being identified. The following question

Supported by National Institute General Medical Sciences Grant GM 15768.

must therefore be posed: does the systemic septic response have any necessary relation to sepsis, or is sepsis simply the systemic response to continuing severe stress? The systemic septic response in patients without organ failure, trauma, or dead tissue is essentially the same as sepsis, except in very depleted patients. These patients can have severe sepsis without the systemic septic response.

Granting the foregoing problems, it seems best to view the systemic septic response as an indication of severe stress that is related in general to necrotic tissue but is not the same as sepsis. This is the same condition that is required for the acute phase hepatic protein response. The systemic septic response requires normal neuroendocrine metabolic responsiveness and may be aborted by steroids, severe protein depletion, and probably agents that interfere severely with the sympathetic nervous system. It appears to be one of the stress catabolic states we have discussed previously [1]. These states in essence mobilize the circulation in multiple ways and mobilize energetic and synthetic substrate so that the body has more blood flow plus a higher concentration of plasma substrates to support the various organs than it has in its normal basal state. This would appear to be particularly important to the local tissue reaction to infections as well as to the systemic antibacterial response. The local tissue reaction plus the systemic antibacterial response are extremely important in preventing systemic sepsis and in localizing areas of sepsis; both reactions are heavily dependent on protein synthesis.

The systemic septic response in essence delivers all the materials required for protein synthesis in high concentrations. This process requires increased and organized activity in the liver, muscle, and adipose tissue. However, there are reasons, developed later, which suggest that, with time and continued stress following injury, the systemic septic response may be altered in a way that limits protein synthesis by endogenous amino acid imbalances but does not limit total delivery of energetic substrate. This limitation in protein synthesis may change the relative proportions of fat and glucose energetic substrates. Clearly, limitations of blood flow or limitations of substrate delivery may decrease the protein synthetic component of the systemic and local septic response and thus enhance the possibility of a local infection becoming a systemic infection. Thus shock and arterial hypoxia reduce the quantity of bacteria required to produce an infection on a systemic basis. The same changes may be produced locally by tourniquets, edema, casts, and vasoconstrictors (see Chapter 12). Both systemic and local factors thus reduce the bacterial contamination required to produce an infection with a given quantity of bacterial nutrient.

Infections following trauma result primarily from local conditions that juxtapose bacterial contamination and bacterial nutrient. The bacterial nutrient results from dead tissue, tissue fluids, hematomas, and secretions. The bacterial contamination results from open wounds, various tubes required for monitoring and life support, or from bacteremias. The multiple trauma patient has particularly favorable local conditions for the onset of infection in several areas. Prevention of infection in these patients is heavily dependent on the management of multiple local problems, and the prevention or treatment of systemic infection is heavily dependent on the management of cardiopulmonary failure and metabolic support.

Local Conditions and Infection

The Organisms

The organisms usually involved are not the extremely invasive organisms that can cross intact skin nor, with the exception of *Streptococcus,* are they locally invasive from an established infection. *Streptococcus* is not usually a significant clinical problem because of its quick response to antibiotics. This response is enhanced by the cellulitis produced, which allows rapid delivery of antibiotics and the systemic antibacterial system from the circulating blood to the area of infections. The organisms usually involved are *Staphylococcus aureus, Pseudomonas, Escherichia coli, Bacteroides,* fungi, yeasts, and several less common but equally noninvasive organisms. In general, these organisms are invasive only if contained in an abscess associated with dead tissue. *Staphylococcus* is very special in its ability to survive prolonged periods of dehydration and to cause airborne contamination. The other bacteria, in general, require hydration and are transferred through wet contacts.

Bacterial Contamination and Bacterial Nutrient

Most open wounds have some degree of bacterial contamination, whether they are surgical or accidental. Few such wounds get infected if properly managed. Most approaches to the problem have concentrated on eliminating bacterial contamination, since this is a partially measurable factor. However, the conversion of a bacterially contaminated area to one of infection depends on far more than the magnitude of the bacterial contamination unless one is considering massive bacterial contamination (see Chapter 12). The factors involved appear to be local bacterial contamination, bacterial nutrient, and the local factors that permit or restrict access of the systemic response to the infecting agent in the area of infection.

Fat. Subcutaneous fat is commonly infected, probably because all wounds allow bacterial access. Surgical wounds physically divide the fat cells, leaving bacterial nutrient in the form of triglycerides. Traumatic wounds may, by crushing and tearing, produce large amounts of dead fat. Subcutaneous fat has, relative to the bacterial nutrient it contains, very poor vascularity. This problem is accentuated by the additional bacterial nutrient provided by those surgeons who hurriedly clamp all bleeders in this area, thereby inducing necrotic tissue and bacterial nutrient at each hemostatic tie. These problems may be made worse if the operation is conducted with the aid of a tourniquet or vasoconstrictors and if the patient is in shock, or severe arterial hypoxia. These conditions also enhance dehydration necrosis and prevent or restrict blood flow at exactly the time the tissues are most exposed to bacteria; and tissue without blood flow is meat that readily supports bacterial growth. The problem can be alleviated by reducing bacterial contamination as well as by the use of wet sponges, control of bleeding by pressure insofar as possible, the use of very few hemostats, and abandonment of subcutaneous and cutaneous sutures by tissue approximation with suction devices (hemovacs) and surgical tape. Reducing intraoperative bacterial contamination may be materially aided by keeping all the wound that is not actually being used covered with sponges and laparotomy pads and by using preoperative systemic antibiotics and intraoperative antibiotic irrigations.

Muscle. Infections in muscle seldom occur. This is probably related to its good vascularity relative to bacterial nutrient, incisions that do not divide or devitalize muscle, the decreased time of exposure relative to the subcutaneous fat, and the placement of sutures in the avascular fascial sheaths that do not produce bleeding and bacterial nutrient. However, the infections that do occur in muscle are almost always devastating and are related to large volumes of necrotic muscle produced by vascular compromise, secondary to accidental or surgical trauma, or direct crushing injuries to the muscle. Direct crushing injuries to muscle are particularly likely to occur if the muscle is superimposed on flat surfaces of bone (e.g., the pelvis) or large displacements of the fracture fragments have occurred at the instant of injury.

Dehydration necrosis is a very real entity that is best observed during surgery. However, it occurs in all wounds that are left open. The extent of dehydration necrosis depends on the vascularity and physical structure of the tissue. Thus, under normal conditions, it probably involves muscle the least, except during surgery, when high-intensity heat lamps accelerate the process. This may be reduced by proper selection of surgery lighting. In contrast fat, because of its content of triglycerides and their impermeability to water, is probably much less involved by dehydration, while nerve and tendon, because of their very poor vascularity, are very much involved. Cortical bone is very avascular, and therefore dehydration necrosis commonly occurs if the periosteum is stripped. However, because of the physical nature of bone, this necrosis predominantly involves the superficial layers. This necrosis is sufficient to prevent investiture by soft tissue during the healing process and causes bare dry bone to persist, awaiting new infection. Dehydration necrosis is prevented by skin coverage, which probably accounts largely for the extreme attempts that have been made to get skin coverage over nerves, tendons, blood vessels, and bone, using autologous, homologous, or heterologous skin.

Dehydration necrosis occurs in all open wounds. The magnitude of the process depends on the exact tissues involved, the size of the wound, the physical movement and hydration of the air, and the exposure to heat sources. The largest such wounds are burns. The process of dehydration necrosis is best observed in partial thickness excision of burn wounds, where the uncovered viable tissues can be observed to have blood vessels with flowing blood. With time these occlude and are associated with increased tissue necrosis following surgery. Open wounds that are covered with autologous, homologous, or heterologous skin have been observed to have a reduction in the superficial bacterial count beneath the applied skin. This process is utilized to prepare an open wound for autologous skin grafting and for protection of tendons, nerves, bone, and blood vessels. Most results are probably due to a reduction of bacterial nutrient by prevention of dehydration necrosis. Nature's way of dealing with this situation is to form a well hydrated covering layer of granulation tissue. This proceeds at the same time as the dehydration necrosis; thus a combination of the two processes is usually present. As a result, most open wounds close without incident but with inflammation. A consequence of the inflammation is the maturation of the vascular granulation tissue into avascular scar tissue with immobile atrophic skin. In general, all open wounds should be covered not only with sterile dressings but also with a water impermeable barrier so that dehydration necrosis is minimized. This has commonly been done with pigskin. However, this procedure has a defect: If laid over islands of dead tissue, these areas may become abscesses. We have also utilized polyethylene sheets. This simple measure has an amazing effect on the inflammation, thickness, mobility of the skin, and the rapidity of reepithelialization as long as it is not utilized in a way that produces an abscess.

Necrotic Bone. Fractured bone presents special problems. Casts clearly do not produce absolute immobilization of the fracture site. The fracture ends, grating together in a cast, can produce additional dead tissue that will support bacterial growth. Whether this phenomenon is important or not depends on the degree of bacterial contamination and the degree of soft tissue damage. Thus most class 1 open fractures can be managed with thorough debridement and plaster casts, because they have minimal contamination and necrotic tissue. This clearly does not necessarily imply the best management, even though it may not be harmful. In contrast, the more severely contaminated injuries with more severe soft tissue trauma require absolute immobilization. Exact reduction aids in preventing postoperative access of bacteria to the marrow cavity as well as in producing absolute immobilization. Tight skin closure of an open fracture after debridement allows collection of blood and fluid that can support bacterial growth and thus encourage infection. The insertion of pins and use of drills to insert screws may also produce, by the heat generated, necrosis of bone to add to the devascularized necrotic bone produced by the original injury. In general, bone receives its blood supply from those areas where muscles, tendons, and ligaments take their origin. Thus bone attached to such areas is in general still vascularized. Devascularized bone that is not involved in infection is usually reincorporated and adds greatly to mechanical stability by its presence as an exactly fitting cortical bone graft; it should not be discarded. The revascularization of such bone proceeds from the edges, where it is in contact with viable bone if there is no motion in the area. Revascularization of the center of a large piece of cortical bone may take many months to years and proceeds long after the edges have united to adjacent viable bone.

Absolute immobility of an open fracture is of the utmost importance in preventing conversion of bacterial contamination to infection. Infection almost always leads to a loss of devascularized cortical fragments if the infected area is allowed to begin as an abscess, whereas the same infection with the wound left open seldom leads to a loss of cortical fragments.

Therefore open fractures require multistage debridement with exploration of every corner of the traumatic cavity, as does any significant wound, to remove all elements that supply bacterial nutrient and to reduce bacterial contamination. In addition, the fracture fragments should be exactly reduced and absolutely immobilized by internal or external fixation. The wound should be very loosely closed or left open, and deep hemovacs should be utilized so that all tissue fluid that can support bacterial growth is removed and viable tissue is brought into approximation. Open wounds should be covered with a sterile dressing plus a loose water-impermeable layer that prevents dehydration, while allowing drainage of overt fluid. Finally, casts that prevent visualization of the earliest signs of deep infection should not be used and the leg should be elevated in such a way that it can be easily observed and edema can be reduced. This procedure also helps marginally viable skin to survive. The presence of inflammation in the wound after surgery suggests the presence of dead tissue (hematoma plus infection) and requires reoperation and re-debridement plus local irrigation with topical antibiotics and systemic antibiotics after culture.

In general, during the initial surgery we use systemic antibiotics started in the emergency room plus irrigation with a solution of antibiotics. Internal fixation that does not involve additional dissection beyond that required for debridement is routinely done. Minor amounts of additional dissection for better internal fixation may be allowed. Intramedullary nails are *never* utilized in open fractures because of the devascularization of bone fragments, produced by nailing, and the possible contamination of the whole marrow cavity. All open fractures are internally fixed with screws or screws and plates. In general, these are placed so that they lie deep to viable muscle and are not placed beneath skin. Fractures that extend beyond the area of debridement or are too comminuted for internal fixation can be immobilized with the use of external fixators. These allow complete immobilization together with elevation and clinical examination for the earliest signs of infection. Steinmann pins usually have a pointed tip with a number of pyramidal flats. Their construction is such that there is no pathway for the bone chips to exit the hole and therefore, when placed, considerable heat may be generated. The heat generated depends on the size of the pin, the rate of rotation, and the thickness of the cortex. In principle, all Steinmann pins should be placed through holes predrilled by drill bits. In practice, the larger pins and thicker cortex absolutely require predrilling to prevent heat necrosis of bone. Pin tract infections, with the pin through viable bone, usually have little consequence other than loosening of the pin, while those through necrotic bone almost always persist until the sequestrum is removed. Heat necrosis is frequently caused by improper use of pins, saws, or dull drills.

Local Antibacterial System Activity

It should be noted that the phagocytic cells that are important in antibacterial activities are also the same cells that scavenge dead tissue. Thus necrotic tissue may not only provide bacterial nutrient but also, in effect, so congest the phagocytic cells that it inhibits antibacterial phagocytosis. In addition, necrotic tissue, by increasing the distance of diffusion from functioning capillaries, can restrict all nutrient supply to the phagocytic cells and thus can inhibit phagocytosis. This problem is further compounded by the additional distance between functioning capillaries and the area of bacterial growth over which both phagocytic cells and all the protein cofactors that enhance phagocytosis must move to reach the bacteria. Thus necrotic tissue not only supplies bacterial nutrient but also interferes in multiple ways with the antibacterial systems that would normally clear the bacteria from the tissues.

Local Prevention of Wound Infections

All trauma patients with open wounds, either traumatic or surgical, should have repeated skin preparation. Since antibacterials used on the skin require time to act, the skin should be scrubbed and prepped before the surgeon scrubs. This allows 10 min for the antibacterial agents to act. Because of the microabrasions produced by shaving, either chemical hair removal preparations should be used or the skin should be minimally shaved in the operating room immediately before surgery. After the surgeon scrubs, the skin should once again be prepped with the antibacterial agent. Patients with open wounds should be started on systemic antibiotics in the emergency room. These patients should be scrubbed in the emergency room and their wound should be initially debrided of obvious dirt and irrigated with an antibiotic solution by one person. This is done compatibly with the pain engendered. The wound is then bandaged and not reopened until the patient is in the operating room. The antibiotics used are basically a blind choice. We use Keflin systemically and Keflin and Kanamycin for local irrigation. In the operating room the skin is again scrubbed and prepped as described above for a closed surgical wound. The patient is then draped, and the wound is debrided of a large volume of necrotic tissue and dirt and is irrigated. All instruments and sterile gear are then discarded. The patient is redraped and reprepped and another exploration, debridement, and irrigation are done. This procedure is conducted in such a way that all cavities of the wound are now explored; it aims at debridement of small masses of tissue. All anatomic structures that cannot be debrided must be identified and preserved. Once again all sterile gear is discarded and the wound is prepped and draped. The exploration this time is very detailed and the debridement consists of very small volumes of tissue with extensive irrigation. Proper debridement consists of a series of progressively more sterile procedures. The number of steps depends on the nature of the wound.

In all wounds the first priority is control of bleeding, the second is prevention of further contamination, the third is removal of present contamination, the fourth is revascularization of unperfused tissue, and the fifth is reconstruction. Thus in a penetrating abdominal wound in the first debridement, all open bowel wounds are closed with rubber-shod clamps to prevent further contamination as soon as bleeding is controlled. The wound is then cleansed in a preliminary fashion and the blood flow to the tissues is checked. Blood flow to the tissues should be reestablished at this time by temporary means either with an extra long saphenous vein graft, a temporary suture, or a polyethylene tube. After blood flow is reestablished the wound is thoroughly and leisurely cleansed with repeated changes of all sterile material, scrubs, preps, debridements, and irrigations. When cleanliness is established, all sterile gear is again discarded, the patient is reprepped and draped, and reconstruction is begun. In the abdomen all bowel anastomoses are done at this time. In the extremities the fractures are reconstructed. When this is done, all sterile gear is once again discarded with reprepping and draping, and formal neurovascular repairs are performed with resection of the edges of lacerations. The reconstruction may or may not be performed through the accidental wound depending on the exposure available. In all stages, wet sponges and laparotomy pads are used and the portion of the wound not being actively used is covered. In the abdomen laparotomy pads are sewn to the fascia so that the subcutaneous fat is always covered. The abdomen is always entered through a midline incision so the wound may be extended upward as a sternal splitting incision for access to the heart or liver. The principal errors in diagnosis that lead to the major postoperative complications and principal causes of technically inadequate surgery are inadequate exposure and attempts to complete the surgery quickly. These errors cannot be permitted. At the end of reconstruction the wound is thoroughly reexamined and redebrided of any dead tissue that may then be recognizable. Hemovacs are then placed commonly in two layers, deep and superficial.

Wounds are always closed loosely and over hemovacs if they are significant wounds. Fascial planes are approximated with a few sutures so that fluid formed in the deep layers can escape and viable tissue is approximated. The midline laparotomy wound is closed with retention sutures for the same reasons; no subcutaneous sutures are placed. The skin is approximated with surgical tape but deliberately left with some gaps. Dressings are allowed for only 48 hours. If the dressings become wet with blood or fluids they are changed in a sterile fashion. Moist dressings cannot be permitted at this stage unless the wound has been left open. Under these conditions, a dry dressing is applied and covered with a polyethylene sheet. This sheet is loosely taped and not occlusive. Hemovacs are removed under sterile conditions when they stop draining. This generally occurs at 48 hours. The hemovac tip is then cultured.

Postoperative Wound Erythema and Swelling Infection

Prevention of Abscesses

The patient who develops postoperative swelling and erythema of the wound is taken to the operating room. The wound is reopened, redebrided, and irrigated with antibiotic. In general, such wounds are left open except for a few sutures or skin tapes to prevent wide gaps. Postoperatively, irrigation is continued from the depths of the wound. In large wounds several irrigation tubes may be placed. The fluid leaving the skin is collected in colostomy bags or through channels made from adhesive surgical plastic. The irrigation is continued for 4 to 7 days. The wound is then inspected and consideration is given to another stage of debridement. In general, most accidental wounds of any magnitude should be closed loosely or left open. Again, dehydration necrosis must be prevented both in the operating room and in the ward.

Established Deep Infections

Most deep infections are probably related to bacterially contaminated hematomas, secondary to inadequate hemostasis or to retained dead tissue. Bacterial contamination may occur in open wounds directly or in such cases as pelvic and retroperitoneal hematomas via the bloodstream or via ruptured hollow viscera, such as the bladder. Pelvic hematomas with sepsis are apt to represent massive infections and lead to death. These results can also occur if large volumes of muscle have been rendered necrotic by crush injury (e.g., gluteal muscles) and have then been contaminated with bacteria from the bloodstream. These types of infections are particularly difficult to localize because they occur without wounds under viable skin in such deep areas that local signs may not be present. It is most important that bacteremias be prevented by vigorous pulmonary and renal support to prevent infection in these areas (see Chapter 14.)

The same considerations apply to deep abdominal and extremity infections, except that there is generally a wound to direct one's attention to the area. Bacteria of the type considered do not grow in viable tissue and therefore infection implies dead tissue, produced either traumatically or by an abscess. The relative proportions of dead muscle and hematoma cannot be judged. Therefore the existence of infections demands that, in addition to drainage and antibiotics, the area be thoroughly debrided of all dead tissue as the major means of treating the infection. This does not apply to the lung, where the nutrient is seldom dead tissue. Since fluids will accumulate after debridement that will also support bacterial growth, the debridement wound must be left open to drain. It is crucial that only living tissue be left behind and that it be approximated. After debridement of a wound to viable tissue, the bacterial contamination is primarily superficial. Therefore these wounds are ideally adapted to treatment with topical antibacterial agents much as burns are. This is given as a different antibiotic from those employed systemically and is generally an agent that cannot be used systemically [2]. These agents should not be given in glucose-containing solutions, since the nutrient will support bacterial growth and the bacteria, not suppressed by the antibiotics, will grow. Clearly irrigation with antibiotics or systemic antibiotics will have no significant effect if dead tissue is left behind to support bacterial growth. The wound that does not quickly improve after systemic antibiotics, debridement, and local, continuous irrigation antibiotics in general has been inadequately debrided or is pooling secretions that support bacterial growth. This applies to peritonitis as well as to extremity wounds.

Intestinal fistulas without distal obstruction and with the bowel wall basically in continuity frequently have active bacterial growth that prevents granulation tissue contracture, probably because of the bacterial nutrient supplied by the intestinal contents. The major advance associated with intravenous hyperalimentation is related not only to better systemic support of protein synthesis but also to decreased fistula drainage and therefore nutrient for bacterial growth.

Chronic Infections

The course of infection is that of hyperemia, ingrowth of well vascularized granulation tissue, and finally maturation of the well vascularized granulation tissue into avascular scar tissue. This last stage limits the blood flow to the area, while simultaneously providing bacterial nutrient, and thus contributes to the chronic nature of the infection. The problem is made worse if this occurs in association with a bony nonunion, where movement of the fracture ends contributes to the production of necrotic tissue to support bacterial growth. In these wounds antibiotics have either no, or only slight, effects. It is of the utmost importance that the avascular infected scar tissue be resected back to viable tissue as well as that all dead tissue be resected. In bones with chronic infection it is also important that the nonunion be absolutely immobilized. This is best accomplished with external fixators that require no additional dissection for their insertion. Segmental bony defects in the thoroughly debrided wound with good bleeding and absolute immobilization may be easily managed by autologous, pure cancellous bone grafts taken from the iliac crest or greater trochanter [2]. Such wounds must be left open in a way that does not produce dehydration necrosis and allows pus to drain.

These principles have been applied in general to stasis ulcers, chronic osteomyelitis, and intestinal fistulas. Chronic osteomyelitis presents the special problem of a noncollapsing bony cavity. This may now be easily managed by insertion of cancellous bone autografts. These grafts take very nicely in infected cavities as long as the infection is not actively invasive and the infected cavity is well vascularized with good bleeding during the debridement.

Tube Sepsis: Nutrient and Contamination

The trauma patient therefore has, in terms of direct accidental and operative trauma, the combinations of bacterial contamination and local bacterial nutrient that readily produces infections. These local changes also occur in other organs in relation to the various tubes employed for monitoring and systemic support. Bacterial contamination through tubes may be considered in terms of luminal and extraluminal contamination.

Luminal Contamination

Luminal contamination occurs through contaminated intravenous and intramuscular solutions and through contaminated air in the respirator. The system of having a busy nurse on the surgical floor mix intravenous solutions is almost certain to lead to bacterial contamination sooner or later. The insistence that has come with intravenous hyperalimentation that intravenous solutions be mixed by trained pharmacists under laminar-flow hoods is certain to benefit not only the patient on intravenous hyperalimentation but all patients. A major portion of this advance lies in restricting the number of people allowed to do the procedure and in giving them time and training so that it is done correctly. The same advances have occurred with the use of respirators and the development of inhalation therapists. This has been greatly reinforced by the realization that bacteria in water grow well in the heated humidifier and the tubing leading to the patient. Thus changing the humidifier and tubing for new sterilized ones every 8 hours has been a major contribution to reducing luminal bacterial contamination, just as it has for intravenous solutions.

Extraluminal Contamination and Nutrient

Extraluminal tube bacterial contamination creates different problems. It is clear that the key problems are bacteria on the surface of the skin, physical motion of the tube, and bacterial nutrient around the tube. Thus certain areas of the body, because of their content of sebaceous and sweat glands, support particularly high resident colonies of bacteria that are available for contamination of the tube. This problem is greatly aggravated by burns and abrasions. Some areas of the body, such as those related to the joints and neck, have particularly mobile skin, so the tube may move in and out with each movement of the joint or neck, causing bacteria to be conducted into the tissues. Still other areas are particularly apt to supply bacterial nutrient around or at the end of the tube so that a small amount of bacterial contamination may produce an infection. Thus an intravascular tube that occludes blood flow in the vessel, causing a stagnant column of blood that is susceptible to a few bacteria, is particularly apt to lead to infections because of the nutrient available. In general, intravenous catheters for prolonged use should not be placed in moving skin, small peripheral vessels, or through areas with high residual skin bacteria. The area of skin through which an intravascular catheter passes should be maintained continuously sterile, the catheter should be completely immobilized, and it should enter a vessel with a large volume of blood flow. The best location is the subclavian; the worst are the groin, neck, antecubital space, wrist, and ankle. Maintaining sterility around the cutaneous puncture requires an occlusive dressing at all times together with a daily antibacterial prep of the area.

The extraluminal contamination that occurs around Foley catheters and endotracheal tubes is particularly difficult because these tubes exist in areas of physical motion, high cutaneous bacterial contamination, and high bacterial nutrient. The problem is made worse if the tubes are so large or their cuffs inflated so strongly that necrotic tissue is also produced. Essentially nothing can be done about the location of these tubes, their motion, or their bacterial contamination. However, much can be done about dead tissue and a phenomenon best described as "washout" of bacteria. Thus oliguric urine flows, by reducing the rate of bacterial washout, must contribute to conversion of contamination to infection. This may be partially reversed by high urine flows or by the use of a three-way Foley catheter with irrigation. Clearly, small Foley catheters should be used to prevent direct tissue damage insofar as possible. An endotracheal tube produces tissue necrosis by virtue of physical motion and inflation of the cuff. Physical motion with respect to the trachea may be reduced by increasing the size of the tube, by insisting that the weight of the airway tubes not be borne by the trachea, by use of a flexible connecting piece from the endotracheal tube to the more rigid tubes of the ventilator, and by drugs to prevent the patient from thrashing about wildly. Tissue necrosis may also be reduced by use of the large cuffs that require low pressure and by insistence that the cuff always be inflated so that there is a 100 to 200 ml leak with each tidal volume. This procedure demands an expiratory spirometer to measure tidal volume, but it has the great advantage that the patient can talk with each tidal volume. Thus it helps reduce the psychological stress element of the metabolic response as well as local tissue necrosis.

The Lungs and Bacterial Nutrient

Essentially all trauma patients on ventilators have bacterial contamination of their airways. In addition, they have atelectasis, enhanced secretions, and may have pulmonary contusions, edematous lungs, airway obstruction by retained secretions, aspiration of blood or gastric contents, and areas of regional hypoventilation secondary to airway obstruction, diaphragm, or chest wall disorders. The normal lung is protected against bacterial contamination by the filtering hydrating action of the upper airways, by the action of the mucosal cilia in transporting mucus and its entrapped contents up the airway, by secretion of mucosal antibodies, and by a physical distribution pattern of the airways that prevents access of particulate material to the alveoli. The remaining material that reaches the alveoli is readily phagocytized by alveolar macrophages.

The patient with trauma on ventilatory support is ideally set up for bacterial contamination of the lungs and the nutrient support required for conversion of contamination to infection. Local alveolar gas hypoxia may also reduce the activity of the antibacterial system. The reduction of luminal bacterial contamination through management of the ventilator and extraluminal contamination through management of the endotracheal tube have already been discussed. The major problem now resides in management of the lung to reduce bacterial nutrient and to improve the local antibacterial system by preventing regional hypoxia. One hundred percent humidification of the inspired gases is of the utmost importance to maintain the secretions in as liquid a state as possible, so they may be readily transported via the cilia from the small to large airways and removed by suction. Retained secretions not only impair pulmonary function, but also help support bacterial growth. Straight suction catheters inserted through a long endotracheal tube tend to routinely go only into the right mainstem bronchus. This is particularly true if the tip of the endotracheal tube screens the left mainstem bronchus or if oral or nasal endotracheal tubes are used. If effective tracheal suctioning is to occur in the left mainstem bronchus, the air must be 100% humidified, and a short tracheostomy endotracheal tube and a curved Caude [1] suction tube must be used. A major problem with the tracheostomy endotracheal tube is the placement through too low a tracheostomy wound. This is particularly true in the patient with a short, thick neck. The trachea should always be approached through a vertical wound that comes down on the larynx. The pretracheal space is then entered and all tissues are divided over a finger so digital control of bleeding is possible and a minimal wound is made. The tracheostomy wound is then made in the second ring. Oral and nasal endotracheal tubes should never be utilized for more than 1 to 2 days unless the patient is rapidly improving. The transport of the multiple trauma patient to the operating room for tracheostomy is a highly hazardous procedure because of the time off the ventilator and the different characteristics of the operating room ventilator. Therefore we do all such tracheostomies in the intensive care unit so the patient is not removed from the ventilator that has been adapted to his needs. The patient with large-volume secretions or intratracheal bleeding should be placed in the Trendelenberg position and the weight of the diaphragm should be taken by additional positive and expiratory pressure so effective suctioning can be done. This generally requires an increased central venous pressure and therefore increased blood volume.

Proper ventilatory support to reduce pulmonary failure also in effect debrides the lungs by reversing and preventing atelectasis, removing secretions, reversing regional hypoventilation, and decreasing intraalveolar edema. Thus it reduces the nutrient available for bacterial growth, while enhancing the alveolar antibacterial system. However, this will not reverse true pulmonary contusions that represent a particularly good source of bacterial nutrient. These patients are therefore particularly at risk for pneumonia. Intraabdominal conditions that produce elevated diaphragms also place the patient at risk for pneumonia by producing basal regional hypoventilation and atelectasis. These include intestinal distention, peritonitis, ascites, and the obese abdomen in the supine patient. The upright position of the chest with decompression of the abdomen is of great importance. In general, any crisis is associated with enhanced tracheal secretions, which also contribute to the risk of pulmonary infection and to a recurrence of pulmonary failure [2].

The Systemic Response to Infection
The area of infection is surrounded by a zone of hyperemia. The hyperemia is found first in existing vessels, but with time there is capillarization of the area by new capillaries and formation of granulation tissue. This local response is very important in preventing systemic sepsis by delivery of enhanced blood flow to the still viable tissue and by delivery of the specific antibacterial systems of the blood to the area of infection. The local response is supplemented by a systemic response that is associated with increased cardiac output and increased energetic and synthetic substrate mobilization. This response mobilizes substrates from areas of lesser demand to areas of greater demand and thus supports a multitude of synthetic activities that appear to be very important in the ability to survive the septic insult. One of these activities is the formation of new capillaries in the area of sepsis. This is undoubtedly very important but, relative to the whole body, very small. The major synthetic activities that occur quantitatively are located in the liver, bone marrow, lymph nodes, and macrophages [1].

Tissue Oxygen Tension
It appears clear that a reduction in arterial oxygen tension decreases the amount of bacterial contamination required to produce infection [4]. This pattern almost routinely occurs in the unsupported patient with significant sepsis. The same effect may be produced by local tissue edema or necrosis that is secondary to trauma. Increasing the tissue oxygen tension appears to be important in preventing conversion of bacterial contamination to infection. Reduced tissue oxygen tensions may be produced by reduced hemoglobin, a left shift of the oxyhemoglobin dissociation curve, reduced cardiac output, arterial hypoxia secondary to pulmonary failure, and by local tissue edema and necrosis. Therefore it appears important in preventing or treat-

ing infection to maintain the hematocrit close to normal, to maintain oxygen tension at normal or above normal levels, to prevent left shift of the oxyhemoglobin curve by preventing alkalemia and using fresh blood, to deliberately run the cardiac output above normal, and to prevent edema. Edema may be greatly minimized in extremity trauma by elevation and in all traumatic wounds by gentle tissue technique. Because of the preceding considerations, all multiple trauma patients are operated on with a volume-cycled ventilator with positive end expiratory pressure and with repeated arterial and central venous blood gases. They are left on the ventilator after surgery until they prove they do not need it. Reduced cardiac output that is secondary to positive end expiratory pressure indicates hypovolemia that requires correction. These patients are deliberately run at an arterial oxygen tension of 140 to 150 and a central venous oxygen tension of 45 to 50 with a normal pH and Pco_2. These measures are maintained, if sepsis develops, until the sepsis is cleared. The severely septic patient should not be removed from the ventilator even if he has normal pulmonary function, because recurrent pulmonary failure and arterial hypoxia almost inevitably occur. In general these patients require much higher central venous pressures than normal to obtain the required central venous oxygen tension. The central venous catheter must be carefully placed in the right atrium to be reliable in terms of venous oxygen tensions.

The central venous pressure that can be generated becomes increasingly dependent on colloid osmotic pressure, because higher central venous pressures are required for a given cardiac output. The major upturn probably occurs as central venous pressure begins to exceed the normal capillary hydrostatic pressure of 12 to 15 torr. This commonly occurs in the severely septic patient. Therefore it is most important to measure daily the plasma albumin and to take measures to maintain it above 3 g per 100 ml. The measures available include infusion of exogenous albumin and increased use of a complete mixture of amino acids.

Summary
The major problem in the trauma patient, in terms of increased susceptibility to infection, is related to the multiple local conditions that juxtapose bacterial contamination and bacterial nutrient. These local conditions simultaneously interfere with the access and the function of the systemic antibacterial systems in response to bacteria. Both systemic and local conditions that reduce the oxygen tension at which the phagocytic cells must operate will also increase the susceptibility of the trauma patient to infection for a given load of bacterial contamination and bacterial nutrient. Both the preoperative use of systemic antibiotics and intraoperative use of irrigation antibiotics can be used to reduce bacterial contamination or at least to reduce bacterial multiplication.

The primary means of preventing acute sepsis in the trauma patient is the reduction of bacterial contamination and removal of dead tissue or fluids that allow multiplication of bacteria to a colony large enough to produce infection. Both endeavors are equally important. In most clean surgical wounds the reduction in bacterial nutrient is probably much more important than further reduction in bacterial contamination. This needs to be done intraoperatively by prevention of the multiple factors that produce tissue necrosis and postoperatively by prevention of accumulation of the tissue fluids and blood that support bacterial growth and prevention of dehydration necrosis.

The magnitude of the bacterial load carried by a patient contributes significantly to the risk of infection. Therefore every effort must be made to reduce this risk by vigorous pulmonary support to prevent pneumonia, vigorous fluid support to give high urine outputs, and vigorous wound care to maintain all open wounds as sterile as possible and to prevent formation of abscesses.

An inadequate supply of nutrient to the wound clearly reduces the bacterial contamination required to produce infection in the presence of a given supply of bacterial nutrient. This may occur because of local or systemic conditions. The local conditions include vascular injury, tourniquets, edema, tight casts, and local use of vasoconstrictors. The systemic conditions are primarily related to limitations of circulatory, pulmonary, or hepatic function. It is of utmost importance that these secondary factors be vigorously managed so that adequate nutrient, including oxygen and blood flow, reaches the wound to increase the local resistance to infection and is supplied to the systemic body to enhance the systemic response to infection.

The traumatic wound is special only in that it is much more heavily contaminated with bacteria and contains much more necrotic tissue. It may be very special if in addition there is occluded blood flow to the tissues. Traumatic wounds require a multistage series of debridements, with each stage progressively more sterile until a clean wound without necrotic tissue is produced. Blood flow needs to be reestablished very early by temporary means when it is occluded with a permanent neurovascular repair as the final stage of reconstruction. This sort of wound management requires considerable time and is impossible to do properly if done hastily or through inadequate incisions. We feel strongly that since movement at the fracture site can produce dead tissue to support infection, all open fractures should be internally fixed as long as this can be done through the debridement wound and the metallic devices can be placed deep to viable muscle.

Closed-space infections have much worse consequences than open wound infections. We therefore feel very strongly that no wound should be closed tightly. Sutures should be used only to approximate tissues, not to produce water-tight closures. Hemovacs should be placed in all significant wounds. Wounds should be made insofar as possible so they can drain by gravity and the skin closure should be made with surgical tape to encourage drainage.

References

1. Border, J. R. Metabolic response to starvation, sepsis and trauma. In J. Mac-Credie (Ed.), *Basic Surgery*. New York: Macmillan, 1976.
2. Border, J. R. Cardiopulmonary failure. In J. MacCredie (Ed.), *Basic Surgery*. New York: Macmillan, 1976.
3. Burri, C. *Post traumatic osteomyelitis*. Bern: Hans Huber, 1974.
4. Hunt, T. K., et al. Oxygen tension and wound infection. *Surg. Forum* 23:47, 1972.

16. Trauma and Delayed Sepsis

John R. Border, R. Seibel, J. LaDuca, R. H.McMenamy,
R. H. Birkhahn, R. Sorkness,
and L. L. Bernardis

The Clinical Problem

The patient who remains chronically, critically ill with multiple organ failures typically develops in time delayed sepsis with organisms that are normally noninvasive and commonly associated with bacteremias. The organ failures typically consist of a cumulative sequence of organ failures, beginning with pulmonary failure, continuing with right ventricle failure, and then with more time several signs of hepatic dysfunction. This state occurs in some multiple trauma patients, particularly those in whom the diagnosis of pulmonary failure has not been quickly made and therapy begun. It is also particularly apt to occur in the patient with multiple injuries, whose condition ranges from lethargic to comatose, who is supine because of traction and is obese. The statistical probability is increased in the patient with preexisting cirrhosis or malnutrition, the patient who has been in prolonged deep shock, or the patient who is severely apprehensive.

The state of multiple organ failures with infection caused by organisms that are normally noninvasive essentially does not occur in the young, healthy, previously active patient, whose organ failures are quickly reversed, in whom pain and anxiety are alleviated, and who is quickly gotten into the sitting position with active movement of all extremities, assuming that the wounds have been managed as previously discussed. The major exception to this rule is the patient who develops postoperative hematomas. To state it differently, injured patients do extremely well with severe short-term stress but do extremely poorly with chronic stress. This fact is discussed by Border as the difference between the hypercatabolic and stress catabolic states [1].

The time required in the state of multiple organ failure to develop sepsis with organisms that are normally noninvasive also has certain clinical correlations. Thus the more severe and prolonged the initial shock, even if reversed, the shorter the period of time to sepsis with organisms that are normally noninvasive. The more severe the pulmonary failure, the sooner sepsis with normally noninvasive organisms occurs. The greater the muscle mass, the longer the time required to develop such sepsis. The use of intravenous hyperalimentation delays the onset of sepsis but does not prevent it and prolongs the time to death once multiple organ system failure occurs. The use of much larger quantities of amino acids than customarily given, either alone or in conjunction with hyper-alimentation (a lowered calorie-nitrogen ratio) seems to further delay and make more manageable sepsis with organisms that are normally noninvasive.. Acute sepsis that is not quickly reversed predisposes greatly to the development of multiple organ system

Supported by the National Institute of General Medical Sciences Grant GM 15768.

failure and sepsis in other areas with organisms that are normally noninvasive.

The sepsis with organisms that are normally noninvasive that occurs is particularly apt to be associated with several other signs of inadequate protein synthesis relative to protein breakdown. Thus these patients are particularly apt to have wounds that do not heal. This category includes patients with anastomotic breakdown, laparotomy wounds that dehisce, the formation of decubital ulcers, late gastric stress ulceration (clearly different from that that occurs in the first few days), hypoalbuminemia, tracheoesophageal or tracheoinnominate artery fistulas, and inadequate local granulation tissue response to sepsis to wall off the area as an abscess. There is clearly a defect in one of the principal mechanisms that localize sepsis, and the wounds may look much like those described for children with congenital cellular immunologic deficiency, since there is an area of sepsis with virtually no local response (see Chapter 8). These patients are also particularly apt to develop bacteremias that are persistent and are caused by the type of organism normally cleared quickly by the reticuloendothelial system. (See Chapter 6.) The predominant blood-exposed reticuloendothelial system is that of the Kupfer cells located in the sinusoids of the liver. We therefore presume they have limited phagocytic activity. These patients are also apt to have clotting difficulties with high prothrombin times, partial thromboplastin times, reduced platelets, and reduced fibrinogen. These same patients are also apt to develop pneumonias and urinary tract infections, which also lead to bacteremias.

The deduction has commonly been made that many of these patients have inadequate gastrointestinal anastomoses for technical reasons and therefore develop intraabdominal sepsis that leads to their deaths. Equally possible is that the same conditions that limit protein synthesis generally also prevent anastomotic healing and therefore contribute to the production of anastomotic leaks and intraabdominal sepsis.

The Deduction from the Clinical Observations
The deduction from the clinical observations is that there is a generalized limitation of protein synthesis relative to protein breakdown that takes time to develop. This scheme must be modified for a number of specific local conditions. The time required for development of an altered relation between protein synthesis and breakdown is related to muscle protein mass, exogenous amino acids, and the severity and duration of the organ failures, particularly cardiopulmonary. It must be clearly stated that the limitation of protein synthesis is relative to the exact physiologic condition prevailing and is not absolute. Thus since the rate of hepatic albumin output is normally carefully matched to the peripheral rate of albumin consumption and the plasma albumin is maintained, constant hypoalbuminemia is considered to be a condition with an inadequate rate of hepatic albumin output

and synthesis for the physiologic state existing, even though the rate of albumin output may be accelerated relative to an overnight fasting state. The overnight fasting state is, in any event, not an adequate reference state, since it is now realized that the rate of hepatic albumin synthesis and output is very responsive to the amino acid and calorie load presented to the liver under normal conditions.

It also must be made clear that the first 2 or 3 days following trauma with good cardiopulmonary function have been carefully excluded, since it appears relatively clear that during this period there is a grossly accelerated protein synthesis, particularly in the liver secondary to muscle amino acid release and the effects of glucocorticoids on muscle and liver [2].

General Analysis and Modification of the
Limited Protein Synthesis Hypothesis

Cellular protein synthesis in vivo depends on the delivery of energetic and synthetic substrate and a number of cofactors by the blood in addition to neuroendocrine regulation of relative intracellular enzymatic activities. The controls of cellular protein breakdown are much more poorly understood but appear to be largely independent of the controls of protein synthesis and under different controls.

Any limitation of protein synthesis is apt to be recognized most flagrantly by concentration changes in those proteins with rapid turnovers. These include the proteins of the liver, pancreas, and gastrointestinal mucosa; wound healing; the heart under conditions of increased load (right ventricle with increased pulmonary artery pressure and increased cardiac output); and the antibacterial system in terms of granulation tissue localization of sepsis, phagocytic activity and bactericidal activity.

The Liver

The expression of such a generalized limitation of protein synthesis in the different organs would be expected to be widely different in magnitude, although in the same direction. Thus the liver, because of its portal circulation and normal architecture, normally has a marginal oxygen supply. This may be further impaired by inadequate cardiac output, inadequate arterial oxygen tension, left shift of oxyhemoglobin oxygen dissociation curves, and increased central venous pressure that produces hepatic edema, which would allow hepatocyte hypoxia in the presence of normal hepatic vein oxygen tension. In addition to these peculiarities of the liver, the liver normally obtains a large element of its nutritional support from the oral ingestion of food, and its metabolism is closely controlled by insulin, glucagon, and the autonomic nervous system [1].

All these elements may go awry in the chronically, critically ill patient. Thus the absence of oral intake deprives both the liver and gastrointestinal mucosa of their normal regional hypernutrition. In the absence of oral intake the nutrient support of the liver and gastrointestinal mucosa is provided by the mobilization of amino acids from the periphery, particularly from muscle, peripheral breakdown of plasma proteins, and long-chain fatty acids from adipose tissue. The normal function of this system is heavily dependent on the plasma glucose and the systemic plasma insulin. The plasma glucose can be elevated by intravenous glucose infusions or can be abnormally controlled at hyperglycemic levels by the neuroendocrine systems. In addition, the hypothalamic override of the normal systems may produce, via an increase in glucagon relative to insulin and the sympathetic hepatic innervation relative to parasympathetic innervation, a situation in which more of the amino acids delivered to the liver are diverted in glucose and away from hepatic protein synthesis. Then the hepatic protein already present is broken down to amino acids for similar uses. These intrahepatic alterations may be magnified if the liver does not properly clear insulin and a relative systemic hyperinsulinemia occurs that limits peripheral release of fat and a complete mixture of amino acids.

The net result is that less of the complete mixture of amino acids required for protein synthesis is delivered from the periphery and more of that delivered is converted to glucose, so hepatic protein synthesis is limited on the basis of several mechanisms in addition to the postulated generalized mechanism that limits protein synthesis. In addition to these mechanisms, which limit hepatic protein synthesis, it is also clear that there are mechanisms that enhance the peripheral consumption of hepatic plasma proteins. Thus it is clear that the quantity of exogenous albumin required in these patients to maintain a normal plasma albumin is grossly increased and that this amount is quantitatively much greater than current known rates of hepatic albumin output. This mechanism probably cannot be extrapolated to the other hepatic plasma transport proteins because of the very specific controls of proteolysis. However, it is clear in very ill persons that not only is the plasma albumin reduced but the plasma vitamin A binding protein is also reduced. Both these observations are typically reversed when oral intake is resumed and nutrient is supplied directly to the liver, independent of the controls of peripheral amino acid and long-chain fatty acid mobilization. However, the ability to eat implies not only gut motility but also a complete anabolic set to the neuroendocrine apparatus. This observation therefore cannot be simply interpreted. Our observations on feeding the elemental diet through a jejunostomy tube with gastric decompression in the chronically, critically ill would suggest that the requirements for exogenous albumin are reduced, that stress ulceration is much less frequent, and that bacteremias are uncommon. It should be noted that this process supplies nutrient not only to the hepatocyte but also to the Kupfer cells that constitute the great bulk of blood-exposed phagocytes in the body. Thus, these nutrients would be expected to support not only hepatocyte function but also Kupfer cell clearance of bacteria and the maintenance of the gastrointestinal mucosa.

Therefore there are a number of very specific factors that modulate protein synthesis and function in the splanchnic complex apart from the hypothesized generalized limitation of protein synthesis. However, because this is an area of rapid protein synthesis, where the rate is particularly susceptible to manipulation (by manipulating the rate of supply of a complete mixture of amino acids), this area would be expected to reflect quickly any generalized limitation of protein synthesis. This limitation would be expected to be superimposed on other specific insults to this area. The picture is not simple, but, it may be manipulated if gastrointestinal feeding can be given to eliminate altered supplies of nutrient on a muscle or adipose tissue basis.

The Gut
The acute gastrointestinal stress ulceration that occurs following trauma appears to be secondary to changes in the circulation of the blood to the mucosa. The delayed stress ulceration that occurs 10 to 14 days later probably has different mechanisms and may reflect, in part, the postulated generalized limitation of protein synthesis. Once again, there are special considerations superimposed. Thus adequate circulation may not have been restored and it may be a continuation of the original mechanism. In addition, since vitamin A is an essential cofactor it may, in part, be a reflection of inadequate hepatic synthesis of vitamin A binding protein, and therefore inadequate transport of vitamin A from the liver stores to the gastrointestinal mucosa. It may also reflect absent oral intake and therefore limited luminal gastrointestinal mucosal nutritional support. Finally, it may also reflect the postulated generalized limitation of protein synthesis.

Wound Healing
Wound healing may be considered a general process. This also probably includes the formation of granulation tissue around areas of infection to produce localization. Again, the generalized limitation of protein synthesis must be extensively qualified. Thus it is clear that the supplies of oxygen to the healing wound probably limit metabolism. The oxygen supply may be modulated by cardiac output, arterial hypoxia, left shifted oxyhemoglobin dissociation curve, local factors influencing blood flow, local edema, sutures that are too tight and limit blood flow, sutures that are too loose and permit too much motion, sepsis, and probably numerous other factors. In addition, there is evidence that severe trauma may produce a state of physiologic scurvy that requires high doses of vitamin C for reversal. Finally, all the amino acids and energetic nutrients must be supplied to support protein synthesis as are required in any organ.

Bacterial Immunity, Phagocytosis, and Bacterial Growth
The delayed sepsis that occurs in these patients has several characteristics that suggest decreased cellular immunity. This is a complex process that, for evaluation, requires separate evaluation of the in vivo rate of bacterial

growth, the factors that modulate phagocytosis, the number of cells active in phagocytosis, the difference between granulocyte and macrophage phagocytosis, and the activity of the T cells that modulate cellular immunity.

The growth of bacteria in vivo seems in significant part to be limited by the supply of free iron available. Two events may occur that would increase the supply of iron. The hematoma with its degenerating hemoglobin presents a local atmosphere for bacterial growth that is not only rich in nutrient generally but is also rich in iron. These areas therefore are particularly good for bacterial growth in the trauma patient. The free iron in the plasma depends largely on transferrin iron binding. Any factor that limits the plasma transferrin may be expected to increase the plasma-free iron to the extent that the percent of transferrin iron binding sites occupied is increased. Thus factors that limit hepatic protein synthesis to the extent they reduce the plasma transferrin may be expected to increase in vivo bacterial growth. These problems may be compounded by the intravenous administration of chelated iron.

A number of factors that modulate in vivo phagocytosis are also observed to change in the chronically, critically ill patient apart from those related directly to humoral immunity. Thus these patients are hyperglycemic. Hyperglycemia has been demonstrated to interfere with phagocytosis by altering the shape of the phagocyte. This has been studied in granulocytes but probably also applies to macrophages. It would be most expected to affect the macrophages of the liver since this blood would be most hyperglycemic. The systemic factors that limit amino acid and energetic supplies to the hepatocytes would also be expected to limit the activity of the Kupfer cell macrophages.

The liver participates in the synthesis of acute phase proteins. Two of these proteins have been studied in the trauma patient. α_1 glycoprotein rises in the trauma patient and interferes with phagocytosis. This, also, since it is released by the liver, would be expected to be in greatest concentration in the hepatic sinusoids and therefore to affect Kupfer cell macrophage activity the most. α_2 glycoprotein is released by the liver and stimulates phagocytosis. This substance was present in unchanged concentrations in our trauma patients doing well with sepsis and reduced in those doing poorly with sepsis. Again, altered hepatic function seems to be related to delayed sepsis with organisms that are normally noninvasive.

Cellular immunity depends on phagocytosis of bacteria with intracellular killing of the organism. This is usually associated with the inflammatory response and the formation of granulation tissue. The response is biphasic in time and the acute response is due to the granulocytes, whose function is largely modulated by the complement system and the proteins of humoral immunity. The delayed response involves the elements of cellular immunity with T cell modulation of macrophage function. All components are heavily dependent on protein synthesis. This includes the humoral antibody and complement response, macrophage processing of antigenic components for both humoral and cellular immune responses, intracellular synthesis of bactericidal components, and the act of phagocytosis itself. It is clear that the immune system can be stimulated acutely following burns, but not at a later time. Thus the use of a polyvalent *Pseudomonas* vaccine acutely reduces the incidence of later *Pseudomonas sepsis* (see Chapter 6). Unfortunately, the burn wound is then invaded by other organisms. It is also clear that protein malnutrition induced by a high carbohydrate intake is associated with reduced antibacterial systems activity [18]. The patient with malnutrition and cancer clearly has reduced cellular immunity [7]. (See Chapter 9).

The patient with reduced plasma albumin usually has reduced immune responses [8]. Repletion of the protein reserves in the protein depleted animal or man usually restores immune competence to normal [7, 12]. These observations are probably linked to the concepts developed in the next section, which are related to the effect of a glucose consumption state over a prolonged period of time, inducing an endogenous amino acid imbalance with a deficiency of leucine and isoleucine that limits protein synthesis. In addition to these changes there may be a release of humoral agents that suppress the immune system [6], consumption of specific opsonins and complement [17], and altered synthesis or function of the bactericidal system in the granulocyte, both as a result of intracellular changes [5] and as a result of the environment in which the cell functions [11].

There are therefore a large number of factors that change in the patient who is chronically, critically ill, which in turn may enhance in vivo bacterial growth, interfere with phagocytosis and intracellular killing, and in general interfere with both cellular and humoral immunity. Some of these may be organ specific, as with the liver, but most are general in nature. Many of these changes are compatible with a generalized limitation of protein synthesis. A specific mechanism for this, which might apply to most ill patients, will be discussed in the next section.

Limited Protein Synthesis Hypothesis: An Endogenous Amino Acid Imbalance

Starvation

The chronically, critically ill patient in the stress catabolic state has a different set of plasma concentrations than the starved patient. Thus, in general, relative to starvation, the patient who is chronically, critically ill is hyperglycemic and hypoalbuminemic, has low plasma long-chain fatty acids, and has low plasma ketone bodies. The amino acids are also abnormal relative to starvation. Thus with starvation all essential amino acids are elevated. In contrast, in the chronically, critically ill, the essential amino acids leucine and isoleucine are typically very low and tryptophan and phenylalanine are elevated [14, 15, 16]. The fall in leucine and isoleucine in association with increased alanine occurs first in time, with the elevation of phenylalanine and tryptophan occurring later in time [14]. The patient with pure starvation oxidizes fatty acids either directly or indirectly as ketone bodies for essentially all energy needs except for about one-half of the brain's energy needs, which are provided by glucose. The rate of gluconeogenesis is very carefully controlled in starvation, largely by the rate of muscle release of the gluconeogenic amino acids alanine to the liver and glutamine to the kidney. This is achieved by muscle interconversion of amino acids, during which these two amino acids are released in gross excess of their muscle content. One exception to this process is apparent in leucine and isoleucine, which are consumed within the muscle as ketone bodies. To preserve a balanced amino acid mixture, leucine and isoleucine must be consumed by muscle in proportion to the alanine and glutamine released by muscle and consumed by the liver and kidney.

This system of starvation is highly interrelated and controlled. Thus with the beginning of starvation, the supply of gluconeogenic substrate to the liver, the rate of hepatic gluconeogenesis, the hepatic glycogen, and the rate of hepatic glucose output are reduced. With time the plasma glucose is also reduced. As this occurs, the plasma insulin falls and the hypothalamic monitor of glucose perceives hypoglycemia. Secondary to these factors the plasma glucagon rises, the sympathetic nervous system is stimulated, and the parasympathetic nervous system is inhibited. These changes are associated with enhanced mobilization of glycogen from the liver as glucose and enhanced hepatic clearance of gluconeogenic amino acids in addition to enhanced mobilization of long-chain fatty acids from adipose tissue. Secondary to these changes the liver begins to partially oxidize long-chain fatty acids for energy with a release of ketone bodies. The rest of the body is then presented with very little glucose relative to large amounts of long-chain fatty acids and ketone bodies. Because of a mitochondrial preference for these fuels relative to glucose, the whole body, other than the brain, begins to burn fat and fat products. As this occurs, intracellular enzyme adaptations also occur that limit even the synthetic utilization of glucose. These processes are aided and abetted by increased hepatic synthesis of carnitine, which then increases the tissue stores. Carnitine is required for the transport of long-chain fatty acids from the cytoplasm through the mitochondrial wall for use in beta oxidation and production of the fuel substrate acetyl-coenzyme A. The increased carnitine stores thus allow enhanced long-chain fatty acid oxidation relative to the plasma concentration of long-chain fatty acids.

Muscle is very special in this adaptation because in the resting state it can either burn very little or no glucose. It may utilize glucose in the glycolytic cycle during exercise. In contrast, liver and heart can burn almost any fuel. At the beginning of starvation muscle burns predominantly long-chain fatty acids and ketone bodies. The ketone bodies do not require carnitine to enter the mitochondria and probably initially are derived predominantly from leucine and isoleucine. All leucine and isoleucine so burned release equivalent quantities of gluconeogenic amino acids, and these stimulate hepatic gluconeogenesis. The amino acids that are in excess as a result of the consumption of leucine and isoleucine are interconverted by the extensive amino acid enzymatic system within the muscle cells and are released as alanine or glutamine. Thus the only plasma sign of muscle leucine and isoleucine oxidation is that of a rise in plasma alanine and glutamine in muscle venous blood. The change in systemic plasma alanine and glutamine depends on the balance between muscle production and liver and kidney consumption. It appears clear under these conditions that the plasma alanine largely modulates the rate of hepatic gluconeogenesis. Thus muscle oxidation of leucine and isoleucine largely modulates the rate of hepatic (alanine) and renal (glutamine) gluconeogenesis. With time the plasma ketone bodies rise because of hepatic ketogenesis and more and more ketone bodies are consumed by muscle from the plasma with less and less derived from leucine and isoleucine. As this occurs the liver synthesizes carnitine, and the muscle burns more and more long-chain fatty acids from plasma and less and less ketone bodies of all types. During this time the liver requires the same amount of energy and continues with the same rate of ketogenesis. Since the ketone bodies are consumed by muscle at a lesser rate but are produced at the same rate, the plasma concentration of ketone bodies continues to rise. Two factors result: in one, the leucine and isoleucine required for muscle ketone body oxidation are further reduced; in the other, eventually the plasma ketone bodies become high enough that even the brain begins to utilize this water-soluble fat as an energy source. The net effect of these two results is that the delivery of gluconeogenic amino acids to the liver and kidney by muscle is further reduced because of reduced muscle oxidation of leucine and isoleucine, and in the other the systemic need for glucose is reduced. The sum of all these results is to conserve muscle protein from oxidation. While all these factors are occurring the plasma proteins are maintained at essentially normal levels, but the hepatic protein mass and glycogen content are reduced [1]. The maintenance of plasma proteins at normal levels occurs in the face of reduced hepatic protein synthesis, which is matched at least for albumin by reduced peripheral albumin consumption. With prolonged starvation the plasma proteins do fall. Eventually, just before death, when essentially all fat stores have been consumed, the body mobilizes amino acids for gluconeogenesis and reconverts for the short period of remaining survival time to a glucose economy.

The Chronically, Critically Ill

These patients have an hepatic glucose output that is elevated and appears unresponsive to the normal controls [13, 14, 15]| Secondary to this elevated output they oxidize more glucose, utilize more glucose synthetically, and have a much decreased ketone body response. In addition, they do not increase their muscle carnitine stores as the starved patient or animal does [3]. This maintained glucose economy in the face of inadequate calorie intake appears to reflect, in large part, altered hypothalamic function relative to perceived organ failure, pain, and anxiety, but may be accentuated by intravenous glucose infusion [1]. In association with these changes there is acutely a very low plasma leucine and isoleucine and an increased alanine [14].

Given normal physiology the system has gone awry in a way that can only encourage the consumption of the essential amino acids leucine and isoleucine. The absence of the rise in plasma ketone bodies seen in starvation prevents muscle from obtaining ketone bodies from plasma at the same rate it normally would. The lack of increase in muscle carnitine simultaneously interferes with long-chain fatty acid oxidation at a rate that would normally be achieved for a given plasma concentration of long-chain fatty acids. This problem may be further accentuated if, simultaneously, glucose infusion produces a lower concentration of plasma fatty acids.

The net results of these changes can only be an accelerated muscle consumption of the essential amino acids leucine and isoleucine as a source of ketone bodies. However consumption of two essential amino acids produces an endogenous amino acid imbalance in which all other amino acids are present in relative excess. The normal result of such an amino acid imbalance is that the amino acids present in excess are cleared by the liver and converted to glucose. As long as this is only a muscle process, the amino acids released in excess will be alanine and glutamine. This further prevents hepatic ketogenesis and accentuates hepatic glucose and urea output. In fact, this would probably produce exactly what has been observed in that it would produce an hepatic glucose output that is not sensitive to the normal controls with accelerated glucose oxidation and utilization of glucose for synthetic purposes.

Eventually the muscle becomes depleted of leucine and isoleucine and begins to draw these two amino acids from other organs in the body. In part, during this period, the low plasma leucine and isoleucine could be overcome for intracellular protein synthesis by enhanced cellular transport of these amino acids, so normal intracellular concentrations could be maintained in the presence of reduced plasma concentrations. It should be noted that all amino acids are required to be present in the proper concentration at the same instant in time for protein synthesis to occur. The cellular transport mechanisms during this period of time could account for proteins being moved from organs with less vigorous amino acid transport mechanisms to those with more vigorous transport mechanisms. This would limit protein synthesis in some organs but not in others. Eventually protein synthesis must be generally limited because of inadequate supplies of leucine and isoleucine. The time required to achieve this would depend on the magnitude of the total body leucine and isoleucine pool, the rate of oxidation of leucine and isoleucine, and the rate of exogenous supply of leucine and isoleucine.

When the muscle sources of leucine and isoleucine become sufficiently depleted in the presence of inadequate plasma ketone bodies and limited long-chain fatty acid oxidation, muscle will begin to draw leucine and isoleucine from other organs and proteins. Albumin is a protein that is clearly consumed throughout the body; it not only has its usually well known functions, but also acts as a transport form for amino acids from the liver to the systemic body [13]. The gross increase in albumin consumption at this time may be related to its utilization as a donor of ketone bodies to muscle. Unfortunately, albumin, although rich in leucine, is deficient in isoleucine. Thus although albumin infusion can supply ketone bodies to muscle for oxidation, it will increase the relative deficiency of this amino acid but will not alleviate the limitation in protein synthesis because of its isoleucine deficiency. The infusion of a complete mixture of amino acids may also not restore protein synthesis if the two amino acids leucine and isoleucine are infused at the rate they are consumed by muscle.

The consumption of leucine and isoleucine by muscle leads to a plasma amino acid concentration imbalance that is acutely only of alanine and glutamine, because all other amino acids are interconverted within the muscle cell to alanine and glutamine and are not released to the plasma. This may or may not occur in other organs or with the consumption of albumin. Clearly, if protein synthesis is limited but proteolysis continues, the other amino acids will also be released and, if not consumed within the cell, will appear in the plasma. Under these conditions the concentrations of the other amino acids would rise in the plasma until their rate of destruction is equal to the rate of consumption of leucine and isoleucine by muscle. This, in general, would not apply to the nonessential amino acids, since they can be interconverted within most cells, but would apply to the essential amino acids that can be catabolized only in muscle or in liver.

Thus the fact that the low concentration phase of leucine and isoleucine is followed by a rise in plasma tryptophan, phenylalanine, and lysine is not surprising. This observation would indicate limited protein synthesis in organs other than muscle with continued proteolysis. Granted the activities of the protein synthetic apparatus in the liver and the fact that it can be observed, this would be expected to be the first organ to show such a change.

Our observations in the severely traumatized patient who later becomes septic and in the dog with induced peritonitis are completely compatible with the preceding pathophysiology [14, 15, 16, 19]. One patient, because of renal failure, was maintained on glucose and albumin. In association with the albumin the plasma leucine, although low, was high relative to the isoleucine. The low isoleucine was associated with a high alanine, pyruvate, and plasma glucose [14]. The patient developed a high plasma tryptophan and phenylalanine in the basal state as time went on [14]. These changes were associated over time with a progressive reduction in splanchnic clearance of all amino acids, except tryptophan and alanine [15]. The observations in septic dogs show hepatic clearance of all amino acids in the controlled fasting state and release of all amino acids in the severely septic

238.

state [19]. This is associated in the dog, where the function of the organs can be separated with normal gut metabolism in the same animals that had grossly abnormal hepatic function [19].

The first amino acid to become abnormal after leucine, isoleucine, and alanine in the septic dog is tryptophan [19]. In man, administration of isotonic Freamine did not change splanchnic clearance, but administration of a much larger dose of Freamine was associated with increased plasma leucine and isoleucine, a gross increase in splanchnic clearance of all amino acids, and a reduction in plasma tryptophan. The observations in the dog show a gross increase in the rate of hepatic gluconeogenesis, hepatic glucose output, and glucose and alanine oxidation.

It should be noted that hepatic coma is also associated with low plasma leucine and isoleucine and high tryptophan and phenylalanine. This change in plasma amino acid concentration has been shown to be associated with alterations in brain neurotransmitters. Thus it is known to be associated with increased brain serotonin, reduced brain norepinephrine, and the presence of the false neurotransmitter octopamine. Fischer and associates have shown that animals can be brought out of hepatic coma by an amino acid mixture that is rich in leucine and isoleucine but deficient in tryptophan and phenylalanine [10]. This is exactly the mixture one would predict should be used for the chronically, critically ill patient on the basis of our observations. The additional prediction would be that it would enhance protein synthesis generally and would enhance both local and systemic resistance to sepsis.

Summary: Pathophysiology
A clinical description of the chronically, critically ill patient who develops delayed sepsis has been given. The deduction has been made that not only does such a patient have reduced local and systemic resistance to sepsis, but he also has a generalized limitation of protein synthesis relative to protein breakdown. The various organs and the specific insults present in such a patient that can limit protein synthesis have been discussed. It is pointed out that the liver has a large number of specific insults present that can limit protein synthesis independent of an endogenous amino acid imbalance. All such hepatic stresses must be managed independently. The liver is particularly at risk because of its limited oxygen supplies from any cardiopulmonary stress.

The normal balance of substrates between liver, muscle, and adipose tissue with starvation has been discussed. Hepatic ketogenesis and carnitine synthesis are particularly important in stimulating fat and ketone body oxidation in muscle and therefore in conserving muscle leucine and isoleucine and limiting amino acid gluconeogenic substrate. These processes therefore conserve muscle protein. The stress catabolic response and intravenous glucose, by producing hyperglycemia and therefore limiting hepatic ketogenesis and carnitine synthesis, interfere seriously with muscle oxidation of fat and ketone bodies and therefore stimulate muscle oxidation of the essential amino acids leucine and isoleucine, and amino acids gluconeogenesis and ureagenesis. This phenomenon, when prolonged, eventually leads to a total body deficiency of leucine and isoleucine that limits protein synthesis generally, while enhancing hepatic gluconeogenesis. In the end, this disorder is associated with a low plasma leucine and isoleucine as well as with elevated concentrations of plasma tryptophan, phenylalanine, and methionine. These are the amino acid concentration changes associated with hepatic coma.

Implications for Therapy
The best therapy is clearly immediate reversal of all organ failures, aggressive treatment of sepsis, alleviation of pain and anxiety, and internal fixation of all fractures so the patient can quickly be sat up and all extremities begun on a cycle of active movements. Under these conditions the metabolic-nutritional support offered to the patient really does not matter.

When the preceding cannot be accomplished, the nature of the metabolic nutritional support offered becomes critical, largely in terms of its effects on hepatic protein synthesis and indirectly through its effects on muscle. These effects are of great importance in preventing delayed sepsis and enhancing the body's response to sepsis. Clearly pure intravenous glucose, because of its effects on hepatic ketogenesis, fat mobilization, and hepatic protein synthesis should never be used for more than a few days. Intravenous amino acids, because they are directly cleared by the liver and may be utilized for protein synthesis, gluconeogenesis, or liponeogenesis, are a great improvement over intravenous glucose. The amount required to achieve protein synthesis depends on the amount of leucine and isoleucine consumed by muscle as ketone bodies and the amount of the other amino acids consumed by the liver for gluconeogenesis. It seems clear that, the more ill the patient, the greater the quantity of exogenous amino acids consumed in these two processes and therefore the greater the quantity of exogenous amino acids required to achieve protein synthesis.

Amino acids given intravenously provide hepatic nutritional support because they are largely cleared by the liver. However, they do not provide luminal gastrointestinal mucosal nutritional support, nor do they provide the specific high concentrations of nutrients normally received by the liver. Thus, as a general principle, the gastrointestinal route of nutritional support is preferred to the intravenous route, because it provides luminal gastrointestinal mucosal nutrition and the normal high concentrations of nutrient to the liver. Gastrointestinal feeding may be used in the critically ill patient with an ileus if the elemental diet is given into the jejunum and the stomach is placed on suction. This may be accomplished by use of a Cantor tube or jejunostomy tube in association with a nasogastric tube.

The nutrient content of the solution administered should not produce stools and should have a high nitrogen content. In general, these should be designed so they contain not only a complete mixture of amino acids with relative excesses of leucine and isoleucine, but also so they provide carnitine and ketone bodies or for at least part of the day are ketogenic.

Carnitine is a normal component of meats and soups. The Jewish mother's idea of chicken soup for her ill children examined in this light proves almost ideal, since it provides water, salt, carnitine, and a complete mixture of amino acids that are largely the same as human muscle. Given the lability of tryptophan, it is probably deficient in or lacking this amino acid. However, this is another point in its favor, since high plasma tryptophans contribute to hepatic coma. Also, chicken soup provides some fat, but is basically glucose free and therefore ketogenic. Thus many of the components of the ideal mixture considered in the light of inadequate calories are present in chicken soup. Inadequate calories probably present no real problem so long as there are adequate fat reserves.

The elemental diet typically utilized (e.g., Vivonex-HN) has a basic caloric support medium of carbohydrates; it contains no carnitine; and it has an essential amino acid content based on the feeding of healthy animals. It therefore is ideally set up to inhibit hepatic ketogenesis and to limit the peripheral utilization of long-chain fatty acids both by glucose interference of long-chain fatty acid mobilization and by producing a muscle carnitine deficient state. In contrast to these deficiencies with respect to muscle, it does provide good hepatic nutritional support. Muscle nutritional support could be improved by addition of carnitine to the elemental diet by increasing the content of leucine and isoleucine, by adding ketone bodies, or by adding muscle metabolizable short-chain fatty acids either per se or as glycerides. A better caloric support medium for the elemental diet in terms of the joint requirements of muscle and liver would probably be one in which the calories are supplied by a mixture of short- and long-chain fatty acid glycerides, in which the glucose required by the brain is provided by gluconeogenesis from the glycerol provided by breakdown of the glycerides. The short-chain fatty acids should be short enough so they can be metabolized oxidatively by muscle independent of carnitine (e.g., octanoic, hexanoic, butyric, and acetoacetate).

Intravenous long-chain fatty acid triglycerides, if administration is accompanied by hepatic ketogenesis and carnitine, should provide a good caloric support medium. If administration is not associated with ketogenesis and carnitine, the only action of this medium would be to replenish adipose tissue fat stores and to provide glycerol for hepatic gluconeogenesis. This appears largely to be the case since the reduction in urinary nitrogen observed is largely associated with the glycerol administered [4].

Intravenous glucose and albumin have commonly been utilized, particularly with multiple organ failures, including renal failure. This probably should not be utilized because of the expense of albumin and also because albumin is deficient in isoleucine. Thus under these conditions hepatic ketogenesis is compromised, while enhancing the use of leucine and isoleucine's fuel and providing a support medium deficient in isoleucine. A much better choice would be a complete mixture of amino acids or of just the essential amino acids plus albumin sufficient to maintain the plasma albumin between 3 and 4 g per 100 ml for circulatory support.

At present one must deal, for practical reasons, largely with a choice between intravenous amino acids, intravenous hyperalimentation, and the elemental diet through the gastrointestinal tract. The more ill the patient, the greater the quantity of amino acids required, regardless of the route, and in general, the greater the number of total calories required. However, because the need for amino acids increases much more than the need for calories, in general the more ill the patient, the lower the calorie-to-nitrogen ratio required. Intravenous hyperalimentation has 150 cal per gram of nitrogen. A starved, healthy person burns on the order of 400 to 600 cal per gram of nitrogen. Pure protein or amino acids have a calorie-to-nitrogen ratio of 25. The calorie-to-nitrogen ratio of hyperalimentation fluid is excellent for someone who is not very ill (e.g., the intestinal fistula patient, where formation of the fistula has also drained the only abscess). However, it is not adequate for the patient who still has undrained abscesses or pneumonias, who is in severe cardiopulmonary failure, or who is severely apprehensive with pain. These patients require a lower calorie-to-nitrogen ratio with more amino acids probably to provide more leucine and isoleucine. This may be achieved by doubling or tripling the amino acids relative to the basic calorie support medium. This is required whether one is utilizing the gastrointestinal (preferred) or intravenous route.

References

1. Border, J. R. The metabolic response to starvation, sepsis and trauma. In J. McCredie (Ed.), *Basic Surgery*. New York: Macmillan, 1976.
2. Border, J. R. Metabolic response to short term starvation, sepsis and trauma. In P. Cooper, and L. M. Nyhus (Eds.), *Surgery Annual*. New York: Appleton-Century-Crofts, 1970.
3. Border, J. R., et al. Carnitine levels in severe infection and starvation: A possible key to the catabolic state. *Surgery* 68:175, 1970.
4. Brennan, M. F., Fitzpatrick, G. F., and Moore, F. D. Glycerol: Major contributor to the protein sparing effects of fat emulsions in normal man. Paper presented at the American Surgical Association meeting, Quebec City, Quebec, May 7–9, 1975.
5. Cole, W. O., Cook, J. J., and Grogan, J. B. In vitro neutrophil function and lysosomal enzyme levels in patients with sepsis. *Surg. Forum* 26:79, 1975.
6. Constantian, M. B., et al. A method of assessing impairment of immunity after trauma. *Surg. Forum* 26:1, 1975.
7. Copeland, E. M., et al. Hyperalimentation and immune competence in cancer. *Surg. Forum* 26:138, 1975.
8. Dhillon, K. S., MacLean, L. D., and Meakins, J. L. Neutrophile function in surgical patients: Correlation of neutrophile bacteriocidal function. Serum albumin and sepsis. *Surg. Forum* 26:27, 1975.

9. Elwyn, D. The role of the liver in regulation of amino acid and protein metabolism. In H. N. Munro (Ed.), *Mammalian Protein Metabolism,* Vol. 4. New York: Academic Press, 1970.

10. Fischer, J. E., et al. The role of plasma amino acids in hepatic encephalopathy. *Surgery* 78:276, 1975.

11. Hohn, D. C., and Hunt, T. K. Oxidative metabolism and microbicidal activity of rabbit phagocytes: Cells from wounds and from peripheral blood. *Surg. Forum* 26:85, 1975.

12. Law, D. K., Dudrick, S. J., and Abdow, H. I. Effects of protein calorie malnutrition on immune competence of surgical patients. *Surg. Gynecol. Obstet.* 139:257, 1974.

13. Long, C. L., et al. Carbohydrate metabolism in man: Effect of elective operation and major injury. *J. Appl. Physiol.* 31:110, 1971.

14. McMenamy, R. H., et al. Plasma concentrations and splanchnic uptake of amino acids and other substances in the basal state: Report I of a trauma case. In preparation.

15. McMenamy, R. H., et al. Effects of infusates on plasma concentrations and splanchnic uptake and release of glucose, amino acids, and other substances. Report II of a trauma case. In preparation.

16. McMenamy, R. H., et al. Relationships between plasma tryptophan and fatty acid concentrations and their effects on other substances: Report III of a trauma patient study. In preparation.

17. Ogle, C. K., et al. Determination of serum opsonin and opsonization in patients with sepsis. *Surg. Forum* 26:6, 1975.

18. Scrimshaw, N. S. Protein deficiency and infective disease. In H. N. Munro and J. R. Allison (Eds.), *Mammalian Protein Metabolism,* Vol. II. New York: Academic Press, 1964.

19. Vaidyanath, N., et al. Plasma concentrations and tissue uptake of free amino acids in sepsis and starvation: Effects of glucose infusion. *J. Trauma* 16:125, 1976.

Index

AC. *See* Anticomplementary activity
AMCI. *See* Immunity, cellular, antibody-mediated
Abscesses, postoperative, prevention of, 217
Actin, in neutrophil locomotion, 4–5
Adrenalin, and staphylococcal contamination, 178, 179
Agammaglobulinemia, as B cell deficiency, 28
Aggressin, and virulence of *S. aureus*, 86
Albumin, as transport for amino acids, 237
Amino acids
  in chronically ill, 235–238
  and critically ill, 241
  in delaying sepsis, 227
  endogenous imbalance, and limited protein synthesis, 233–238
  intravenous, in therapy for sepsis, 239
  in protein synthesis, in critically ill, 230, 231
  in starvation, 233–235
Amniotic fluid, contaminated, in neonatal sepsis, 82
Amphotericin B, in prophylactic regimens, 146
Ampicillin
  and cancer surgery, 197
  in *E. coli* infection, 87
Antibacterial immunity, acquired, 21–22
Antibiotic prophylaxis
  in acute leukemia, 143, 145, 146, 147
  in deep wound sepsis prevention, 188, 189, 190
  parenteral vs. oral, 148, 149–150
  use in surgery, 193, 195, 197–199, 200
Antibiotic therapy
  high-dose, and deficient neutrophils, 1
  and neonatal susceptibility, 80–81
  postoperative, in cancer patients, 195, 196–197
  preventive
    effective time period, 179
    in surgery, 180
  protected environment–prophylactic programs, 147–155
  for septic neonate, 87
Antibiotics
  implantation of, in hip replacement, 190
  systemic, in trauma patient, 214, 215, 223
  topical, in deep wound infection, 189–190
  wide-spectrum, in cancer surgery, 197, 198
  in wound fluid, postoperative concentrations of, 198–199
Antibody(ies)
  anti-idiotype, 33

humoral, in immunosuppressive therapy, 166
negative feedback by, 32
passive, as preventive measure, 103, 106
role in preventing infection, 27–28
  in resistance to *Pseudomonas aeruginosa*, 35–40
transplacental, and neonatal immune responses, 81
Antibody-antigen combination, in specific immune response, 76
Anticomplementary activity (AC), 138–139
Antigen(s)
  effect on bone marrow B cell competence, 32
  response to, in PCM, 132
  and suppression of immunity, 30–32
  as susceptibility to T cell killing, 27
Anti-lymphocyte serum, and cellular immunity, 162–163
Antimicrobial agents, 106. *See also* Antibiotic prophylaxis; Antibiotic therapy; Antibiotics
  prophylactic, 112, 115
Antithymocyte serum, and cellular immunity, 162–163
Arabinosyl cytosine, in remission consolidation therapy, for acute leukemia, 152
Aspiration, preoperative, in hip replacement, 187
Assays, to measure transfer factor, 45
Azathioprine
  and antibody production, 164, 165
  effect on host defenses, 157, 158, 160
  effect on polymorph function, 169
  and K cell activity, 168, 169
  and reticuloendothelial system, 170
  and skin-test reactions, 162

B lymphocytes (B cells). *See also* T lymphocytes
  differentiation of, 30, 31
  and immunosuppressive therapy, 158–159
  specialization among, 28–30
  and specific immune response, 76
  tests of function
    in infection-proneness, 59
    in PCM, 123
Bacteria. *See also* Organisms *and names of specific species,* as *Pseudomonas aeruginosa*
  and antibody immunodeficiency, 99
  effect of prophylactic measures on, 146
  gram-negative, in hospital environment, 199, 200